The Renal Drug Handbook

Edited by

Ray Bunn and Caroline Ashley

UK Renal Pharmacy Group

Foreword by

Professor John Moorhead

Centre for Nephrology
Royal Free and University
College Medical School, London

©1999 UK Renal Pharmacy Group

Radcliffe Medical Press Ltd
18 Marcham Road, Abingdon, Oxon OX14 1AA

British Library Cataloguing in Publication Data

ISBN 1 85775 115 9

Typeset by Advance Typesetting Ltd, Oxfordshire
Printed and bound by Biddles Ltd, Guildford and King's Lynn

Contents

Preface

Welcome to the first edition of *The Renal Drug Handbook*. The information contained in this book has been compiled from a wide range of sources and from the clinical experience of the editorial board of the UK Renal Pharmacy Group, all of whom are involved in the pharmaceutical care of renally impaired patients. As such, some of the information contained in the monographs may not be in accordance with the licensed indications or use of the drug.

The Handbook aims to:

• provide healthcare professionals with a single reference of easily retrievable, practical information relating to drug use, sourced from the practical experience of renal units throughout the UK. By referring to the monographs, the user is guided in how to prescribe, prepare and administer the drug with due regard to potentially serious drug interactions and any renal replacement therapy the patient may be undergoing;

• provide a practice-based review of drug utilisation in renal units across the UK indicating, where appropriate, any local methods of use, licensed or otherwise.

The Handbook is **not** intended to offer definitive advice or guidance on how drugs should be used in patients with renal impairment, nor is it a comprehensive and complete list of all drugs licensed in the UK. The range of drugs covered will continue to grow with subsequent editions. The Handbook is not a guide to diagnosis or an indication of a drug's side-effect profile, except where adverse drug events are more pronounced in the presence of renal impairment. For a full account of the drug, users are advised to refer to the Summary of Product Characteristics, *British National Formulary*, package inserts or other product data for more in-depth information.

The use of drugs in patients with impaired renal function can give rise to problems for several reasons.

• Altered pharmacokinetics of some drugs, i.e. changes in absorption, tissue distribution, extent of plasma protein binding, metabolism and excretion. In renal impairment these parameters are often variable and interrelated in a complex manner. This may be further complicated if the patient is undergoing renal replacement therapy.

For many drugs, some or even all of the altered pharmacokinetic parameters and modified interrelationships are unknown. In such circumstances, the informed professional judgement of clinicians and pharmacists must be used to predict drug disposition. This must be based on knowledge of the drug, its class, chemistry and pharmacokinetics in patients with normal renal function.

• Sensitivity to some drugs is increased, even if elimination is unimpaired.

• Many side-effects are particularly poorly tolerated by renally impaired patients.

• Some drugs are ineffective when renal function is reduced.

• Renal function generally declines with age, and many elderly patients have a GFR less than 50 mL/min which, because of reduced muscle mass, may not be reflected by an elevated creatinine. Consequently, one can justifiably assume mild renal impairment when prescribing for the elderly.

Many of these problems can be avoided by careful choice and use of drugs. This Handbook seeks to assist healthcare professionals in this process.

Using the monographs

• **Drug name**: the approved (generic) name is usually stated.

• **Clinical use**: a brief account of the more common indications in renally impaired patients is given. Where an indication is unlicensed, this is usually stated.

• **Dose in normal renal function**: the doses quoted for patients with normal renal function are generally the licensed dosage recommendations stated in the summary of product characteristics for each drug. Where a product is not licensed in the UK, dosage guidelines are provided by the relevant drug company.

• **Pharmacokinetics**: basic pharmacokinetic data such as molecular weight, half-life, percentage protein-binding, volume of distribution and percentage excreted unchanged in the urine are quoted, to assist in predicting drug handling in both renal impairment and renal replacement therapy. '–' denotes 'not known' or 'no data available'.

• **Dose in renal impairment**: the level of renal function below which the dose of a drug must be reduced depends largely on the extent of renal metabolism and elimination, and on the drug's toxicity. Most drugs are relatively well tolerated, have a broad therapeutic index or are metabolised and excreted hepatically, so precise dose modification is unnecessary. In such cases, the user is instructed to 'dose as in normal renal function'.

For drugs which are renally excreted, with a narrow therapeutic index, the total daily maintenance dose may be reduced either by reducing the dose or by increasing the dosing interval, or sometimes by a combination of both. Dosing guidelines for varying degrees of renal impairment are stated accordingly.

- **Dose in renal replacement therapy**: details are given for dosing in continuous ambulatory peritoneal dialysis (CAPD), intermittent haemodialysis (HD), and continuous arterio-venous/veno-venous haemodiafiltration (CAV/VVHD), where known. Drugs are categorised into dialysable/not dialysable/dialysability unknown, to aid the practitioner in making an informed decision for dosing within a particular form of renal replacement therapy. No specific guidelines are given for dosing in continuous arterio-venous/veno-venous haemofiltration (CAV/VVH). In general, dosing schedules are the same as for those quoted for CAV/VVHD, although it should be borne in mind that CAV/VVH may have a lower drug clearance capacity. Thus the clinician or pharmacist should use informed professional judgement, based on knowledge of the drug and its pharmacokinetics, whether to further modify dosing regimens.

- **Important drug interactions**: these are specifically given for cyclosporin. The interactions with other drugs listed are those identified by a black spot in Appendix 1 of the *British National Formulary*. They are defined as those interactions which are potentially serious, and where combined administration of the drugs involved should be avoided, or only undertaken with caution and appropriate monitoring. Users of the monographs are referred to Appendix 1 of the *British National Formulary* for a more comprehensive list of interactions deemed to be not so clinically significant.

- **Administration**: information on reconstitution, route and rate of administration, and any additional comments are given. Much of the information relates to local practice, since the avoidance of the administration of large volumes of fluids is paramount. Only the most commonly used and compatible reconstitution and dilution solutions are stated.

- **Other information**: details given here are only relevant to the use of that particular drug in patients with impaired renal function or on renal replacement therapy. For further, more general information, please refer to the Summary of Product Characteristics for that drug.

Your contribution to future editions is vital. Any ideas, comments, corrections, requests, additions, local practices, etc. on the drugs in the Handbook should be put in writing to the editor-in-chief: Caroline Ashley, Pharmacy Department, Royal Free Hospital, Hampstead, London NW3 2QG.

Ray Bunn

Caroline Ashley

November 1998

The following texts have been used as reference sources for the compilation of the monographs in this book:

- *ABPI Compendium of Data Sheets and Summaries of Product Characteristics* (1998/99).

- *British National Formulary No. 34* (1997). Pharmaceutical Press.

- *Martindale: The Extra Pharmacopoeia* (31st ed). (1996) Pharmaceutical Press.

- Bennett WM *et al.* (1994) *Drug Prescribing in Renal Failure: Dosing Guidelines for Adults* (3rd ed). American College of Physicians.

- *American Hospital Formulary Service* (1997).

- Knoben JE and Anderson PO (1993) *Clinical Drug Handbook* (7th ed). Drug Intelligence Publications Inc.

- Schrier RW and Gambertoglio JG (1991) *Handbook of Drug Therapy in Liver and Kidney Disease*. Little, Brown and Co.

- Dollery C (1991) *Therapeutic Drugs*. Churchill Livingstone.

- Seyffart G (1991) *Drug Dosage in Renal Insufficiency*. Kluwer Academic Publishers.

- *Cyclosporin Interaction File* (Novartis Pharmaceuticals UK).

- *Drugdex Database*. Micromedex Inc., USA.

- Drug company information.

Foreword

Great advances have been made in recent years in the understanding of renal disease and renal failure. Despite the rapid growth of information technology there is still a scarcity of information in drug prescribing in patients with renal impairment, or those who are undergoing some form of renal replacement therapy. Moreover, the data that does exist are often difficult to access.

This book is unique in that it is both comprehensive in range and easy to use. Each of the enormous range of drugs covered is monographed so as to facilitate clinical interpretation of the data according to the needs of the individual patient. Perhaps most importantly, it is the only British reference source of its type, and as such, includes many drugs not found in the standard American texts.

This long-awaited handbook fulfils a real need and will be an invaluable aid to practising clinicians, pharmacists and other healthcare professionals involved in the treatment of renal patients.

John Moorhead FRCP
Emeritus Professor, Centre for Nephrology
Royal Free and University College
Medical School, London
November 1998

UK Renal Pharmacy Group

Acknowledgements

Our thanks go to the numerous members of the
UK Renal Pharmacy Group who assisted with the
compilation of the monographs in this handbook.

Acebutolol

Clinical use

Beta-adrenoreceptor blocker for hypertension, angina, arrhythmias

Dose in normal renal function

Hypertension:
400 mg once a day or 200 mg twice daily increased after 2 weeks to 400 mg twice daily if necessary
Angina:
400 mg once a day or 200 mg twice daily initially. Increase up to 300 mg 3 times daily (max 1200 mg)
Arrhythmias:
400–1200 mg/day (in divided doses)

Pharmacokinetics

Molecular weight (daltons)	372.9 (as hydrochloride)
% Protein binding	20
% Excreted unchanged in urine	55
Volume of distribution (L/kg)	1.2
Half-life – normal/ESRF (hrs)	7–9/unchanged

Dose in renal impairment GFR (mL/min)

20–50	Dose as in normal renal function, but frequency should not exceed once daily in renal impairment
10–20	50% of normal dose, but frequency should not exceed once daily in renal impairment
<10	30–50% of normal dose, but frequency should not exceed once daily in renal impairment

Dose in patients undergoing renal replacement therapies

CAPD	Unknown dialysability. Dose as in GFR = <10 mL/min
HD	Dialysed. Dose as in GFR = <10 mL/min
CAV/VVHD	Dialysed. Dose as in GFR = 10–20 mL/min

Important drug interactions

CYCLOSPORIN

–

POTENTIALLY HAZARDOUS INTERACTIONS WITH OTHER DRUGS

- Enhanced hypotensive effect with anaesthetics
- Increased risk of myocardial depression and bradycardia with antiarrhythmics. With amiodarone increased risk of bradycardia + AV block
- Enhanced hypotensive effect with antihypertensives. Increased risk of first-dose hypotensive effect with post-synaptic alpha-blockers such as prazosin
- Increased risk of bradycardia + AV block with diltiazem. Severe hypotension and heart failure occasionally with nifedipine. Asystole, severe hypotension and heart failure with verapamil
- Severe hypertension with adrenaline and noradrenaline (especially with non-selective beta-blockers)
- Increased AV block and bradycardia with cardiac glycosides

Administration

RECONSTITUTION

–

ROUTE

- Oral

RATE OF ADMINISTRATION

- N/A

COMMENTS

Other information

- Administration of high doses in severe renal failure cautioned due to accumulation
- Dose frequency should not exceed once daily in renal impairment

Acetazolamide

Clinical use

Glaucoma, diuretic, epilepsy

Dose in normal renal function

Glaucoma/epilepsy:
0.25–1 g daily in divided doses
Diuretic: 250–375 mg daily

Pharmacokinetics

Molecular weight (daltons)	222.2
% Protein binding	70–95
% Excreted unchanged in urine	100
Volume of distribution (L/kg)	0.2
Half-life – normal/ESRF (hrs)	1.7–8/34

Dose in renal impairment GFR (mL/min)

20–50	250 mg up to four times a day
10–20	250 mg up to twice a day
<10	250 mg daily

Dose in patients undergoing renal replacement therapies

CAPD	Unknown dialysability. Dose as in GFR = <10 mL/min
HD	Dialysed. Dose as in GFR = <10mL/min
CAV/VVHD	Unknown dialysability. Dose as in GFR = 10–20 mL/min

Important drug interactions

CYCLOSPORIN

–

POTENTIALLY HAZARDOUS INTERACTIONS WITH OTHER DRUGS

• Aspirin reduces excretion of acetazolamide (risk of toxicity)
• Increased toxicity of cardiac glycosides if hypokalaemia occurs
• Lithium excretion increased
• Increased risk of osteomalacia with phenytoin

Administration

RECONSTITUTION

• Add at least 5 mL of water for injection

ROUTE

• Oral, IM, IV

RATE OF ADMINISTRATION

• Give slow IV

COMMENTS

• Avoid IM due to alkaline pH
• Monitor for signs of extravasation and skin necrosis during administration

Other information

• Use cautioned in severe renal failure
• Acetazolamide sodium (Diamox) parenteral contains 2.36 millimoles of sodium per vial
• Severe metabolic acidosis may occur in the elderly and in patients with reduced renal function

Acetylcysteine

Clinical use

Treatment of paracetamol overdose

Dose in normal renal function

IV infusion:

initially 150 mg/kg in 200 mL glucose 5% over 15 min followed by 50 mg/kg in 500 mL glucose 5% over 4 hrs, then 100 mg/kg in 1000 mL over 16 hrs

Pharmacokinetics

Molecular weight (daltons)	163
% Protein binding	50
% Excreted unchanged in urine	30
Volume of distribution (L/kg)	0.33–0.47
Half-life – normal/ESRF (hrs)	2.3–6/–

Dose in renal impairment GFR (mL/min)

20–50	Dose as in normal renal function
10–20	Dose as in normal renal function
<10	Dose as in normal renal function. See 'Other information'

Dose in patients undergoing renal replacement therapies

CAPD	Unknown dialysability. Dose as in normal renal function
HD	Unknown dialysability. Dose as in normal renal function
CAV/VVHD	Unknown dialysability. Dose as in normal renal function

Important drug interactions

CYCLOSPORIN

–

POTENTIALLY HAZARDOUS INTERACTIONS WITH OTHER DRUGS

–

Administration

RECONSTITUTION

• Glucose 5%

ROUTE

• IV, oral (oral route unlicensed in the UK)

RATE OF ADMINISTRATION

• See dose

COMMENTS

• Children should be treated with the same doses and regimen as adults; however, the quantity of IV fluid should be modified to account for age and weight

• Acetylcysteine has been administered neat or in a 1 to 1 dilution using an infusion pump. These are unlicensed methods of administration

Other information

• Bennett recommends administering 75% of dose for patients with severe renal impairment. However, Evans Medical does not recommend a dose reduction and, from their records, neither do the National Poisons Centre

Aciclovir (IV)

Clinical use

Antiviral agent for herpes simplex and herpes zoster infection

Dose in normal renal function

Herpes simplex treatment:
normal or immunocompromised 5 mg/kg every 8 hrs

Recurrent varicella zoster infection:

normal immune status 5 mg/kg every 8 hrs

Primary and recurrent varicella zoster infection:
immunocompromised 10 mg/kg every 8 hrs

Herpes simplex encephalitis:

normal or immunocompromised 10 mg/kg every 8 hrs.

Pharmacokinetics

Molecular weight (daltons)	225
% Protein binding	15–30
% Excreted unchanged in urine	40–70
Volume of distribution (L/kg)	0.7
Half-life – normal/ESRF (hrs)	2.1–3.8/20 (dialysis: 6)

Dose in renal impairment GFR (mL/min)

25–50	5–10 mg/kg every 12 hrs
10–25	5–10 mg/kg every 24 hrs (some units use 3.5–7 mg/kg every 24 hrs)
<10	2.5–5 mg/kg every 24 hrs

Dose in patients undergoing renal replacement therapies

CAPD	Not dialysed. Dose as in GFR = <10 mL/min
HD	Dialysed. Dose as in GFR = <10 mL/min
CAV/VVHD	Dialysed. Dose as in GFR = 10–25 mL/min

Important drug interactions

CYCLOSPORIN

• Reports of increased and decreased cyclosporin levels.

POTENTIALLY HAZARDOUS INTERACTIONS WITH OTHER DRUGS

• Higher plasma levels of aciclovir with concomitant administration of mycophenolate mofetil

Administration

RECONSTITUTION

• Sodium chloride 0.9% or water for injection; 10 mL to each 250-mg vial; 20 mL to 500-mg vial (resulting solution contains 25 mg/mL)

ROUTE

• IV

RATE OF ADMINISTRATION

• 1 hr. Can worsen renal impairment if injected too rapidly

COMMENTS

• Reconstituted solution may be further diluted to concentrations not greater than 5 mg/mL
• Compatible with sodium chloride 0.9% and glucose 5%
• Do not refrigerate
• Do not use turbid or crystal-containing solutions
• Reconstituted solution very alkaline (pH 11)

Other information

• Aciclovir clearance in CAVHD is approximately equivalent to urea clearance, i.e. lower clearance than in intermittent haemodialysis
• Monitor aciclovir levels in critically ill patients. **Reports of neurological toxicity at maximum recommended doses**
• Renal impairment developing during treatment with aciclovir usually responds rapidly to rehydration of the patient and/or dosage reduction or withdrawal of the drug. Adequate hydration of the patient should be maintained

Aciclovir (oral)

Clinical use

Antiviral agent for herpes simplex and herpes zoster infection

Dose in normal renal function

Simplex treatment:

200–400 mg 5 times daily

Prophylaxis:

200 mg every 6 hrs

Suppression:

200 mg every 6 hrs, or 400 mg every 12 hrs

Zoster:

800 mg 5 times a day for 7 days

Pharmacokinetics

Molecular weight (daltons)	225
% Protein binding	15–30
% Excreted unchanged in urine	40–70
Volume of distribution (L/kg)	0.7
Half-life – normal/ESRF (hrs)	2.1–3.8/20 (dialysis: 6)

Dose in renal impairment GFR (mL/min)

20–50	Dose as in normal renal function
10–20	Simplex: dose as in normal renal function
	Zoster: 800 mg every 8 hrs
<10	Simplex: 200 mg every 12 hrs
	Zoster: 800 mg every 12 hrs

Dose in patients undergoing renal replacement therapies

CAPD	Not dialysed. Dose as in GFR = <10 mL/min
HD	Dialysed. Dose as in GFR = <10 mL/min. Give dose after dialysis
CAV/VVHD	Dialysed. Dose as in GFR = 10–20 mL/min

Important drug interactions

CYCLOSPORIN

• Reports of increase and decrease in cyclosporin levels.

POTENTIALLY HAZARDOUS INTERACTIONS WITH OTHER DRUGS

• Higher plasma levels of aciclovir with concomitant administration of mycophendate mofetil

Administration

RECONSTITUTION

–

ROUTE

• Oral

RATE OF ADMINISTRATION

–

COMMENTS

• Dispersible tablets may be dispersed in a minimum of 50 mL of water or swallowed whole with a little water

Other information

• Consider IV therapy for zoster infection if patient is severely immunocompromised
• Monitor aciclovir levels

Acitretin

Clinical use

Severe extensive psoriasis, palmoplantar pustular psoriasis, severe congenital ichthyosis, severe Darier's disease

Dose in normal renal function

Initially 25–30 mg daily (Darier's disease 10 mg daily) for 2–4 weeks adjusted according to response. Usually 25–50 mg/day (maximum 75 mg) for a further 6–8 weeks (in Darier's disease and ichthyosis not more than 50 mg daily for up to 6 months)

Pharmacokinetics

Molecular weight (daltons)	326.4
% Protein binding	Highly bound. Less than 0.1% present as unbound drug in pooled human plasma
% Excreted unchanged in urine	Excreted as metabolites
Volume of distribution (L/kg)	9
Half-life – normal/ESRF (hrs)	47/–

Dose in renal impairment GFR (mL/min)

20–50	No data available. Assume dose as in normal renal function
10–20	No data available. Assume dose as in normal renal function
<10	No data available. Assume dose as in normal renal function

Dose in patients undergoing renal replacement therapies

CAPD	Unknown dialysability. Dose as in normal renal function
HD	Unknown dialysability. Dose as in normal renal function
CAV/VVHD	Unknown dialysability. Dose as in normal renal function

Important drug interactions

CYCLOSPORIN

–

POTENTIALLY HAZARDOUS INTERACTIONS WITH OTHER DRUGS

• Possible antagonism of the anticoagulant effect of warfarin
• Increased plasma concentration of methotrexate (also increased risk of hepatotoxicity)

Administration

RECONSTITUTION

–

ROUTE

• Oral

RATE OF ADMINISTRATION

–

COMMENTS

• Take once daily with meals or with milk

Other information

• Manufacturer's literature contraindicates the use of acitretin in renal failure

Acrivastine

Clinical use

Antihistamine – symptomatic relief of allergy such as hay fever and urticaria

Dose in normal renal function

8 mg 3 times a day

Pharmacokinetics

Molecular weight (daltons)	348.4
% Protein binding	50
% Excreted unchanged in urine	–
Volume of distribution (L/kg)	0.6–0.7
Half-life – normal/ESRF (hrs)	1.4–2.1/–

Dose in renal impairment GFR (mL/min)

20–50	8 mg twice a day
10–20	8 mg once or twice a day
<10	8 mg daily

Dose in patients undergoing renal replacement therapies

CAPD	Unknown dialysability. Dose as in GFR = <10 mL/min
HD	Unknown dialysability. Dose as in GFR = <10 mL/min
CAV/VVHD	Unknown dialysability. Dose as in GFR = 10–20 mL/min

Important drug interactions

CYCLOSPORIN

–

POTENTIALLY HAZARDOUS INTERACTIONS WITH OTHER DRUGS

• MAOIs and tricyclics increase the antimuscarinic and sedative effects. Increased risk of ventricular arrhythmias with tricyclics
• Concomitant use of astemizole and terfenadine not recommended (risk of hazardous arrhythmias)
• Increased risk of ventricular arrhythmias with sotalol

Administration

RECONSTITUTION

–

ROUTE

• Oral

RATE OF ADMINISTRATION

–

COMMENTS

–

Other information

• Manufacturer does not recommend use in patients with significant renal impairment

Adenosine

Clinical use

Rapid reversion to sinus rhythm of paroxysmal supraventricular tachycardias. Diagnosis of broad or narrow complex supraventricular tachycardias

Dose in normal renal function

Initially: 3 mg over 2 sec with cardiac monitoring followed, if necessary, by 6 mg after 1–2 min and then by 12 mg after a further 1–2 min

Pharmacokinetics

Molecular weight (daltons)	267.2
% Protein binding	0
% Excreted unchanged in urine	<5
Volume of distribution (L/kg)	–
Half-life – normal/ESRF	<10 sec/ unchanged

Dose in renal impairment GFR (mL/min)

20–50	Dose as in normal renal function
10–20	Dose as in normal renal function
<10	Dose as in normal renal function

Dose in patients undergoing renal replacement therapies

CAPD	Not dialysed. Dose as in normal renal function
HD	Not dialysed. Dose as in normal renal function
CAV/VVHD	Not dialysed. Dose as in normal renal function

Important drug interactions

CYCLOSPORIN

–

POTENTIALLY HAZARDOUS INTERACTIONS WITH OTHER DRUGS

• Effect is enhanced and extended by dipyridamole; therefore, if use of adenosine is essential, dosage should be reduced by a factor of 4 (i.e. initial dosage of 0.5–1 mg)

• Theophylline and other xanthines are potent inhibitors of adenosine

Administration

RECONSTITUTION

–

ROUTE

• IV

RATE OF ADMINISTRATION

• Rapid IV bolus (see dose)

COMMENTS

• Do not refrigerate

• Administer into central vein, large peripheral vein, or into an IV line. If IV line is used, follow the dose with rapid sodium chloride 0.9% flush

Other information

• Neither the kidney nor the liver are involved in the degradation of exogenous adenosine, so dose adjustments are not required in hepatic or renal insufficiency

• Unlike verapamil, adenosine may be used in conjunction with beta-blockers

• Common side-effects: facial flushing, chest pain, dyspnoea, bronchospasm, nausea and lightheadedness; the side-effects are short-lived

Adrenaline

Clinical use

Sympathomimetic and inotropic agent

Dose in normal renal function

1–20 micrograms/min

Pharmacokinetics

Molecular weight (daltons)	183.2
% Protein binding	50
% Excreted unchanged in urine	1
Volume of distribution (L/kg)	–
Half-life – normal/ESRF	Phase 1: 3 min; phase 2: 10 min

Dose in renal impairment GFR (mL/min)

20–50	Dose as in normal renal function
10–20	Dose as in normal renal function
<10	Dose as in normal renal function

Dose in patients undergoing renal replacement therapies

CAPD	Not dialysed. Dose as in normal renal function
HD	Not dialysed. Dose as in normal renal function
CAV/VVHD	Not dialysed. Dose as in normal renal function

Important drug interactions

CYCLOSPORIN

–

POTENTIALLY HAZARDOUS INTERACTIONS WITH OTHER DRUGS

- Risk of arrhythmias if given with volatile anaesthetics
- Risk of arrhythmias and hypertension if given with tricyclic antidepressants
- Risk of severe hypertension if given with beta-blockers

Administration

RECONSTITUTION

- 1 mg in 100 mL glucose 5%
- 6 mL/hr = 1 microgram/min – according to local protocol

ROUTE

- Central line

RATE OF ADMINISTRATION

- Monitor blood pressure and adjust dose according to response

COMMENTS

–

Other information

- Catecholamines have a high non-renal systemic clearance, therefore the effect of any renal replacement therapy is unlikely to be relevant

Alcuronium

Clinical use

A competitive neuromuscular blocker used to produce skeletal muscle relaxation during surgical procedures

Dose in normal renal function

Initially 100–250 micrograms/kg IV. Supplementary doses of ⅙–¼ of the initial dose provide relaxation for additional periods of similar duration to the first

Pharmacokinetics

Molecular weight (daltons)	827.9
% Protein binding	40
% Excreted unchanged in urine	80–85
Volume of distribution (L/kg)	0.28–0.36
Half-life – normal/ESRF (hrs)	3–3.5/16

Dose in renal impairment GFR (mL/min)

20–50	100–150 micrograms/kg
10–20	100–150 micrograms/kg
<10	100–150 micrograms/kg

Dose in patients undergoing renal replacement therapies

CAPD	Unknown dialysability. Dose as in GFR = <10 mL/min
HD	Unknown dialysability. Dose as in GFR = <10 mL/min
CAV/VVHD	Unknown dialysability. Dose as in GFR = 10–20 mL/min

Important drug interactions

CYCLOSPORIN

–

POTENTIALLY HAZARDOUS INTERACTIONS WITH OTHER DRUGS

- The neuromuscular block of botulinum toxin may be enhanced by non-depolarising muscle relaxants (increased risk of toxicity)
- The effect of non-depolarising muscle relaxants can be enhanced by aminoglycosides, azlocillin, clindamycin and colistin
- Procainamide and quinidine can enhance the muscle relaxant effect

Administration

RECONSTITUTION

–

ROUTE

- IV

RATE OF ADMINISTRATION

- Variable

COMMENTS

- Neuromuscular blocking agents are generally incompatible with alkaline solutions, such as thiopentone sodium

Other information

- With usual doses the onset of muscle relaxation is about 2 min and lasts about 20–30 min
- Doses of 160 micrograms/kg have been used without any problems in patients with chronic renal failure undergoing renal transplantation. The average duration of action of this dose was 37 min
- Respiratory acidosis and hypokalaemia may increase the effects of alcuronium
- Any residual neuromuscular blockade at the end of surgery can be reversed using atropine and neostigmine

Alfacalcidol

Clinical use

Vitamin D analogue. Increase in serum calcium levels, inhibition of parathyroid hormone release and suppression of PTH production

Dose in normal renal function

0.25–1 micrograms daily according to response. Alternatively, up to 4 micrograms PO/IV 3 times a week

Pharmacokinetics

Molecular weight (daltons)	400.6
% Protein binding	Extensive plasma protein binding
% Excreted unchanged in urine	19–41
Volume of distribution (L/kg)	–
Half-life – normal/ESRF	16–30 days

Dose in renal impairment GFR (mL/min)

20–50	Dose as in normal renal function
10–20	Dose as in normal renal function
<10	Dose as in normal renal function

Dose in patients undergoing renal replacement therapies

CAPD	Not dialysed. Dose as in normal renal function
HD	Not dialysed. Dose as in normal renal function
CAV/VVHD	Not dialysed. Dose as in normal renal function

Important drug interactions

CYCLOSPORIN

–

POTENTIALLY HAZARDOUS INTERACTIONS WITH OTHER DRUGS

• Carbamazepine, phenytoin, phenobarbitone and primidone may increase metabolism of alfacalcidol, necessitating larger doses than normal to produce the desired effect

Administration

RECONSTITUTION

–

ROUTE

• Oral, IV

RATE OF ADMINISTRATION

• IV over 30 sec

COMMENTS

–

Other information

• Adjust dose according to response. Serum calcium reference range 2.1–2.6 mmol/L (total)
• An IV preparation (2 micrograms/mL) and an oral solution (0.2 micrograms/mL) are also available
• Doses of 1 microgram daily for 5 days may need to be given immediately prior to parathyroidectomy. Alternatively, 5 micrograms can be given immediately prior to parathyroidectomy
• Capsules of One-Alpha (Leo) contain sesame oil

Alfentanil

Clinical use

Opioid analgesic – used for short surgical procedures or intensive care sedation

Dose in normal renal function

IV injection:

spontaneous respiration up to 500 micrograms over 30 sec; supplemental dose = 250 micrograms

assisted ventilation 30–50 micrograms/kg; supplemental dose = 15 micrograms/kg

By IV infusion with assisted ventilation:

loading dose 50–100 micrograms/kg as bolus or fast infusion over 10 min followed by 0.5–1 micrograms/kg/min. Discontinue infusion 30 min before anticipated end of surgery

For analgesia and suppression of respiratory activity during intensive care with assisted ventilation:

by IV infusion 30 micrograms/kg/hr adjusted according to response (usual range 0.5–10 mg/hr)

For more rapid initial control give 5 mg IV in divided portions over 10 min (slower if hypotension or bradycardia develop); additional doses of 0.5–1 mg may be given by IV injection during short painful procedures

Pharmacokinetics

Molecular weight (daltons)	453.0
% Protein binding	88–95
% Excreted unchanged in urine	<1
Volume of distribution (L/kg)	0.3–1.0
Half-life – normal/ESRF (hrs)	1–4/unchanged

Dose in renal impairment GFR (mL/min)

20–50	Dose as in normal renal function
10–20	Dose as in normal renal function
<10	Dose as in normal renal function

Dose in patients undergoing renal replacement therapies

CAPD	Not dialysed. Dose as in normal renal function
HD	Not dialysed. Dose as in normal renal function
CAV/VVHD	Not dialysed. Dose as in normal renal function

Important drug interactions

CYCLOSPORIN

–

POTENTIALLY HAZARDOUS INTERACTIONS WITH OTHER DRUGS

- Possible CNS excitation or depression (hypertension or hypotension) in patients also receiving MAOIs (including moclobemide)
- Cimetidine or erythromycin can inhibit clearance of alfentanil. This may increase the risk of prolonged respiratory depression
- Beta-blockers and anaesthetics depressing the heart by increasing vagal tone may predispose to bradycardia or hypotension

Administration

RECONSTITUTION

–

ROUTE

- IV bolus, IV infusion

RATE OF ADMINISTRATION

- See dose

COMMENTS

- Alfentanil can be mixed with sodium chloride 0.9%, glucose 5% or compound sodium lactate injection (Hartmann's solution)

Other information

- There is an increase in free fraction of drug in renal failure; hence dose requirements may be reduced
- IV administration: 500 micrograms alfentanil have peak effect in 90 sec and provide analgesia for 5–10 min (in unpremedicated adults)
- Transient fall in BP and bradycardia may occur on administration
- Analgesic potency = ¼ of that of fentanyl
- Duration of action = ⅓ of that of an equianalgesic dose of fentanyl
- Onset of action = 4 times more rapid than an equianalgesic dose of fentanyl

ALG – Merieux (horse) (lymphoglobuline) (unlicensed product)

Clinical use

Prophylaxis and/or treatment of acute or steroid-resistant transplant rejection

Dose in normal renal function

5–10 mg/kg/day for up to 10–14 days

Pharmacokinetics

Molecular weight (daltons)	–
% Protein binding	–
% Excreted unchanged in urine	–
Volume of distribution (L/kg)	–
Half-life – normal/ESRF (hrs)	48–72/–

Dose in renal impairment GFR (mL/min)

20–50	Dose as in normal renal function
10–20	Dose as in normal renal function
<10	Dose as in normal renal function

Dose in patients undergoing renal replacement therapies

CAPD	Not dialysed. Dose as in normal renal function
HD	Not dialysed. Dose as in normal renal function
CAV/VVHD	Not dialysed. Dose as in normal renal function

Important drug interactions

CYCLOSPORIN

• Risk of over-immunosuppression

POTENTIALLY HAZARDOUS INTERACTIONS WITH OTHER DRUGS

• Do not give blood or blood derivatives concomitantly
• Avoid simultaneous infusion of glucose solutions in same line

Administration

RECONSTITUTION

• Dilute total dose in 250 mL sodium chloride 0.9% (maximum concentration 1 mg/mL)

ROUTE

• IV centrally: if there is no central access, via peripheral vein with good blood flow rates

RATE OF ADMINISTRATION

• 4–16 hrs

COMMENTS

• To minimise risk of adverse effects, chlorpheniramine (10 mg IV) and hydrocortisone (100 mg IV) may be given 15–60 min before administration of full ALG dose
• Chlorpheniramine, hydrocortisone and adrenaline should be immediately available in case of severe anaphylaxis

Other information

• Dose may be modified to optimise immunosuppression. Aim to keep total lymphocyte count below 3% of total white cell count or 50 cells/µL. Alternatively, keep absolute T-cell count below 50 cells/µL, and only dose when above this
• Avoid simultaneous transfusions of blood or blood derivatives and infusions of other solutions, particularly lipids
• A test dose is advised in accordance with manufacturer's literature
• ALG should not be administered in the presence of fluid overload, allergy to horse protein, or pregnancy

Allopurinol

Clinical use

Gout prophylaxis, hyperuricaemia

Dose in normal renal function

100–900 mg/day (usually 300 mg/day)

Pharmacokinetics

Molecular weight (daltons)	136.1
% Protein binding	<5
% Excreted unchanged in urine	30
Volume of distribution (L/kg)	0.5
Half-life – normal/ESRF (hrs)	2–8/unchanged

Dose in renal impairment GFR (mL/min)

20–50	200–300 mg daily
10–20	100–200 mg daily
<10	100 mg daily/alternate days

Dose in patients undergoing renal replacement therapies

CAPD	Dialysed. Dose as in GFR = <10 mL/min
HD	Dialysed. Dose as in GFR = <10 mL/min
CAV/VVHD	Dialysed. Dose as in GFR = 10–20 mL/min

Important drug interactions

CYCLOSPORIN

• Isolated reports of raised cyclosporin levels (risk of nephrotoxicity)

POTENTIALLY HAZARDOUS INTERACTIONS WITH OTHER DRUGS

• Effects of azathioprine, cyclophosphamide and mercaptopurine enhanced with increased toxicity
• Increased risk of toxicity with captopril

Administration

RECONSTITUTION

–

ROUTE

• Oral

RATE OF ADMINISTRATION

–

COMMENTS

• In all grades of renal impairment commence with 100 mg/day and increase if serum and/or urinary urate response is unsatisfactory. Doses less than 100 mg/day may be required in some patients
• Take as a single daily dose, preferably after food

Other information

• A parenteral preparation is available from Wellcome on a 'named patient' basis
• HD patients may be given 300 mg post dialysis, i.e. on alternate days
• There is an increased incidence of skin rash in patients with renal impairment
• Efficient dialysis usually controls serum uric acid levels
• If the patient is prescribed azathioprine or 6-mercaptopurine concomitantly, reduce azathioprine or 6-mercaptopurine dose by 75%
• Occasionally prescribed concurrently with colchicine in patients with impaired renal function, unable to have NSAIDs during severe gout episodes
• Main active metabolite oxypurinol renally excreted; % plasma protein binding 17%; half-life – normal/ESRF = 13–18/>125 hrs–1 week

Alteplase (t-Pa) (recombinant human tissue-type plasminogen activator)

Clinical use

Fibrinolytic drug used for acute myocardial infarction and pulmonary embolism

Dose in normal renal function

Myocardial infarction:

accelerated regimen (initiated within 6 hrs) 15 mg IV bolus, 50 mg over 30 min, then 35 mg over 1 hr (total dose 100 mg); or (if initiated within 6–12 hrs) 10 mg over 1–2 min followed by IV infusion of 50 mg over 1 hr, then 40 mg over subsequent 2 hrs (total dose 100 mg over 3 hrs)

Pulmonary embolism:

total dose of 100 mg should be administered in 2 hrs. Total dose should not exceed 1.5 mg/kg in patients who weigh <65 kg

Pharmacokinetics

Molecular weight (daltons)	64497.8 (non-glycosylated protein)
% Protein binding	–
% Excreted unchanged in urine	–
Volume of distribution (L/kg)	0.1
Half-life – normal/ESRF (hrs)	0.5

Dose in renal impairment GFR (mL/min)

20–50	Dose as in normal renal function
10–20	Dose as in normal renal function
<10	Dose as in normal renal function

Dose in patients undergoing renal replacement therapies

CAPD	Not dialysed. Dose as in normal renal function
HD	Not dialysed. Dose as in normal renal function
CAV/VVHD	Not dialysed. Dose as in normal renal function

Important drug interactions

CYCLOSPORIN

–

POTENTIALLY HAZARDOUS INTERACTIONS WITH OTHER DRUGS

• Risk of haemorrhage can be increased by the use of coumarine derivatives, platelet aggregation inhibitors, heparin and other agents influencing coagulation

Administration

RECONSTITUTION

• 50-mg vial – dissolve in 50 mL water for injection; 20-mg vial – dissolve in 20 mL water for injection. The reconstituted solutions can be further diluted (minimum concentration 0.2 mg/mL) with sterile sodium chloride 0.9%

ROUTE

• IV

RATE OF ADMINISTRATION

• See dose

COMMENTS

• Water or glucose solution must NOT be used for dilution
• 50-mg vial = 29 mega-units/vial
• 20-mg vial = 11.6 mega-units/vial

Other information

• Patients weighing less than 65 kg should receive a total dose of 1.5 mg/kg according to dose schedule
• Allergic reactions are less likely with alteplase than streptokinase and repeated administration is possible
• 1.7 g arginine in the 50-mg vial, 0.7 g arginine in 20-mg vial – may lead to hyperkalaemia in renal failure
• Pay attention to potential bleeding sites during treatment

Aluminium hydroxide

Clinical use

Phosphate-binding agent

Dose in normal renal function

As Alu-Caps:
4–20 capsules daily in divided doses
As mixture:
30–120 mL daily in divided doses in accordance
with response

Pharmacokinetics

Molecular weight (daltons)	78
% Protein binding	70–90
% Excreted unchanged in urine	–
Volume of distribution (L/kg)	–
Half-life – normal/ESRF (hrs)	–

Dose in renal impairment
GFR (mL/min)

20–50	Dose as in normal renal function
10–20	Dose as in normal renal function
<10	Dose as in normal renal function

Dose in patients undergoing renal replacement therapies

CAPD	Dose as in normal renal function
HD	Dose as in normal renal function
CAV/VVHD	Dose as in normal renal function

Important drug interactions

CYCLOSPORIN

–

POTENTIALLY HAZARDOUS INTERACTIONS WITH
OTHER DRUGS

–

Administration

RECONSTITUTION

–

ROUTE

• Oral

RATE OF ADMINISTRATION

–

COMMENTS

–

Other information

• End-stage renal failure patients on chronic therapy
may develop aluminium toxicity, therefore best
avoided in all but short-term therapy (calcium
carbonate can be used in chronic therapy)

• Take/administer with, or immediately before, meals

• In patients undergoing chronic therapy with
aluminium hydroxide, serum aluminium levels
should be monitored using the desferrioxamine
test (5 mg/kg) (see local protocol)

• Suspension available (not prescribable by GPs)

Amantidine

Clinical use

Parkinson's disease (but not drug-induced
extrapyramidal symptoms), herpes zoster,
prophylaxis and treatment of influenza A

Dose in normal renal function

Parkinson's disease:

100 mg once a day increased after 1 week to
100 mg twice a day

Herpes zoster:

100 mg twice a day for 14 days

Influenza A:

treatment – 100 mg once a day for 4–5 days;
prophylaxis – 100 mg once a day

Pharmacokinetics

Molecular weight (daltons)	187.7
% Protein binding	67
% Excreted unchanged in urine	90
Volume of distribution (L/kg)	4–5
Half-life – normal/ESRF (hrs)	12/500

Dose in renal impairment GFR (mL/min)

20–50	100 mg every 24–48 hrs
10–20	100 mg every 48–72 hrs
<10	100 mg every 7 days

Dose in patients undergoing renal replacement therapies

CAPD	Unknown dialysability. Dose as in GFR = <10 mL/min
HD	Unknown dialysability. Dose as in GFR = <10 mL/min
CAV/VVHD	Unknown dialysability. Dose as in GFR = 10–20 mL/min

Important drug interactions

CYCLOSPORIN

–

POTENTIALLY HAZARDOUS INTERACTIONS WITH
OTHER DRUGS

–

Administration

RECONSTITUTION

–

ROUTE

• Oral

RATE OF ADMINISTRATION

–

COMMENTS

–

Other information

• Peripheral oedema may occur in some patients,
which should be considered when the drug is
prescribed for those with congestive heart failure

• Side-effects are often mild and transient. They
usually appear within 2–4 days of treatment and
disappear 24–48 hrs after discontinuation of the
drug

• Due to extensive tissue binding, <5% of a dose is
removed by a 4-hr haemodialysis session

• A reduction in creatinine clearance to 40mL/min
may result in a 5-fold increase in elimination
half-life

Amikacin

Clinical use

Antibacterial agent

Dose in normal renal function

15 mg/kg/day in two divided doses (maximum dose: 1.5 g/day, maximum total dose: 15 g)

Pharmacokinetics

Molecular weight (daltons)	585.6
% Protein binding	<5
% Excreted unchanged in urine	95
Volume of distribution (L/kg)	0.22–0.29
Half-life – normal/ESRF (hrs)	1.4–2.3/17–150

Dose in renal impairment GFR (mL/min)

20–50	5–6 mg/kg every 12 hrs
10–20	3–4 mg/kg every 24 hrs
<10	2 mg/kg every 24–48 hrs

Dose in patients undergoing renal replacement therapies

CAPD	Dialysed. Dose as in GFR = <10 mL/min
HD	Dialysed. Give 5 mg/kg after dialysis
CAV/VVHD	Dialysed. Dose as in GFR = 10–20 mL/min and monitor levels

Important drug interactions

CYCLOSPORIN

• Increased risk of nephrotoxicity

POTENTIALLY HAZARDOUS INTERACTIONS WITH OTHER DRUGS

• Botulinum toxin: neuromuscular block enhanced risk of toxicity
• Cholinergics: antagonism of effect of neostigmine and pyridostigmine

• Cytotoxics: increased risk of nephrotoxicity and possibly of ototoxicity with cisplatin
• Diuretics: increased risk of ototoxicity with loop diuretics
• Muscle relaxants: effects of non-depolarising muscle relaxants such as tubocurarine enhanced

Administration

RECONSTITUTION

–

ROUTE

• IM, IV

RATE OF ADMINISTRATION

• IV bolus – slow over 2–3 min; infusion – at concentration of 2.5 mg/mL over 30 min (diluents: sodium chloride 0.9%, glucose 5% and others)

COMMENTS

• May be used intraperitoneally
• Do not mix physically with any other antibacterial agents

Other information

• Nephrotoxic and ototoxic. Toxicity no worse when hyperbilirubinemic
• Serum levels must be measured for efficacy and toxicity
• Peritoneal absorption increases with presence of inflammation
• Volume of distribution increases with oedema, obesity and ascites
• Peak serum concentration should not exceed 30 mg/L
• Trough serum concentration should be less than 10 mg/L
• Amikacin affects auditory function to a greater extent than gentamicin

Aminophylline

Clinical use

Reversible airway obstruction

Dose in normal renal function

Oral:

200–400 mg every 12 hrs, maximum 900 mg daily

IV loading dose:

5 mg/kg

Maintenance dose:

0.5 mg/kg/hr

Pharmacokinetics

Molecular weight (daltons)	420.4
% Protein binding	40–60 (theophylline)
% Excreted unchanged in urine	<10
Volume of distribution (L/kg)	0.4–0.7 (theophylline)
Half-life – normal/ESRF (hrs)	4–12/unchanged (theophylline)

Dose in renal impairment GFR (mL/min)

20–50	200–400 mg every 12 hrs
10–20	200–300 mg every 12 hrs and adjust in accordance with blood levels
<10	200–300 mg every 12 hrs and adjust in accordance with blood levels

Dose in patients undergoing renal replacement therapies

CAPD	Not dialysed. Dose as in GFR = <10 mL/min. Monitor blood levels
HD	Not dialysed. Dose as in GFR = <10 mL/min. Monitor blood levels
CAV/VVHD	Not dialysed. Dose as in GFR = 10–20 mL/min. Monitor blood levels

Important drug interactions

CYCLOSPORIN

–

POTENTIALLY HAZARDOUS INTERACTIONS WITH OTHER DRUGS

- Plasma concentration increased by ciprofloxacin, erythromycin, clarithromycin and norfloxacin. Also by diltiazem, verapamil, cimetidine and combined oral contraceptives
- Plasma concentrations reduced by carbamazepine, phenobarbitone, phenytoin, primidone and rifampicin
- Antagonism of anti-arrhythmic effect of adenosine

Administration

RECONSTITUTION

–

ROUTE

- IV, oral

RATE OF ADMINISTRATION

- Loading dose over 20 min by slow IV injection

COMMENTS

–

Other information

- Optimum response obtained at plasma theophylline levels of 10–20 mg/L (55–110 mmol/L)
- Increased incidence of gastrointestinal and neurological side-effects in renal impairment at plasma levels above optimum range
- Aminophylline: 80% theophylline + 20% ethylenediamine

Amiodarone

Clinical use

Cardiac arrhythmias

Dose in normal renal function

Oral:

200 mg three times a day for 1 week, then twice a day for 1 week, then 200 mg daily maintenance dose or minimum required to control arrhythmia

IV:

via central catheter: 5 mg/kg
(maximum 1.2 g in 24 hrs)

Pharmacokinetics

Molecular weight (daltons)	645.3
% Protein binding	96
% Excreted unchanged in urine	<5
Volume of distribution (L/kg)	70–140
Half-life – normal/ESRF	14–120 days/ unchanged

Dose in renal impairment GFR (mL/min)

20–50	Dose as in normal renal function
10–20	Dose as in normal renal function
<10	Dose as in normal renal function

Dose in patients undergoing renal replacement therapies

CAPD	Not dialysed. Dose as in normal renal function
HD	Not dialysed. Dose as in normal renal function
CAV/VVHD	Not dialysed. Dose as in normal renal function

Important drug interactions

CYCLOSPORIN

• Increased levels of cyclosporin possible

POTENTIALLY HAZARDOUS INTERACTIONS WITH OTHER DRUGS

• Other anti-arrhythmics: additive effect and increased risk of myocardial depression

• Warfarin: metabolism inhibited (increased anticoagulant effect)

• Phenytoin: metabolism inhibited (increased plasma concentration)

• Beta-blockers and calcium-channel blockers: increased risk of bradycardia, AV block and myocardial depression

• Digoxin: increased plasma concentration (halve digoxin maintenance dose)

• Terfenadine and astemizole: increased risk of ventricular arrhythmias

• Phenothiazines: increased risk of ventricular arrhythmias

Administration

RECONSTITUTION

• Add dose to 250 mL glucose 5%

ROUTE

• IV via central catheter or peripherally in veins with good blood flow

RATE OF ADMINISTRATION

• 20–120 min (max. 1.2 g in up to 500 mL glucose 5% in 24 hrs)

COMMENTS

• Solutions containing less than 300 mg in 500 mL glucose 5% should not be used, as unstable

• Volumetric pump should be used as amiodarone can reduce drop size

Other information

• Amiodarone and desethylamiodarone levels can be monitored to assess compliance

• In extreme clinical emergency may be given by slow IV bolus using 150–300 mg in 10–20 mL glucose 5% over a minimum of 3 min with close patient monitoring. This should not be repeated for at least 15 min

• Incompatible with sodium chloride 0.9%

• Rapid IV administration has been associated with anaphylactic shock, hot flushes, sweating and nausea

Amitriptyline

Clinical use

Tricyclic antidepressant used especially where sedation is required

Dose in normal renal function

Oral:

initially 75 mg/day, increased gradually to maximum of 150 mg. Usual maintenance: 50–100 mg daily

IM/IV:

10–20 mg 4 times a day

Pharmacokinetics

Molecular weight (daltons)	277.4
% Protein binding	96
% Excreted unchanged in urine	<10
Volume of distribution (L/kg)	6–36
Half-life – normal/ESRF (hrs)	24–40/unchanged

Dose in renal impairment GFR (mL/min)

20–50	Dose as in normal renal function
10–20	Dose as in normal renal function
<10	Dose as in normal renal function

Dose in patients undergoing renal replacement therapies

CAPD	Not dialysed. Dose as in normal renal function
HD	Not dialysed. Dose as in normal renal function
CAV/VVHD	Not dialysed. Dose as in normal renal function

Important drug interactions

CYCLOSPORIN

–

POTENTIALLY HAZARDOUS INTERACTIONS WITH OTHER DRUGS

- Anaesthetics: risk of arrhythmias and hypotension increased
- Interaction with anti-arrhythmics: increased risk of ventricular arrhythmias with drugs which prolong QT interval
- MAOIs: CNS excitation and hypertension
- Antagonism with anti-epileptics: convulsive threshold lowered. Also anti-epileptics may lower plasma concentration of some tricyclics
- Antihistamines: increased antimuscarinic and sedative effects; increased risk of ventricular arrhythmias with astemizole and terfenadine
- Antimalarials: increased risk of ventricular arrhythmias with halofantrine
- Hypertension and arrhythmias with adrenaline
- Hypertension with noradrenaline

Administration

RECONSTITUTION

–

ROUTE

- Oral, IM, IV

RATE OF ADMINISTRATION

–

COMMENTS

–

Other information

- Introduce treatment gradually in renal impairment due to dizziness and postural hypotension
- Withdraw treatment gradually
- Anticholinergic side-effects – causes urinary retention, drowsiness, dry mouth, blurred vision and constipation

Amlodipine

Clinical use

Calcium-channel-blocker for hypertension, angina prophylaxis

Dose in normal renal function

5–10 mg daily

Pharmacokinetics

Molecular weight (daltons)	567.1
% Protein binding	>95
% Excreted unchanged in urine	<10
Volume of distribution (L/kg)	21
Half-life – normal/ESRF (hrs)	35–50/50

Dose in renal impairment GFR (mL/min)

20–50	Dose as in normal renal function
10–20	Dose as in normal renal function
<10	Dose as in normal renal function

Dose in patients undergoing renal replacement therapies

CAPD	Not dialysed. Dose as in normal renal function
HD	Not dialysed. Dose as in normal renal function
CAV/VVHD	Not dialysed. Dose as in normal renal function

Important drug interactions

CYCLOSPORIN

–

POTENTIALLY HAZARDOUS INTERACTIONS WITH OTHER DRUGS

• Antihypertensives: enhanced hypotensive effect, increased risk of first-dose hypotensive effect of pre-synaptic alpha-blockers

Administration

RECONSTITUTION

–

ROUTE

• Oral

RATE OF ADMINISTRATION

–

COMMENTS

–

Other information

• Amlodipine is extensively metabolised to inactive metabolites

Amoxycillin

Clinical use

Antibacterial agent

Dose in normal renal function

250–500 mg every 8 hrs (maximum 6 g per day)

Pharmacokinetics

Molecular weight (daltons)	365.4
% Protein binding	15–25
% Excreted unchanged in urine	50–70
Volume of distribution (L/kg)	0.26
Half-life – normal/ESRF (hrs)	0.9–2.3/5–20

Dose in renal impairment GFR (mL/min)

20–50	Dose as in normal renal function
10–20	Dose as in normal renal function
<10	250 mg every 8 hrs

Dose in patients undergoing renal replacement therapies

CAPD	Dialysed. Dose as in GFR = <10 mL/min
HD	Dialysed. Dose as in GFR = <10 mL/min
CAV/VVHD	Dialysed. Dose as in normal renal function

Important drug interactions

CYCLOSPORIN

–

POTENTIALLY HAZARDOUS INTERACTIONS WITH OTHER DRUGS

• Amoxycillin can reduce the excretion of methotrexate (increased risk of toxicity)

Administration

RECONSTITUTION

• IV: dissolve each 250 mg in 5 mL water for injection
• IV infusion: dilute in 100 mL glucose 5% or sodium chloride 0.9%
• IM: dissolve 250 mg in 1.5 mL water for injection; 500 mg in 2.5 mL water for injection; 1 g in 2.5 mL water for injection or 1% sterile lignocaine hydrochloride

ROUTE

• Oral, IV, IM

RATE OF ADMINISTRATION

• Slow bolus IV over 3–4 min
• Infusion over 30–60 min

COMMENTS

• Stability in infusion depends upon diluent

Other information

• Sodium – 3.3 mmol/g vial of Amoxil
• Do not mix with aminoglycosides

Amphotericin IV

Clinical use

Antifungal agent for systemic fungal infections (yeasts and yeast-like fungi including candida albicans)

Dose in normal renal function

250 micrograms–6 mg/kg/day (usually in range 500 micrograms–1.5 mg/kg/day) (see individual product data sheet)

Liposomal amphotericin dosages:

1–5 mg/kg/day (see individual product data sheet)

Pharmacokinetics

Molecular weight (daltons)	924
% Protein binding	90
% Excreted unchanged in urine	5
Volume of distribution (L/kg)	4
Half-life – normal/ESRF (hrs)	24/unchanged

Dose in renal impairment GFR (mL/min)

20–50	250 micrograms–6 mg/kg every 24 hrs
10–20	250 micrograms–6 mg/kg every 24 hrs
<10	250 micrograms–6 mg/kg every 24–36 hrs

Dose in patients undergoing renal replacement therapies

CAPD	Not dialysed. Dose as in GFR = <10 mL/min
HD	Not dialysed. Dose as in GFR = <10 mL/min
CAV/VVHD	Not dialysed. Dose as in GFR = 10–20 mL/min

Important drug interactions

CYCLOSPORIN

• Increased nephrotoxicity

POTENTIALLY HAZARDOUS INTERACTIONS WITH OTHER DRUGS

• Increased risk of nephrotoxicity with aminoglycosides

Administration

RECONSTITUTION

• See individual data sheet. Prepare intermittent infusion in glucose 5% (incompatible with sodium chloride 0.9%, electrolytes or other drugs)

• Reconstitute vial contents with water for injection. pH should be adjusted to >4.2

ROUTE

• Peripheral or central IV

RATE OF ADMINISTRATION

• Over 6 hrs (liposomal amphotericin over1 hr)

COMMENTS

• Infusions of total dose over 2–4 hrs have been reported without adverse events (unlicensed)

• Higher rates of infusion are associated with greater risk of adverse reactions

• Paracetamol and parenteral pethidine may alleviate rigors associated with amphotericin administration

• Flush existing IV line with glucose 5% before and after infusion administration

• For patients on CAV/VVHD, amphotericin should be given into the venous return of the dialysis circuit

Other information

• **AMPHOTERICIN IS HIGHLY NEPHROTOXIC** – it can cause distal tubular acidosis

• May cause polyuria, hypovolaemia, hypokalaemia and acidosis. Enhancement of nephrotoxicity of amphotericin by other drugs is possible, e.g. aminoglycosides. Concomitant administration of corticosteroids may increase hypokalaemia

• Amphotericin and flucytosine act synergistically when co-administered, enabling lower doses to be used effectively

• A test dose of amphotericin is recommended at the beginning of a new course

• Monitor renal function, full blood count, potassium, magnesium and calcium levels

• Liposomal amphotericin is considerably less nephrotoxic compared to amphotericin, but is considerably more expensive

• There are reports of the use of amphotericin in 20% lipid solution being as well tolerated as liposomal amphotericin

Ampicillin

Clinical use

Antibacterial agent

Dose in normal renal function

Oral:
250 mg–1 g every 6 hrs
IM/IV:
500 mg–2 g every 6 hrs

Pharmacokinetics

Molecular weight (daltons)	349
% Protein binding	20
% Excreted unchanged in urine	30–90
Volume of distribution (L/kg)	0.17–0.31
Half-life – normal/ESRF (hrs)	0.8–1.5/7–20

Dose in renal impairment
GFR (mL/min)

20–50	Dose as in normal renal function
10–20	250–500 mg every 6 hrs
<10	250 mg every 6 hrs

Dose in patients undergoing renal replacement therapies

CAPD	Dialysed. Dose as in GFR = <10 mL/min
HD	Dialysed. Dose as in GFR = <10 mL/min
CAV/VVHD	Dialysed. Dose as in GFR = 10–20 mL/min

Important drug interactions

CYCLOSPORIN

• May increase cyclosporin levels

POTENTIALLY HAZARDOUS INTERACTIONS WITH OTHER DRUGS

• Reduces excretion of methotrexate (increased risk of toxicity)

Administration

RECONSTITUTION

• Use water for injection: 5 mL for each 250 mg (1.5 mL for 250 mg or 500 mg for IM administration)

ROUTE

• Oral, IV, IM

RATE OF ADMINISTRATION

• Slow IV bolus over 3–4 min. Doses greater than 500 mg should be given by infusion at a rate not exceeding 500 mg/min

COMMENTS

–

Other information

• Rashes are more common in patients with renal impairment
• Can cause nephrotoxicity if dose is not reduced in renal impairment
• Sodium content of injection 2.7 mmol/g
• Ampicillin may be used in peritoneal dialysis fluids for treatment of peritonitis
• Do not mix with aminoglycosides

Ascorbic acid

Clinical use

Acidification of urine, vitamin C deficiency

Dose in normal renal function

Up to 4 g daily in divided doses

Pharmacokinetics

Molecular weight (daltons)	176
% Protein binding	24
% Excreted unchanged in urine	<10
Volume of distribution (L/kg)	–
Half-life – normal/ESRF (hrs)	3–4/unchanged

Dose in renal impairment GFR (mL/min)

20–50	Dose as in normal renal function
10–20	Dose as in normal renal function
<10	Dose as in normal renal function

Dose in patients undergoing renal replacement therapies

CAPD	Dialysed. Dose as in normal renal function
HD	Dialysed. Dose as in normal renal function
CAV/VVHD	Dialysed. Dose as in normal renal function

Important drug interactions

CYCLOSPORIN

–

POTENTIALLY HAZARDOUS INTERACTIONS WITH OTHER DRUGS

–

Administration

RECONSTITUTION

–

ROUTE

• Oral

RATE OF ADMINISTRATION

–

COMMENTS

–

Other information

• No scientific evidence in clinical trial of efficacy in reducing incidence of urinary tract infections via acidification of urine

Aspirin

Clinical use

Prophylaxis of cerebrovascular disease or myocardial infarction

Dose in normal renal function

75–300 mg daily

Pharmacokinetics

Molecular weight (daltons)	180
% Protein binding	72–95
% Excreted unchanged in urine	5 (acidic urine); 85 (alkaline urine)
Volume of distribution (L/kg)	0.1–0.2
Half-life – normal/ESRF (hrs)	2–3/unchanged

Dose in renal impairment GFR (mL/min)

20–50	Dose as in normal renal function
10–20	Dose as in normal renal function
<10	Dose as in normal renal function

Dose in patients undergoing renal replacement therapies

CAPD	Dialysed. Dose as in normal renal function
HD	Dialysed. Dose as in normal renal function
CAV/VVHD	Dialysed. Dose as in normal renal function

Important drug interactions

CYCLOSPORIN

–

POTENTIALLY HAZARDOUS INTERACTIONS WITH OTHER DRUGS

• Anticoagulants: increased risk of bleeding due to antiplatelet effect
• Cytotoxics: reduced excretion of methotrexate. Risk of increased toxicity

Administration

RECONSTITUTION

–

ROUTE

• Oral

RATE OF ADMINISTRATION

–

COMMENTS

–

Other information

• Aspirin at analgesic/antipyretic dose is best avoided in patients with renal impairment, especially if severe
• Antiplatelet effect may add to uraemic, gastrointestinal and haematological symptoms
• Degree of protein binding reduced in ESRD

Astemizole

Clinical use

Antihistamine – symptomatic relief of allergy such as hay fever and urticaria

Dose in normal renal function

10 mg once a day

Pharmacokinetics

Molecular weight (daltons)	458.6
% Protein binding	97
% Excreted unchanged in urine	0
Volume of distribution (L/kg)	–
Half-life – normal/ESRF	20 days/unchanged

Dose in renal impairment GFR (mL/min)

20–50	Dose as in normal renal function
10–20	Dose as in normal renal function
<10	Dose as in normal renal function

Dose in patients undergoing renal replacement therapies

CAPD	Not dialysed. Dose as in normal renal function
HD	Not dialysed. Dose as in normal renal function
CAV/VVHD	Not dialysed. Dose as in normal renal function

Important drug interactions

CYCLOSPORIN

POTENTIALLY HAZARDOUS INTERACTIONS WITH OTHER DRUGS

- Increased risk of ventricular arrhythmias with anti-arrhythmic drugs
- Metabolism of astemizole inhibited by erythromycin and other macrolides (risk of hazardous arrhythmias)
- Itraconazole, ketoconazole and possibly other imidazoles (and triazoles) inhibit astemizole metabolism (cardiac toxicity reported)
- Concomitant use of astemizole and terfenadine not recommended (risk of hazardous arrhythmias)
- Increased risk of ventricular arrhythmias with halofantrine, quinine, antipsychotics, sotalol and tricyclic antidepressants
- Diuretics: hypokalaemia increases risk of ventricular arrhythmias with astemizole

Administration

RECONSTITUTION

–

ROUTE

- Oral

RATE OF ADMINISTRATION

–

COMMENTS

- Give at least 1 hr before or 2 hrs after a meal

Other information

- Do not exceed recommended dose
- Avoid in significant hepatic impairment
- Ventricular arrhythmias (including QT prolongation and *torsades de pointes*) have occurred at high doses

Atenolol

Clinical use

Beta-adrenoreceptor blocker for hypertension,
angina, arrhythmias

Dose in normal renal function

50–100 mg daily

Pharmacokinetics

Molecular weight (daltons)	266.3
% Protein binding	3
% Excreted unchanged in urine	>90
Volume of distribution (L/kg)	0.5–1.5
Half-life – normal/ESRF (hrs)	6.7/15–35

Dose in renal impairment
GFR (mL/min)

20–50	Dose as in normal renal function
10–20	Dose as in normal renal function
<10	50 mg once a day

Dose in patients undergoing renal replacement therapies

CAPD	Dialysed. Dose as in GFR = <10 mL/min
HD	Dialysed. Dose as in GFR = <10 mL/min
CAV/VVHD	Dialysed. Dose as in normal renal function

Important drug interactions

CYCLOSPORIN

–

POTENTIALLY HAZARDOUS INTERACTIONS WITH OTHER DRUGS

- Anaesthetics: enhanced hypotensive effect
- Anti-arrhythmics: increased risk of myocardial depression and bradycardia
- Calcium-channel blockers: increased risk of bradycardia and AV block with diltiazem. Hypotension and heart failure possible with nifedipine. Asystole, severe hypertension and heart failure with verapamil
- Sympathomimetics: severe hypertension with adrenaline and noradrenaline
- Cardiac glycosides: increased risk of bradycardia and AV block

Administration

RECONSTITUTION

–

ROUTE

- Oral

RATE OF ADMINISTRATION

–

COMMENTS

–

Other information

- IV injection available
- CSM advise that beta-blockers are contraindicated in patients with asthma or history of obstructive airway disease

ATG – Merieux (rabbit) (thymoglobuline) (unlicensed product)

Clinical use

Prophylaxis and treatment of acute (or steroid-resistant) transplant rejection

Dose in normal renal function

2.5–5 mg/kg/day for up to 10–14 days

Pharmacokinetics

Molecular weight (daltons)	–
% Protein binding	–
% Excreted unchanged in urine	–
Volume of distribution (L/kg)	–
Half-life – normal/ESRF (hrs)	48–72/–

Dose in renal impairment GFR (mL/min)

20–50	Dose as in normal renal function
10–20	Dose as in normal renal function
<10	Dose as in normal renal function

Dose in patients undergoing renal replacement therapies

CAPD	Not dialysed. Dose as in normal renal function
HD	Not dialysed. Dose as in normal renal function
CAV/VVHD	Not dialysed. Dose as in normal renal function

Important drug interactions

CYCLOSPORIN

–

POTENTIALLY HAZARDOUS INTERACTIONS WITH OTHER DRUGS

• Risk of over-immunosuppression

Administration

RECONSTITUTION

• Dilute dose in 250 mL sodium chloride 0.9%, maximum concentration 5 mg/mL

ROUTE

• IV via central line or via peripheral vein with good blood flow rates

RATE OF ADMINISTRATION

• 4–16 hrs

COMMENTS

• To minimise risk of adverse effects, chlorpheniramine (10 mg IV) and hydrocortisone (100 mg IV) may be given 15–60 min before administration of full-dose ATG

• Chlorpheniramine, hydrocortisone and adrenaline should be immediately available in case of severe anaphylaxis

Other information

• Dosage may be modified to optimise immunosuppression. Aim to keep total lymphocyte count below 3% of total white cell count or 50 cells/μL. Alternatively, keep absolute T-cell count below 50 cells/μL, and only dose when above this

• Avoid simultaneous transfusions of blood or blood derivatives and infusions of other solutions, particularly lipids

• A test dose is advised in accordance with the manufacturer's literature

• ATG should not be administered in the presence of fluid overload, allergy to rabbit protein, pregnancy or acute viral illness

• Local experience at Oxford: ATG is always given centrally and the maximum concentration (1 mg/2 mL) recommended by the company has often been exceeded. Concentrations of 1mg/mL have been given over 8 hrs with no problems. In addition, local in-house data is available to support a 28-day expiry of drug when reconstituted in Pharmacy CIVA

Atracurium

Clinical use

A non-depolarising muscle relaxant of short to medium duration

Dose in normal renal function

0.3–0.6 mg/kg depending on duration of full block required. Full block can be prolonged with supplementary doses of 0.1–0.2 mg/kg as required

Pharmacokinetics

Molecular weight (daltons)	1243.5
% Protein binding	82
% Excreted unchanged in urine	0
Volume of distribution (L/kg)	0.15–0.18
Half-life – normal/ESRF (hrs)	0.3–0.4/unchanged

Dose in renal impairment GFR (mL/min)

20–50	Dose as in normal renal function
10–20	Dose as in normal renal function
<10	Dose as in normal renal function

Dose in patients undergoing renal replacement therapies

CAPD	Not dialysed. Dose as in normal renal function
HD	Not dialysed. Dose as in normal renal function
CAV/VVHD	Not dialysed. Dose as in normal renal function

Important drug interactions

CYCLOSPORIN

–

POTENTIALLY HAZARDOUS INTERACTIONS WITH OTHER DRUGS

• Procainamide and quinidine enhance muscle relaxant effect
• Aminoglycosides, azlocillin, clindamycin, colistin and piperacillin enhance effect of atracurium
• Atracurium enhances the neuromuscular block produced by botulinum toxin (risk of toxicity)

Administration

RECONSTITUTION

–

ROUTE

• IV bolus, IV infusion

RATE OF ADMINISTRATION

• IV infusion: initial bolus dose of 0.3–0.6 mg/kg over 60 sec, then administer as a continuous infusion at rates of 0.3–0.6 mg/kg/hr

COMMENTS

• Stable in sodium chloride 0.9% for 24 hrs and glucose 5% for 8 hrs when diluted to concentrations of 0.5 mg/mL or above

Other information

–

Auranofin

Clinical use

Active progressive rheumatoid arthritis in adults when NSAIDs are inadequate alone

Dose in normal renal function

6 mg daily (maximum 9 mg)

Pharmacokinetics

Molecular weight (daltons)	678.5
% Protein binding	60–80
% Excreted unchanged in urine	50
Volume of distribution (L/kg)	–
Half-life – normal/ESRF	70–80 days/–

Dose in renal impairment GFR (mL/min)

20–50	3–6 mg daily
10–20	3 mg daily
<10	Avoid

Dose in patients undergoing renal replacement therapies

CAPD	Unknown dialysability. Dose as in GFR = <10 mL/min
HD	Not dialysed. Dose as in GFR = <10 mL/min
CAV/VVHD	Not dialysed. Dose as in GFR = 10–20 mL/min

Important drug interactions

CYCLOSPORIN

–

POTENTIALLY HAZARDOUS INTERACTIONS WITH OTHER DRUGS

–

Administration

RECONSTITUTION

–

ROUTE

• Oral

RATE OF ADMINISTRATION

–

COMMENTS

• Take with food
• Start initially with morning and evening dose – if well tolerated, patient can take dose once a day

Other information

• Warn patients to tell the doctor immediately if sore throat, mouth ulcers, bruising, fever, malaise, rash, diarrhoea or non-specific illness develop
• Blood tests should be carried out monthly and treatment should be withdrawn if the platelets fall below 100 000/µL or if signs and symptoms suggestive of thrombocytopenia appear
• Gold can produce nephrotic syndrome or less severe glomerular disease with proteinuria and haematuria, which are usually mild and transient. If persistent or clinically significant proteinuria develops, treatment with gold should be discontinued. Minor transient changes in renal function may also occur
• Urine tests should be carried out monthly to test for proteinuria and haematuria

Azathioprine

Clinical use

Immunosuppression for prophylaxis of transplant rejection

Dose in normal renal function

Oral and IV: 1–2.5 mg/kg/day

Pharmacokinetics

Molecular weight (daltons)	277.3
% Protein binding	20–30
% Excreted unchanged in urine	<2
Volume of distribution (L/kg)	0.55–0.8
Half-life – normal/ESRF (hrs)	0.16–1/increased

Dose in renal impairment GFR (mL/min)

20–50	Dose as in normal renal function
10–20	75–100%
<10	50–75%

Dose in patients undergoing renal replacement therapies

CAPD	Dialysable. Dose as in GFR = <10 mL/min
HD	Dialysable – 40–50% removed. Dose as in normal renal function
CAV/VVHD	Dialysable. Dose as in GFR = 10–20 mL/min

Important drug interactions

CYCLOSPORIN

• ? Decreased cyclosporin absorption and bioavailability

POTENTIALLY HAZARDOUS INTERACTIONS WITH OTHER DRUGS

• Allopurinol enhances effect with increased toxicity. Reduce azathioprine dose by 50–75% if administered concomitantly
• Cytotoxic agents may be additive or synergistic in producing toxicity, particularly in the bone marrow

Administration

RECONSTITUTION

• Add 5 mL water for injection to each vial (50 mg)

ROUTE

• IV bolus peripherally, preferably in the side arm of a fast-running infusion

RATE OF ADMINISTRATION

• Over not less than 1 min

COMMENTS

• **Very irritant to veins.** Flush with 50 mL sodium chloride 0.9% after administration
• Take tablets with or after food

Other information

• Extensively metabolised to mercaptopurine
• 1 mg by IV injection is equivalent to 1 mg by oral route
• 6-Mercaptopurine levels can be monitored in patients with low urate clearance
• Monitor white cell and platelet counts
• Can be given as an intermittent infusion (up to 250 mg in 100 mL)

Azithromycin

Clinical use

Antibacterial agent

Dose in normal renal function

Genital chlamydial infections:
1 g as single dose
All other indications:
500 mg daily for 3 days

Pharmacokinetics

Molecular weight (daltons)	785
% Protein binding	8–50
% Excreted unchanged in urine	6–12
Volume of distribution (L/kg)	18
Half-life – normal/ESRF (hrs)	10–60/–

Dose in renal impairment GFR (mL/min)

20–50	Dose as in normal renal function
10–20	Dose as in normal renal function
<10	Dose as in normal renal function

Dose in patients undergoing renal replacement therapies

CAPD	Unknown dialysability. Dose as in normal renal function
HD	Unknown dialysability. Dose as in normal renal function
CAV/VVHD	Unknown dialysability. Dose as in normal renal function

Important drug interactions

CYCLOSPORIN

• May inhibit the metabolism of cyclosporin (increased plasma cyclosporin levels)

POTENTIALLY HAZARDOUS INTERACTIONS WITH OTHER DRUGS

• The effect of digoxin may be enhanced
• Azithromycin and ergot derivatives should not be co-administered due to possibility of ergotism
• Effect of nicoumalone and warfarin may be enhanced
• May inhibit the metabolism of astemizole and terfenadine (risk of hazardous arrhythmias)

Administration

RECONSTITUTION

• Powder for oral suspension to be reconstituted with water (200 mg/5 mL strength)

ROUTE

• Oral

RATE OF ADMINISTRATION

–

COMMENTS

• Administer as a once daily dose 1 hr before food or 2 hrs after food

Other information

• ESRD dosing is based on extrapolation as no data are yet available

Azlocillin (sodium)

Clinical use

Antibacterial agent

Dose in normal renal function

2–5 g every 8 hrs

Pharmacokinetics

Molecular weight (daltons)	483.5
% Protein binding	30
% Excreted unchanged in urine	50–75
Volume of distribution (L/kg)	0.18–0.27
Half-life – normal/ESRF (hrs)	0.8–1.5/5–6

Dose in renal impairment GFR (mL/min)

20–50	Dose as in normal renal function
10–20	Dose as in normal renal function
<10	2 g every 12 hrs

Dose in patients undergoing renal replacement therapies

CAPD	Dialysed. Dose as in GFR = <10 mL/min
HD	Dialysed. Dose as in GFR = <10 mL/min
CAV/VVHD	Dialysed. Dose as in normal renal function

Important drug interactions

CYCLOSPORIN

–

POTENTIALLY HAZARDOUS INTERACTIONS WITH OTHER DRUGS

• Penicillins cause reduced excretion of methotrexate (increased risk of toxicity)

Administration

RECONSTITUTION

–

ROUTE

• IV bolus or infusion

RATE OF ADMINISTRATION

• For doses of 2 g or less: give as slow bolus over 5 min;
doses >2 g: infuse over 20–30 min

COMMENTS

• Compatible with glucose 5% and sodium chloride 0.9%

Other information

• Azlocillin is compatible with aminoglycosides, ciprofloxacin and metronidazole
• Sodium: 2.17 mEq for each 1 g dose
• Hypokalaemia may occur at high doses

Aztreonam

Clinical use

Antibacterial agent

Dose in normal renal function

1–8 g daily (usually 3–4 g daily) in divided doses, i.e. 0.5–2.0 g every 6–12 hrs

Pharmacokinetics

Molecular weight (daltons)	435.4
% Protein binding	55
% Excreted unchanged in urine	75
Volume of distribution (L/kg)	0.1–2.0
Half-life – normal/ESRF (hrs)	1.7–2.9/6–8

Dose in renal impairment GFR (mL/min)

20–50	100% of appropriate normal dose
10–20	50% of appropriate normal dose
<10	25% of appropriate normal dose

Dose in patients undergoing renal replacement therapies

CAPD	Dialysed. Dose as in GFR = <10 mL/min
HD	Dialysed. Dose as in GFR = <10 mL/min
CAV/VVHD	Dialysed. Dose as in GFR = 10–20 mL/min

Important drug interactions

CYCLOSPORIN

–

POTENTIALLY HAZARDOUS INTERACTIONS WITH OTHER DRUGS

• Possibly enhanced anticoagulant effect of nicoumalone and warfarin

Administration

RECONSTITUTION

–

ROUTE

• IM, IV bolus, IV infusion

RATE OF ADMINISTRATION

• IM injection: give by deep injection into a large muscle mass
• IV: slowly inject directly into the vein over a period of 3–5 min
• IV infusion: give over 20–60 min

COMMENTS

• Suitable infusion solutions: glucose 5%, sodium chloride 0.9%, compound sodium lactate
• Once reconstituted, aztreonam can be stored in a refrigerator for 24 hrs
• IV route recommended for single doses >1 g

Other information

• Manufacturer recommends that patients with renal impairment be given the usual initial dose followed by a maintenance dose adjusted according to creatinine clearance. The normal dose interval should not be altered

Baclofen

Clinical use

Chronic severe spasticity of voluntary muscles

Dose in normal renal function

5 mg 3 times a day, increased gradually up to
100 mg/day

Pharmacokinetics

Molecular weight (daltons)	213.7
% Protein binding	30
% Excreted unchanged in urine	70
Volume of distribution (L/kg)	–
Half-life – normal/ESRF (hrs)	3–4/–

Dose in renal impairment GFR (mL/min)

20–50	5 mg 3 times a day and titrate according to response
10–20	5 mg twice a day and titrate according to response
<10	5 mg/day

Dose in patients undergoing renal replacement therapies

CAPD	Unknown dialysability. Dose as in GFR = <10 mL/min
HD	Unknown dialysability. Dose as in GFR = <10 mL/min
CAV/VVHD	Unknown dialysability. Dose as in GFR = 10–20 mL/min

Important drug interactions

CYCLOSPORIN

–

POTENTIALLY HAZARDOUS INTERACTIONS WITH OTHER DRUGS

• Procainamide, quinidine and tricyclic antidepressants enhance muscle relaxant effect
• Antihypertensives and ACE inhibitors enhance hypotensive effect

Administration

RECONSTITUTION

–

ROUTE

• Oral – tablets or liquid

RATE OF ADMINISTRATION

–

COMMENTS

• Take after food
• Baclofen can be given intrathecally (at doses greatly reduced compared with oral dose) by bolus injection or continuous infusion. Individual titration of dosage is essential due to variability in response. Test doses must be given. Maintenance dose: 10–1200 micrograms/day

Other information

• Withdraw treatment gradually over 1–2 weeks to avoid anxiety and confusional state, etc.
• Drowsiness and nausea are frequent at the start of therapy

Benzylpenicillin

Clinical use

Antibacterial agent

Dose in normal renal function

600 mg–14.4 g daily in 2–6 divided doses

Pharmacokinetics

Molecular weight (daltons)	334
% Protein binding	50
% Excreted unchanged in urine	60–85
Volume of distribution (L/kg)	0.3–0.42
Half-life – normal/ESRF (hrs)	0.5/6–20

Dose in renal impairment GFR (mL/min)

20–50	Dose as in normal renal function
10–20	75%
<10	20–50%

Dose in patients undergoing renal replacement therapies

CAPD	Dialysed. Dose as in GFR = <10 mL/min
HD	Dialysed. Dose as in GFR = <10 mL/min
CAV/VVHD	Dialysed. Dose as in GFR = 10–20 mL/min

Important drug interactions

CYCLOSPORIN

–

POTENTIALLY HAZARDOUS INTERACTIONS WITH OTHER DRUGS

• Reduced excretion of methotrexate

Administration

RECONSTITUTION

• IV bolus: 600 mg in 5 mL water for injection
• IV infusion: 600 mg in at least 10 mL sodium chloride 0.9%
• IM: 600 mg in 1.6 mL water for injection. 600 mg displaces 0.4 mL

ROUTE

• IV bolus, IV infusion, IM

RATE OF ADMINISTRATION

• Over 3–4 min

COMMENTS

• IV doses in excess of 1.2 g must be given slowly at a minimum rate of 300 mg/min

Other information

• Dose in *normal* renal function: meningitis up to 14.4 g daily, bacterial endocarditis 4.8 g daily
• Maximum dose in severe renal impairment: 2.4–3.6 g per day
• 600 mg (1 mega-unit) contain 1.68 mmol of sodium and 1.7 mmol of potassium
• Increased incidence of neurotoxicity in renal impairment (seizures)
• False-positive urinary protein reactions may be caused by benzylpenicillin therapy

Betamethasone

Clinical use

Corticosteroid used for suppression of
inflammatory and allergic disorders

Dose in normal renal function

Oral:

0.5–5 mg daily

Injection:

4–20 mg repeated up to 4 times in 24 hrs

Pharmacokinetics

Molecular weight (daltons)	392.5
% Protein binding	65
% Excreted unchanged in urine	5
Volume of distribution (L/kg)	1.4
Half-life – normal/ESRF (hrs)	5.5/–

Dose in renal impairment
GFR (mL/min)

20–50	Dose as in normal renal function
10–20	Dose as in normal renal function
<10	Dose as in normal renal function

Dose in patients undergoing renal replacement therapies

CAPD	Unknown dialysability. Dose as in normal renal function
HD	Unknown dialysability. Dose as in normal renal function
CAV/VVHD	Unknown dialysability. Dose as in normal renal function

Important drug interactions

CYCLOSPORIN

• Rare reports of convulsions in patients on
  cyclosporin and high-dose corticosteroids

POTENTIALLY HAZARDOUS INTERACTIONS WITH
OTHER DRUGS

• Metabolism accelerated by rifampicin,
  carbamazepine, phenobarbitone, phenytoin and
  primidone
• Enhanced hypokalaemic effects of acetazolamide,
  loop diuretics and thiazide diuretics
• Efficacy of coumarin anticoagulants may be
  enhanced

Administration

RECONSTITUTION

–

ROUTE

• Oral, IV, IM, topical

RATE OF ADMINISTRATION

• IV bolus: over $^1/_2$–1 min

COMMENTS

–

Other information

• 750 micrograms betamethasone
  ≡ 5 mg prednisolone
• Even when applied topically, sufficient
  corticosteroid may be absorbed to give a systemic
  effect
• The effects of betamethasone on sodium and
  water retention are less than those of
  prednisolone, and approximately equal to those of
  dexamethasone

Betaxolol

Clinical use

Beta-adrenoreceptor blocker for hypertension

Dose in normal renal function

20–40 mg daily (elderly patients 10 mg)

Pharmacokinetics

Molecular weight (daltons)	307.4
% Protein binding	45–60
% Excreted unchanged in urine	80–90
Volume of distribution (L/kg)	5–10
Half-life – normal/ESRF (hrs)	15–20/30–35

Dose in renal impairment GFR (mL/min)

20–50	Dose as in normal renal function
10–20	Dose as in normal renal function
<10	10–20 mg daily

Dose in patients undergoing renal replacement therapies

CAPD	Unknown dialysability. Dose as in GFR = <10 mL/min
HD	Unknown dialysability. Dose as in GFR = <10 mL/min
CAV/VVHD	Unknown dialysability. Dose as in normal renal function

Important drug interactions

CYCLOSPORIN

–

POTENTIALLY HAZARDOUS INTERACTIONS WITH OTHER DRUGS

- Use with care in combination with myocardial depressants or drugs which depress AV conduction
- Increased risk of withdrawal hypertension with clonidine
- Enhanced hypotensive effect with anaesthetics
- Increased risk of myocardial depression and bradycardia with anti-arrhythmics
- Increased risk of bradycardia + AV block with amiodarone
- Severe hypertension with adrenaline and noradrenaline

Administration

RECONSTITUTION

–

ROUTE

- Oral (topical for glaucoma)

RATE OF ADMINISTRATION

–

COMMENTS

–

Other information

- Use with caution in patients with asthma or a history of obstructive airways disease or diabetes
- Systemic absorption may follow topical administration to the eye

Bezafibrate

Clinical use

Hyperlipidaemia

Dose in normal renal function

600 mg/day (400 mg in hypertriglyceridaemia)

Pharmacokinetics

Molecular weight (daltons)	361.8
% Protein binding	95
% Excreted unchanged in urine	35–40
Volume of distribution (L/kg)	0.24–0.35
Half-life – normal/ESRF (hrs)	2.1/7.8

Dose in renal impairment GFR (mL/min)

20–50	400 mg daily
10–20	200 mg daily
<10	200 mg every 24–48 hrs

Dose in patients undergoing renal replacement therapies

CAPD	Unknown dialysability. Dose as in GFR = <10 mL/min
HD	Unknown dialysability. Dose as in GFR = <10 mL/min
CAV/VVHD	Unknown dialysability. Dose as in GFR = 10–20 mL/min

Important drug interactions

CYCLOSPORIN

–

POTENTIALLY HAZARDOUS INTERACTIONS WITH OTHER DRUGS

- Enhances effect of nicoumalone, phenindione and warfarin (Dosage of anticoagulant should be reduced by up to 50% and readjusted by monitoring INR)
- Increased risk of myopathy with combination therapy with HMG CoA reductase inhibitors

Administration

RECONSTITUTION

–

ROUTE

- Oral

RATE OF ADMINISTRATION

–

COMMENTS

–

Other information

- Take dose with or after food
- Contraindicated in nephrotic syndrome
- There should be an interval of 2 hrs between intake of ion-exchange resin and bezafibrate

Bisoprolol

Clinical use

Beta-1-adrenoreceptor blocker for hypertension, angina pectoris

Dose in normal renal function

5–10 mg daily (maximum 20 mg daily)

Pharmacokinetics

Molecular weight (daltons)	767
% Protein binding	30
% Excreted unchanged in urine	50
Volume of distribution (L/kg)	–
Half-life – normal/ESRF (hrs)	10–12/–

Dose in renal impairment GFR (mL/min)

20–50	5–20 mg daily
10–20	5–20 mg daily
<10	5–10 mg daily

Dose in patients undergoing renal replacement therapies

CAPD	Unknown dialysability. Dose as in GFR = <10 mL/min
HD	Unknown dialysability. Dose as in GFR = <10 mL/min
CAV/VVHD	Unknown dialysability. Dose as in GFR = 10–20 mL/min

Important drug interactions

CYCLOSPORIN

–

POTENTIALLY HAZARDOUS INTERACTIONS WITH OTHER DRUGS

- Enhanced hypotensive effect with anaesthetics
- Increased risk of myocardial depression + bradycardia with anti-arrhythmics
- Increased risk of bradycardia + AV block with amiodarone
- Increased risk of withdrawal hypertension and bradycardia with clonidine
- Severe hypertension with adrenaline and noradrenaline

Administration

RECONSTITUTION

–

ROUTE

- Oral

RATE OF ADMINISTRATION

–

COMMENTS

–

Other information

Use with caution in patients with chronic obstructive airways disease, asthma or diabetes

Bleomycin

Clinical use

Antineoplastic agent

Dose in normal renal function

- Squamous cell carcinoma and testicular teratoma: range 45–60 x 10^3 IU per week IM/IV (total cumulative dose up to 500 x 10^3 IU), continuous IV infusion 15 x 10^3 IU/24 hrs for up to 10 days, or 30 x 10^3 IU/24 hrs for up to 5 days
- Malignant lymphomas: 15–30 x 10^3 IU/week IM to total dose of 225 x 10^3 IU. Lower doses required in combination chemotherapy
- Malignant effusions: 60 x 10^3 IU in 100 mL sodium chloride 0.9% introduced IP (total cumulative dose of 500 x 10^3 IU)

Pharmacokinetics

Molecular weight (daltons)	Approximately 1500
% Protein binding	1
% Excreted unchanged in urine	60
Volume of distribution (L/kg)	0.3
Half-life – normal/ESRF (hrs)	9/20

Dose in renal impairment GFR (mL/min)

20–50	Dose as in normal renal function
10–20	75% of normal dose (100% for malignant effusions)
<10	50% of normal dose (100% for malignant effusions)

Dose in patients undergoing renal replacement therapies

CAPD	Unknown dialysability. Dose as in GFR = <10 mL/min
HD	Unknown dialysability. Dose as in GFR = <10 mL/min
CAV/VVHD	Unknown dialysability. Dose as in GFR = 10–20 mL/min

Important drug interactions

CYCLOSPORIN

–

POTENTIALLY HAZARDOUS INTERACTIONS WITH OTHER DRUGS

- Bleomycin plus vinca alkaloids can lead to morbus Raynaud's syndrome and peripheral ischaemia

Administration

RECONSTITUTION

- IM: dissolve required dose in up to 5 mL sodium chloride 0.9% (or 1% solution of lignocaine if pain on injection)
- IV: dissolve dose in 5–200 mL sodium chloride 0.9%
- Intra-cavitary: 60 x 10^3 IU in 100 mL sodium chloride 0.9%
- Locally: dissolve in sodium chloride 0.9% to make a 1–3 IU/mL solution

ROUTE

- IM, IV, also intra-arterially, intrapleurally, intraperitoneally, locally into tumour

RATE OF ADMINISTRATION

- Give by slow IV injection or add to reservoir of a running IV infusion

COMMENTS

- Avoid direct contact with the skin

Other information

- Lesions of skin and oral mucosa are common after full course of bleomycin
- Pulmonary toxicity: interstitial pneumonia and fibrosis – most serious delayed effect

Bretylium

Clinical use

Ventricular arrhythmias resistant to other
treatment

Dose in normal renal function

IV bolus:

5 mg/kg – if no response after 5 min repeat dose
or increase to 10 mg/kg

IV infusion:

5–10 mg/kg over 15–30 min repeated at
1–2 hr intervals. Once arrhythmias are controlled,
give this dose every 6 hrs or continuously
infuse at 1–2 mg/min

IM:

5–10 mg/kg given every 6–8 hrs

Pharmacokinetics

Molecular weight (daltons)	414.4
% Protein binding	6
% Excreted unchanged in urine	75
Volume of distribution (L/kg)	8.2
Half-life – normal/ESRF (hrs)	6–13.6/16–32

Dose in renal impairment
GFR (mL/min)

20–50	Dose as in normal renal function
10–20	25–50%
<10	25%

Dose in patients undergoing renal replacement therapies

CAPD	Dialysed. Dose as in GFR = <10 mL/min
HD	Dialysed. Dose as in GFR = <10 mL/min
CAV/VVHD	Dialysed. Dose as in GFR = 10–20 mL/min

Important drug interactions

CYCLOSPORIN

–

POTENTIALLY HAZARDOUS INTERACTIONS WITH
OTHER DRUGS

• Bretylium may exacerbate arrhythmias caused by
  digoxin toxicity

Administration

RECONSTITUTION

• For IV infusion can be diluted with glucose 5% or
  sodium chloride 0.9% to give a final concentration
  of not more than 10 mg/mL

ROUTE

• IV, IM

RATE OF ADMINISTRATION

• IV bolus: undiluted by rapid injection
• IV infusion: infuse diluted dose over at least
  8 min (preferably 15–30 min)
• IV continuous maintenance: infuse at rate of
  1–2 mg/min

COMMENTS

• If bretylium is to be used for less serious
  ventricular rhythm disturbances, give more slowly
  and in diluted form to reduce the risk of vomiting

Other information

• Orthostatic hypotension may occur 20–30 min
  after acute administration

Bromocriptine

Clinical use

Parkinsonism (but not drug-induced extrapyramidal symptoms), endocrine disorders

Dose in normal renal function

Parkinson's disease:

week 1: 1–1.25 mg at night.; week 2: 2–2.5 mg at night; week 3: 2.5 mg twice daily; week 4: 2.5 mg three times daily; then increasing by 2.5 mg every 3–14 days according to response – usual range 10–40 mg daily

Hypogonadism/galactorrhoea, infertility:

1–1.25 mg at night, increased gradually; usual dose 7.5 mg daily in divided doses (maximum 30 mg daily)

Infertility without hyperprolactinaemia:

2.5 mg twice daily

Cyclical benign breast disease and cyclical menstrual disorders:

1–1.25 mg at night increased gradually; usual dose 2.5 mg twice daily

Acromegaly:

1–1.25 mg at night increased gradually to 5 mg every 6 hrs

Prolactinoma:

1–1.25 mg at night increased gradually to 5 mg every 6 hrs (maximum 30 mg daily)

Pharmacokinetics

Molecular weight (daltons)	750.7
% Protein binding	90–96
% Excreted unchanged in urine	2
Volume of distribution (L/kg)	1–3
Half-life – normal/ESRF (hrs)	2–12/–

Dose in renal impairment GFR (mL/min)

20–50	Dose as in normal renal function
10–20	Dose as in normal renal function
<10	Dose as in normal renal function

Dose for patients undergoing renal replacement therapies

CAPD	Not dialysed. Dose as in normal renal function
HD	Not dialysed. Dose as in normal renal function
CAV/VVHD	Not dialysed. Dose as in normal renal function

Important drug interactions

CYCLOSPORIN

–

POTENTIALLY HAZARDOUS INTERACTIONS WITH OTHER DRUGS

–

Administration

RECONSTITUTION

–

ROUTE

• Oral

RATE OF ADMINISTRATION

–

COMMENTS

• Take with food

Other information

• Hypotensive reactions may occur during the first few days of treatment. Tolerance may be reduced by alcohol
• Digital vasospasm can occur
• Concomitant administration of macrolide antibiotics may elevate bromocriptine levels

Brompheniramine

Clinical use

Symptomatic relief of allergy, such as hay fever
and urticaria

Dose in normal renal function

4–8 mg 3–4 times daily

12–24 mg twice daily for modified release
preparation

Pharmacokinetics

Molecular weight (daltons)	435.3
% Protein binding	72
% Excreted unchanged in urine	3
Volume of distribution (L/kg)	2.5–10
Half-life – normal/ESRF (hrs)	6/–

Dose in renal impairment GFR (mL/min)

20–50	Dose as in normal renal function
10–20	Dose as in normal renal function
<10	Dose as in normal renal function

Dose in patients undergoing renal replacement therapies

CAPD	Unknown dialysability. Dose as in normal renal function
HD	Unknown dialysability. Dose as in normal renal function
CAV/VVHD	Unknown dialysability. Dose as in normal renal function

Important drug interactions

CYCLOSPORIN

–

POTENTIALLY HAZARDOUS INTERACTIONS WITH
OTHER DRUGS

–

Administration

RECONSTITUTION

–

ROUTE

• Oral

RATE OF ADMINISTRATION

–

COMMENTS

–

Other information

• Use with care in epileptiform patients
• Drowsiness may occur
• Predominantly hepatically metabolised with renal
  elimination of metabolites

Budesonide

Clinical use

Asthma, allergic and vasomotor rhinitis,
inflammatory skin disorders

Dose in normal renal function

Inhaler/turbohaler:

200–1600 micrograms daily in divided doses

Respules:

1–2 mg twice daily. Half doses for maintenance

Nasal spray:

100 micrograms each nostril twice daily or
200 micrograms each nostril once daily.
Reduce to 100 micrograms each nostril once daily
when symptoms are controlled

Topical preparations:

apply 1–2 times daily

Capsules:

9 mg daily

Pharmacokinetics

Molecular weight (daltons)	430.5
% Protein binding	8.8
% Excreted unchanged in urine	0
Volume of distribution (L/kg)	4.3
Half-life – normal/ESRF (hrs)	2–2.7/–

Dose in renal impairment
GFR (mL/min)

20–50	Dose as in normal renal function
10–20	Dose as in normal renal function
<10	Dose as in normal renal function

Dose in patients undergoing renal replacement therapies

CAPD	Unknown dialysability. Dose as in normal renal function
HD	Unknown dialysability. Dose as in normal renal function
CAV/VVHD	Unknown dialysability. Dose as in normal renal function

Important drug interactions

CYCLOSPORIN

–

POTENTIALLY HAZARDOUS INTERACTIONS WITH
OTHER DRUGS

–

Administration

RECONSTITUTION

• Respules: may be diluted up to 50% with sterile
sodium chloride 0.9%

ROUTE

• Inhalation, topical

RATE OF ADMINISTRATION

–

COMMENTS

–

Other information

• Special care is needed in patients with quiescent
lung tuberculosis or fungal and viral infections in
the airways

Bumetanide

Clinical use

Loop diuretic

Dose in normal renal function

Oral:

I mg in the morning repeated after 6–8 hrs if necessary, severe cases 5 mg or more daily

Injection:

IV 1–2 mg repeated after 20 min; IM, if necessary, I mg then adjust according to response

IV infusion:

2–5 mg over 30–60 min

Pharmacokinetics

Molecular weight (daltons)	364.4
% Protein binding	99
% Excreted unchanged in urine	42–82
Volume of distribution (L/kg)	0.2–0.5
Half-life – normal/ESRF (hrs)	1.2–1.5/1.5

Dose in renal impairment GFR (mL/min)

20–50	Dose as in normal renal function
10–20	Dose as in normal renal function
<10	Dose as in normal renal function

Dose in patients undergoing renal replacement therapies

CAPD	Not dialysed. Dose as in normal renal function
HD	Not dialysed. Dose as in normal renal function
CAV/VVHD	Not dialysed. Dose as in normal renal function

Important drug interactions

CYCLOSPORIN

–

POTENTIALLY HAZARDOUS INTERACTIONS WITH OTHER DRUGS

• Risk of cardiac toxicity with anti-arrhythmics if hypokalaemia occurs

• Increased risk of ototoxicity with aminoglycosides, colistin and vancomycin

• Antihistamines: hypokalaemia increases risk of ventricular arrhythmias with astemizole and terfenadine

• Antihypertensives: enhanced hypotensive effect – increased risk of first-dose hypotensive effect with alpha-blockers, increased risk of hypokalaemia with indapamide

• Antimalarials: electrolyte disturbances increase risk of ventricular arrhythmias with halofantrine

• Cardiac glycosides: increased toxicity if hypokalaemia occurs with bumetanide

• Lithium: risk of toxicity

Administration

RECONSTITUTION

–

ROUTE

• Oral, IV, IM

RATE OF ADMINISTRATION

• IV infusion: 2–5 mg in 50 mL of infusion fluid over 30–60 min

COMMENTS

• Compatible with glucose 5% or sodium chloride 0.9%

Other information

• I mg bumetanide ≡ 40 mg frusemide at low doses, but avoid direct substitution at high doses

• In patients with severe chronic renal failure given high doses of bumetanide there are reports of musculoskeletal pain and muscle spasm

• Orally: diuresis begins within 30 min, peaks after 1–2 hrs and lasts 3 hrs

• IV: diuresis begins within a few minutes and ceases in about 2 hrs

• Use with caution in patients receiving nephrotoxic or ototoxic drugs

• Smaller doses (500 micrograms) may be sufficient in the elderly and in cirrhotic patients

• Use twice daily for higher doses

Buspirone

Clinical use

Anxiolytic

Dose in normal renal function

Initially 5 mg 2–3 times daily. Usual range 15–30 mg daily in divided doses (maximum 45 mg daily)

Pharmacokinetics

Molecular weight (daltons)	422.0
% Protein binding	95
% Excreted unchanged in urine	0
Volume of distribution (L/kg)	5
Half-life – normal/ESRF (hrs)	2–3/5.8

Dose in renal impairment
GFR (mL/min)

20–50	Dose as in normal renal function
10–20	Dose as in normal renal function
<10	Dose as in normal renal function

Dose in patients undergoing renal replacement therapies

CAPD	Not dialysed. Dose as in normal renal function
HD	Not dialysed. Dose as in normal renal function
CAV/VVHD	Not dialysed. Dose as in normal renal function

Important drug interactions

CYCLOSPORIN

–

POTENTIALLY HAZARDOUS INTERACTIONS WITH OTHER DRUGS

• MAOIs: risk of severe hypertension

Administration

RECONSTITUTION

–

ROUTE

• Oral

RATE OF ADMINISTRATION

–

COMMENTS

–

Other information

• Peak plasma levels occur 60–90 min after dosing
• Steady-state plasma concentrations are achieved within 2 days, although response to treatment may take 2 weeks
• Non-sedative
• Do not use in patients with severe hepatic disease
• Use in severe renal impairment not recommended, due to risk of accumulation of active metabolites

Calcitriol

Clinical use

Vitamin D analogue. Promotes intestinal calcium absorption; suppresses PTH production and release

Dose in normal renal function

Orally:

250 nanograms daily or on alternate days, increased if necessary in steps of 250 nanograms at intervals of 2–4 weeks. Usual dose 0.5–1 microgram daily

IV:

treatment of hyperparathyroidism in haemodialysis patients: initially 500 nanograms 3 times a week, increased if necessary in steps of 250–500 nanograms at intervals of 2–4 weeks. Usual dose 0.5–3 micrograms 3 times a week after dialysis

Pharmacokinetics

Molecular weight (daltons)	416.6
% Protein binding	>90
% Excreted unchanged in urine	minimal
Volume of distribution (L/kg)	–
Half-life – normal/ESRF (hrs)	3–6/–

Dose in renal impairment GFR (mL/min)

20–50	Dose as in normal renal function. Titrate to response
10–20	Dose as in normal renal function. Titrate to response
<10	Dose as in normal renal function. Titrate to response

Dose in patients undergoing renal replacement therapies

CAPD	Unknown dialysability. Dose as in normal renal function
HD	Unknown dialysability. Dose as in normal renal function
CAV/VVHD	Unknown dialysability. Dose as in normal renal function

Important drug interactions

CYCLOSPORIN

–

POTENTIALLY HAZARDOUS INTERACTIONS WITH OTHER DRUGS

• The effects of vitamin D may be reduced in patients taking barbiturates or anticonvulsants
• Increased risk of hypercalcaemia if thiazides are given with vitamin D

Administration

RECONSTITUTION

–

ROUTE

• Oral, IV

RATE OF ADMINISTRATION

• Bolus

COMMENTS

–

Other information

• Check plasma calcium concentrations at regular intervals (initially weekly)
• Dose of phosphate-binding agent may need to be modified as phosphate transport in the gut and bone may be affected
• Hypercalcaemia and hypercalciuria are the major side-effects and indicate excessive dosage

Calcium acetate

Clinical use

Phosphate-binding agent

Dose in normal renal function

–

Pharmacokinetics

Molecular weight (daltons)	158.2
% Protein binding	–
% Excreted unchanged in urine	–
Volume of distribution (L/kg)	–
Half-life – normal/ESRF (hrs)	–

Dose in renal impairment GFR (mL/min)

20–50	Dose as in normal renal function. Titrate to response
10–20	Dose as in normal renal function. Titrate to response
<10	Dose as in normal renal function. Titrate to response

Dose in patients undergoing renal replacement therapies

CAPD	Unknown dialysability. Dose as in normal renal function
HD	Unknown dialysability. Dose as in normal renal function
CAV/VVHD	Unknown dialysability. Dose as in normal renal function

Important drug interactions

CYCLOSPORIN

–

POTENTIALLY HAZARDOUS INTERACTIONS WITH OTHER DRUGS

–

Administration

RECONSTITUTION

–

ROUTE

• Oral

RATE OF ADMINISTRATION

–

COMMENTS

• Take tablets with meals

Other information

• Calcium actetate (anhydrous): calcium content per gram = 253 mg (6.3 mmol 12.6 mEq)

Calcium carbonate

Clinical use

Phosphate-binding agent

Dose in normal renal function

420–2500 mg 3 times a day with meals. Dose adjusted according to serum phosphate and calcium levels

Pharmacokinetics

Molecular weight (daltons)	100
% Protein binding	45
% Excreted unchanged in urine	–
Volume of distribution (L/kg)	–
Half-life – normal/ESRF (hrs)	–

Dose in renal impairment GFR (mL/min)

20–50	Dose as in normal renal function. Titrate to response
10–20	Dose as in normal renal function. Titrate to response
<10	Dose as in normal renal function. Titrate to response

Dose in patients undergoing renal replacement therapies

CAPD	Unknown dialysability. Dose as in normal renal function
HD	Unknown dialysability. Dose as in normal renal function
CAV/VVHD	Unknown dialysability. Dose as in normal renal function

Important drug interactions

CYCLOSPORIN

–

POTENTIALLY HAZARDOUS INTERACTIONS WITH OTHER DRUGS

–

Administration

RECONSTITUTION

–

ROUTE

• Oral

RATE OF ADMINISTRATION

–

COMMENTS

• Take with or immediately before meals

Other information

• Monitor for hypercalcaemia particularly if patient is also taking alfacalcidol
• Calcium carbonate impairs absorption of some drugs, e.g. iron, ciprofloxacin
• Titralac contains 420 mg calcium carbonate per tablet (168 mg elemental calcium)
• Calcichew contains 1250 mg calcium carbonate (500 mg elemental calcium)
• Calcium 500 contains 1250 mg calcium carbonate (500 mg elemental calcium)

Calcium gluconate/effervescent

Clinical use

Hypocalcaemia

Dose in normal renal function

–

Pharmacokinetics

Molecular weight (daltons)	448.4
% Protein binding	–
% Excreted unchanged in urine	–
Volume of distribution (L/kg)	–
Half-life – normal/ESRF (hrs)	–

Dose in renal impairment GFR (mL/min)

20–50	Dose as in normal renal function. Titrate to response
10–20	Dose as in normal renal function. Titrate to response
<10	Dose as in normal renal function. Titrate to response

Dose in patients undergoing renal replacement therapies

CAPD	Dialysed. Dose as in normal renal function
HD	Dialysed. Dose as in normal renal function
CAV/VVHD	Dialysed. Dose as in normal renal function

Important drug interactions

CYCLOSPORIN

–

POTENTIALLY HAZARDOUS INTERACTIONS WITH OTHER DRUGS

–

Administration

RECONSTITUTION

–

ROUTE

• Oral, IV, IM

RATE OF ADMINISTRATION

• IV: slow 3–4 min for each 10 mL (2.25 mmol calcium)

COMMENTS

• Acute hypocalcaemia: give 10–20 mL calcium gluconate (2.25–4.5 mmol calcium) slow IV injection over 3–10 min

Other information

• Check patient's magnesium levels
• Monitor calcium and phosphate serum levels
• Calcium Sandoz 400: 10 mmol calcium per tablet; Calcium Sandoz 1000: 25 mmol calcium per tablet
• Calcium levels cannot be corrected until magnesium levels are normal

Calcium resonium

Clinical use

Hyperkalaemia (not for emergency treatment)

Dose in normal renal function

Oral:
15 g 3–4 times daily in water
PR:
30 g in methylcellulose solution retained for 9 hrs

Pharmacokinetics

Molecular weight (daltons)	–
% Protein binding	–
% Excreted unchanged in urine	0
Volume of distribution (L/kg)	–
Half-life – normal/ESRF (hrs)	–

Dose in renal impairment
GFR (mL/min)

20–50	Dose as in normal renal function. Titrate to response
10–20	Dose as in normal renal function. Titrate to response
<10	Dose as in normal renal function. Titrate to response

Dose in patients undergoing renal replacement therapies

CAPD	Not dialysed. Dose as in normal renal function
HD	Not dialysed. Dose as in normal renal function
CAV/VVHD	Not dialysed. Dose as in normal renal function

Important drug interactions

CYCLOSPORIN

–

POTENTIALLY HAZARDOUS INTERACTIONS WITH OTHER DRUGS

–

Administration

RECONSTITUTION

• PR: mix with methylcellulose solution 2%
• Oral: mix with a little water, sweetened if preferred

ROUTE

• Oral or PR

RATE OF ADMINISTRATION

–

COMMENTS

–

Other information

• Ensure a regular laxative is prescribed – one can mix calcium resonium powder with lactulose to be taken orally
• Some units mix the dose with a little water and give PR 4 times a day. Not retained for so long, but still effective

Capreomycin

Clinical use

Antibacterial agent in combination with other drugs; tuberculosis-resistant to first-line drugs

Dose in normal renal function

Deep IM injection:

1 g daily (not more than 20 mg/kg) for 2–4 months, then 1 g 2–3 times each week

Pharmacokinetics

Molecular weight (daltons)	652.7
% Protein binding	–
% Excreted unchanged in urine	50
Volume of distribution (L/kg)	–
Half-life – normal/ESRF (hrs)	2

Dose in renal impairment GFR (mL/min)

20–50	Dose as in normal renal function
10–20	Dose as in normal renal function
<10	1 g every 48 hrs

Dose in patients undergoing renal replacement therapies

CAPD	Not dialysed. Dose as in GFR = <10 mL/min
HD	Not dialysed. Dose as in GFR = <10 mL/min
CAV/VVHD	Not dialysed. Dose as in normal renal function

Important drug interactions

CYCLOSPORIN

–

POTENTIALLY HAZARDOUS INTERACTIONS WITH OTHER DRUGS

• Increased risk of nephrotoxicity and ototoxicity with aminoglycosides and vancomycin

Administration

RECONSTITUTION

• Dissolve in 2 mL of sodium chloride 0.9% or water for injection. 2–3 min should be allowed for complete solution

ROUTE

• Deep IM injection

RATE OF ADMINISTRATION

–

COMMENTS

–

Other information

• Nephrotoxic
• Check potassium levels, as hypokalaemia may occur
• Desired steady-state serum capreomycin level is 10 micrograms/mL
• Dose should not exceed 1 g/day in renal failure
• Capreomycin sulphate 1 000 000 U approximately equivalent to capreomycin base 1 g

Captopril

Clinical use

Angiotensin-converting enzyme inhibitor used for hypertension, heart failure

Dose in normal renal function

6.25–50 mg 1–3 times daily

Pharmacokinetics

Molecular weight (daltons)	217
% Protein binding	25–30
% Excreted unchanged in urine	30–40
Volume of distribution (L/kg)	0.7–3
Half-life – normal/ESRF (hrs)	1.9/21–32

Dose in renal impairment GFR (mL/min)

20–50	Start low, adjust according to response
10–20	Start low, adjust according to response
<10	Start low, adjust according to response

Dose in patients undergoing renal replacement therapies

CAPD	Unknown dialysability. Dose as in GFR = <10 mL/min
HD	Dialysed. Dose as in GFR = <10 mL/min
CAV/VVHD	Dialysed. Dose as in GFR = 10–20 mL/min

Important drug interactions

CYCLOSPORIN

• Increased risk of hyperkalaemia

POTENTIALLY HAZARDOUS INTERACTIONS WITH OTHER DRUGS

• Anaesthetics: enhanced hypotensive effect
• Diuretics: enhanced hypotensive effect, hyperkalaemia with potassium-sparing diuretics
• Lithium: reduced excretion. Possibility of enhanced lithium toxicity
• Potassium salts: hyperkalaemia

Administration

RECONSTITUTION

–

ROUTE

• Oral

RATE OF ADMINISTRATION

–

COMMENTS

• Tablets may be dispersed in water

Other information

• Adverse reactions, especially hyperkalaemia, are more common in patients with renal impairment
• Once-daily dosing in severe renal impairment is effective
• Effective sublingually in emergencies
• As renal function declines a hepatic elimination route for captopril becomes increasingly more significant
• 2-mg tablets are available on a named-patient basis
• Renal failure has been reported in association with ACE inhibitors in patients with renal artery stenosis, post-renal transplant, or in those with congestive heart failure
• A high incidence of anaphylactoid reactions has been reported in patients dialysed with high-flux polyacrylonitrile membranes and treated concomitantly with an ACE inhibitor – this combination should therefore be avoided
• Close monitoring of renal function during therapy is necessary in those with renal insufficiency

Carbamazepine

Clinical use

All forms of epilepsy except absence seizures; trigeminal neuralgia, prophylaxis in manic-depressive illness

Dose in normal renal function

Epilepsy:

oral – initially 100–200 mg 1–2 times daily, increased slowly to a usual dose of 0.8–1.2 g daily in divided doses. Maximum 1.6–2 g daily may be needed

rectal – maximum 1 g daily in 4 divided doses for up to 7 days

Trigeminal neuralgia:

generally start with 100 mg 1–2 times daily. Usual dose 200 mg 3–4 times daily, up to 1600 mg/day. Reduce dose gradually as pain goes into remission

Prophylaxis in manic-depressive illness:

initially 400 mg daily in divided doses – maximum 1600 mg/day. Usually 400–600 mg daily in divided doses

Pharmacokinetics

Molecular weight (daltons)	236.3
% Protein binding	75
% Excreted unchanged in urine	2–3
Volume of distribution (L/kg)	0.8–1.6
Half-life – normal/ESRF (hrs)	4–6

Dose in renal impairment GFR (mL/min)

20–50	Dose as in normal renal function
10–20	Dose as in normal renal function
<10	Dose as in normal renal function

Dose in patients undergoing renal replacement therapies

CAPD	Not dialysed. Dose as in normal renal function
HD	Not dialysed. Dose as in normal renal function
CAV/VVHD	Not dialysed. Dose as in normal renal function

Important drug interactions

CYCLOSPORIN

• Metabolism accelerated (reduced plasma cyclosporin concentration)

POTENTIALLY HAZARDOUS INTERACTIONS WITH OTHER DRUGS

• Analgesics: dextropropoxyphene enhances effect of carbamazepine; carbamazepine decreases effect of tramadol

• Antibacterials: reduced effect of doxycycline, plasma carbamazepine concentration increased by clarithromycin, erythromycin and isoniazid. Increased risk of isoniazid hepatotoxicity

• Anticoagulants: metabolism of nicoumalone and warfarin accelerated (reduced anticoagulant effect)

• Antidepressants: antagonism of anticonvulsant effect. Plasma concentration of carbamazepine increased by fluoxetine, fluvoxamine and viloxazine. Metabolism of mianserin and tricyclics accelerated. Avoid with MAOIs or within 2 weeks of MAOIs

• Other anti-epileptics: concomitant administration of two or more anti-epileptics can enhance toxicity without a corresponding increase in anti-epileptic effect

• Ulcer-healing drugs: cimetidine causes an increase in plasma carbamazepine concentration

• Antipsychotics: antagonism of anticonvulsant effect. Also reduces haloperidol concentration

• Calcium-channel blockers: diltiazem and verapamil enhance effect of carbamazepine. Effect of felodipine, isradipine, nicardipine and nifedipine reduced

• Corticosteroids: reduced effect

• Hormone antagonists: danazol inhibits metabolism of carbamazepine

• Oestrogens and progestogens: carbamazepine accelerates metabolism of oral contraceptives and of gestrinone and tibolone

Administration

RECONSTITUTION

–

ROUTE

• Oral, rectal

RATE OF ADMINISTRATION

–

COMMENTS

- When switching a patient from tablets to liquid the same total dose may be used, but given in smaller more frequent doses
- Oral → rectal: increase the dose by approximately 25%

Other information

- It is important to initiate carbamazepine therapy at a low dose and build this up over 1–2 weeks, as it autoinduces its metabolism
- May cause inappropriate antidiuretic hormone secretion
- The therapeutic plasma concentration range = 4–12 micrograms/mL (17–50 micromol/L at steady state)

Carbidopa

Clinical use

Parkinsonism (but not drug-induced extrapyramidal symptoms), combined with levodopa

Dose in normal renal function

Maintenance dose carbidopa 75–200 mg combined with levodopa 0.75–2 g daily in divided doses

Pharmacokinetics

Molecular weight (daltons)	244.2
% Protein binding	–
% Excreted unchanged in urine	30
Volume of distribution (L/kg)	–
Half-life – normal/ESRF (hrs)	2/–

Dose in renal impairment GFR (mL/min)

20–50	Dose as in normal renal function
10–20	Dose as in normal renal function
<10	Dose as in normal renal function

Dose in patients undergoing renal replacement therapies

CAPD	Unknown dialysability. Dose as in normal renal function
HD	Unknown dialysability. Dose as in normal renal function
CAV/VVHD	Unknown dialysability. Dose as in normal renal function

Important drug interactions

CYCLOSPORIN

–

POTENTIALLY HAZARDOUS INTERACTIONS WITH OTHER DRUGS

Levodopa:

• Anaesthetics: risk of arrhythmias with volatile liquid anaesthetics such as halothane

• Antidepressants: hypertensive crisis with MAOIs (including moclobemide). Avoid for at least 2 weeks after stopping MAOIs

• Iron: absorption of levodopa may be reduced

Administration

RECONSTITUTION

–

ROUTE

• Oral

RATE OF ADMINISTRATION

–

COMMENTS

• Take with or after food

• In patients previously on levodopa: discontinue levodopa at least 12 hrs (24 hrs for slow-release preparations) before starting therapy with levodopa/carbidopa preparation. The initial dose of levodopa should be about 20% of the dose previously being taken as levodopa alone

Other information

• Carbidopa is a peripheral decarboxylase inhibitor with little or no pharmacological activity when given alone in usual doses. It is given with levodopa as Co-careldopa

• Co-careldopa 10/100 (levodopa 100 mg + carbidopa 10 mg): the dose of carbidopa may be insufficient to achieve full inhibition of extracerebral dopa-decarboxylase

• Co-careldopa 25/100 (levodopa 100 mg + carbidopa 25 mg) should then be used so that the daily dose of carbidopa is at least 75 mg

• Also available: co-careldopa 25/250 (25 mg carbidopa + 250 mg levodopa), co-careldopa 12.5/50 (12.5 mg carbidopa + 50 mg levodopa), as well as controlled-release preparations

Carboplatin

Clinical use

Antineoplastic agent used for ovarian carcinoma of epithelial origin, and small-cell carcinoma of the lung

Dose in normal renal function

Dose = target AUC x [GFR (mL/min) + 25]
where AUC is commonly 5 or 6, depending on protocol used

Pharmacokinetics

Molecular weight (daltons)	371.3
% Protein binding	15–24
% Excreted unchanged in urine	50–75
Volume of distribution (L/kg)	0.23–0.28
Half-life – normal/ESRF (hrs)	6/increased

Dose in renal impairment GFR (mL/min)

20–50	Dose as in normal renal function
10–20	Dose as in normal renal function
<10	Dose as in normal renal function

Dose in patients undergoing renal replacement therapies

CAPD	Unknown dialysability. Dose as in GFR = <10 mL/min
HD	Unknown dialysability. Dose as in GFR = <10 mL/min
CAV/VVHD	Unknown dialysability. Dose as in GFR = 10–20 mL/min

Important drug interactions

CYCLOSPORIN

–

POTENTIALLY HAZARDOUS INTERACTIONS WITH OTHER DRUGS

• Concurrent therapy with nephrotoxic drugs may increase toxicity due to carboplatin-induced changes of renal clearance

Administration

RECONSTITUTION

–

ROUTE

• IV

RATE OF ADMINISTRATION

• IV infusion over 15–60 min

COMMENTS

• Therapy should not be repeated until 4 weeks after the previous carboplatin course

• The product may be diluted with glucose 5% or sodium chloride 0.9% to concentrations as low as 0.5 mg/mL

Other information

• Patients with abnormal kidney function or receiving concomitant therapy with nephrotoxic drugs are likely to experience more severe and prolonged myelotoxicity

• Blood counts and renal function should be monitored closely

• Some units still use a dose in normal renal function of 400 mg/m^2. In this instance, the dose should be reduced to 50% of normal for a GFR of 10–20 mL/min, and to 25% of normal for a GFR of <10 mL/min

Carmustine

Clinical use

Myeloma, lymphoma and brain tumours

Dose in normal renal function

200 mg/m^2 every 6 weeks (given as single dose or divided into daily injections)

Pharmacokinetics

Molecular weight (daltons)	214.1
% Protein binding	–
% Excreted unchanged in urine	–
Volume of distribution (L/kg)	3.3
Half-life – normal/ESRF (hrs)	1.5/–

Dose in renal impairment GFR (mL/min)

20–50	Dose as in normal renal function
10–20	Dose as in normal renal function
<10	Dose as in normal renal function

Dose in patients undergoing renal replacement therapies

CAPD	Not dialysed. Dose as in normal renal function
HD	Not dialysed. Dose as in normal renal function
CAV/VVHD	Not dialysed. Dose as in normal renal function

Important drug interactions

CYCLOSPORIN

–

POTENTIALLY HAZARDOUS INTERACTIONS WITH OTHER DRUGS

–

Administration

RECONSTITUTION

- Dissolve carmustine with 3 mL of the supplied diluent (absolute ethanol), and then add 27 mL of sterile water for injection. This solution may be further diluted with sodium chloride for injection or 5% glucose for injection

ROUTE

- IV

RATE OF ADMINISTRATION

- Administer by IV drip over a period of 1–2 hrs

COMMENTS

- Therapy should not be repeated before 6 weeks

Other information

- Renal abnormalities, e.g. a decrease in kidney size, progressive azotaemia and renal failure have been reported in patients receiving large cumulative doses after prolonged therapy
- Carmustine is rapidly metabolised; some metabolites are active and are rapidly excreted in the urine, with approximately 30% of a dose being renally excreted after 24 hrs

Cefaclor

Clinical use

Antibacterial agent

Dose in normal renal function

250 mg every 8 hrs (dose may be doubled for
more severe infections – maximum 4 g daily)

Pharmacokinetics

Molecular weight (daltons)	385.8
% Protein binding	25
% Excreted unchanged in urine	70
Volume of distribution (L/kg)	0.24–0.35
Half-life – normal/ESRF (hrs)	1/3

Dose in renal impairment
GFR (mL/min)

20–50	Dose as in normal renal function
10–20	Dose as in normal renal function
<10	125–250 mg every 8 hrs

Dose in patients undergoing renal replacement therapies

CAPD	Unknown dialysability. 250 mg every 8–12 hrs
HD	Dialysed. 250–500 mg every 8 hrs
CAV/VVHD	Unknown dialysability. Dose as in normal renal function

Important drug interactions

CYCLOSPORIN

–

POTENTIALLY HAZARDOUS INTERACTIONS WITH
OTHER DRUGS

• Anticoagulants: effects of warfarin and
nicoumalone may be enhanced

Administration

RECONSTITUTION

–

ROUTE

• Oral

RATE OF ADMINISTRATION

–

COMMENTS

–

Other information

• Cefaclor is associated with protracted skin
reactions

Cefadroxil

Clinical use

Antibacterial agent

Dose in normal renal function

500 mg–1 g every 12–24 hrs

Pharmacokinetics

Molecular weight (daltons)	381.4
% Protein binding	20
% Excreted unchanged in urine	70–90
Volume of distribution (L/kg)	0.31
Half-life – normal/ESRF (hrs)	1.4–22

Dose in renal impairment GFR (mL/min)

20–50	Dose as in normal renal function
10–20	Dose as in normal renal function
<10	500 mg–1 g every 24–48 hrs

Dose in patients undergoing renal replacement therapies

CAPD	Unknown dialysability. Dose as in GFR = <10 mL/min
HD	Unknown dialysability. Dose as in GFR = <10 mL/min
CAV/VVHD	Unknown dialysability. Dose as in normal renal function

Important drug interactions

CYCLOSPORIN

–

POTENTIALLY HAZARDOUS INTERACTIONS WITH OTHER DRUGS

• Anticoagulants: effects of warfarin and nicoumalone may be enhanced

Administration

RECONSTITUTION

–

ROUTE

• Oral

RATE OF ADMINISTRATION

–

COMMENTS

–

Other information

–

Cefixime

Clinical use

Antibacterial agent

Dose in normal renal function

200–400 mg daily (given as a single dose or in two divided doses)

Pharmacokinetics

Molecular weight (daltons)	507.5
% Protein binding	50
% Excreted unchanged in urine	18–50
Volume of distribution (L/kg)	0.6–1.1
Half-life – normal/ESRF (hrs)	3.1/12

Dose in renal impairment GFR (mL/min)

20–50	Dose as in normal renal function
10–20	150–300 mg/day
<10	100–200 mg/day

Dose in patients undergoing renal replacement therapies

CAPD	Unknown dialysability. Dose as in GFR = <10 mL/min
HD	Dialysed. Dose as in GFR = <10 mL/min
CAV/VVHD	Dialysed. Dose as in GFR = 10–20 mL/min

Important drug interactions

CYCLOSPORIN

–

POTENTIALLY HAZARDOUS INTERACTIONS WITH OTHER DRUGS

• Anticoagulants: effects of warfarin and nicoumalone may be enhanced

Administration

RECONSTITUTION

–

ROUTE

• Oral

RATE OF ADMINISTRATION

–

COMMENTS

–

Other information

• Manufacturer recommends that patients with chronic CAPD or HD should not have dose greater than 200 mg/day

Cefotaxime

Clinical use

Antibacterial agent

Dose in normal renal function

Mild infection:

1 g every 12 hrs

Moderate infection:

1 g every 8 hrs

Severe infection:

2 g every 8 hrs

Life-threatening infection:

up to 12 g daily in 3–4 divided doses

Pharmacokinetics

Molecular weight (daltons)	478.5
% Protein binding	13–37
% Excreted unchanged in urine	60
Volume of distribution (L/kg)	0.15–0.55
Half-life – normal/ESRF (hrs)	1/15

Dose in renal impairment GFR (mL/min)

20–50	Dose as in normal renal function
10–20	Dose as in normal renal function
<10	0.5–1 g every 8–12 hrs

Dose in patients undergoing renal replacement therapies

CAPD	Dialysed. Dose as in GFR = <10 mL/min
HD	Dialysed. Dose as in GFR = <10 mL/min
CAV/VVHD	Not dialysed. 1 g every 12 hrs

Important drug interactions

CYCLOSPORIN

–

POTENTIALLY HAZARDOUS INTERACTIONS WITH OTHER DRUGS

• Anticoagulants: effects of warfarin and nicoumalone may be enhanced

Administration

RECONSTITUTION

• IV bolus/IM: 4 mL water for injection to 1 g
• IV infusion: 1 g in 50 mL sodium chloride 0.9%

ROUTE

• IV, IM

RATE OF ADMINISTRATION

• Bolus over 3–4 min, infusion over 20–60 min

COMMENTS

–

Other information

• 1 g contains 2.09 mmol sodium
• Reduce dose further if there is concurrent hepatic and renal failure

Cefoxitin

Clinical use

Antibacterial agent

Dose in normal renal function

1–2 g every 6–8 hrs (1 g every 12 hrs for uncomplicated urinary tract infections)
Maximum 12 g/day

Pharmacokinetics

Molecular weight (daltons)	449.4
% Protein binding	41–75
% Excreted unchanged in urine	80
Volume of distribution (L/kg)	0.2
Half-life – normal/ESRF (hrs)	1/13–23

Dose in renal impairment GFR (mL/min)

20–50	1–2 g every 8 hrs
10–20	1–2 g every 8–12 hrs
<10	1–2 g every 24–48 hrs

Dose in patients undergoing renal replacement therapies

CAPD	Unknown dialysability. Dose as in GFR = <10 mL/min
HD	Dialysed. Dose as in GFR = <10 mL/min
CAV/VVHD	Unknown dialysability. Dose as in GFR = 10–20 mL/min

Important drug interactions

CYCLOSPORIN

–

POTENTIALLY HAZARDOUS INTERACTIONS WITH OTHER DRUGS

• Anticoagulants: effects of warfarin and nicoumalone may be enhanced

Administration

RECONSTITUTION

• IV: reconstitute with water for injection. 10 mL to 1-g or 2-g vials
• IM: 10 mL water for injection to 1 g (or 0.5% or 1% lignocaine hydrochloride without adrenaline)

ROUTE

• IV, IM

RATE OF ADMINISTRATION

• IV bolus: 1–2 g over 3–5 min

COMMENTS

• IM: give by deep injection into a large muscle mass
• Cefoxitin is stable with aminoglycosides mixed in 200 mL of sodium chloride 0.9% or glucose 5%

Other information

• May falsely increase serum creatinine by interference with assay
• Contains 2.3 mmol sodium/g
• Active against anaerobic bacteria, especially *Bacteroides fragilis*, so may be used for abdominal sepsis such as peritonitis

Cefpodoxime

Clinical use

Antibacterial agent

Dose in normal renal function

100–200 mg every 12 hrs

Pharmacokinetics

Molecular weight (daltons)	557.6
% Protein binding	26
% Excreted unchanged in urine	30
Volume of distribution (L/kg)	0.6–1.2
Half-life – normal/ESRF (hrs)	2.5/26

Dose in renal impairment GFR (mL/min)

20–50	Dose as in normal renal function
10–20	Dose as in normal renal function
<10	100–200 mg every 24–48 hrs

Dose in patients undergoing renal replacement therapies

CAPD	Unknown dialysability. Dose as in GFR = <10 mL/min
HD	Dialysed. Dose as in GFR = <10 mL/min
CAV/VVHD	Unknown dialysability. Dose as in normal renal function

Important drug interactions

CYCLOSPORIN

–

POTENTIALLY HAZARDOUS INTERACTIONS WITH OTHER DRUGS

• Anticoagulants: effects of warfarin and nicoumalone may be enhanced

Administration

RECONSTITUTION

–

ROUTE

• Oral

RATE OF ADMINISTRATION

–

COMMENTS

• Take with food
• Antacids and H_2-blockers should be taken 2–3 hrs after administration of cefpodoxime

Other information

–

Ceftazidime

Clinical use

Antibacterial agent

Dose in normal renal function

1–2 g every 8–12 hrs

Pharmacokinetics

Molecular weight (daltons)	637
% Protein binding	17
% Excreted unchanged in urine	60–85
Volume of distribution (L/kg)	0.28–0.4
Half-life – normal/ESRF (hrs)	1.2/13–25

Dose in renal impairment GFR (mL/min)

31–50	1 g every 12 hrs
16–30	1 g every 24 hrs
6–15	500 mg–1 g every 24 hrs
<5	500 mg–1 g every 48 hrs

Dose in patients undergoing renal replacement therapies

CAPD	Dialysed. 500 mg–1 g every 24 hrs
HD	Dialysed. 500 mg–1 g every 24–48 hrs
CAV/VVHD	Not dialysed. 500 mg–1 g every 12 hrs

Important drug interactions

CYCLOSPORIN

–

POTENTIALLY HAZARDOUS INTERACTIONS WITH OTHER DRUGS

–

Administration

RECONSTITUTION

• Amount of water for injection to be added to vials: 1.5 mL to 500-mg vial for IM administration; 5 mL to 500-mg vial for IV injection; 3 mL to 1-g vial for IM administration; 10 mL to 1-g vial for IV injection

ROUTE

• IV, IM rarely

RATE OF ADMINISTRATION

• 3–4 min bolus, or longer if by infusion

COMMENTS

• May be given IP in CAPD fluid 125–250 mg/2 L fluid

• Reconstituted solutions vary in colour, but this is quite normal

• Compatible with most IV fluids, e.g. sodium chloride 0.9%, glucose saline, glucose 5%

Other information

• Vd increases with infection

• Ceftazidime levels can be monitored in patients requiring high doses with impaired renal function

Ceftriaxone

Clinical use

Antibacterial agent

Dose in normal renal function

1 g daily (severe infections: 2–4 g daily)
Gonorrhoea:
single dose 250 mg IM

Pharmacokinetics

Molecular weight (daltons)	661.6
% Protein binding	90
% Excreted unchanged in urine	30–65
Volume of distribution (L/kg)	0.12–0.18
Half-life – normal/ESRF (hrs)	7–9/12–24

Dose in renal impairment
GFR (mL/min)

20–50	Dose as in normal renal function
10–20	Dose as in normal renal function
<10	Dose as in normal renal function

Dose in patients undergoing renal replacement therapies

CAPD	Unknown dialysability. Dose as in normal renal function
HD	Unknown dialysability. Dose as in normal renal function
CAV/VVHD	Unknown dialysability. Dose as in normal renal function

Important drug interactions

CYCLOSPORIN

–

POTENTIALLY HAZARDOUS INTERACTIONS WITH OTHER DRUGS

–

Administration

RECONSTITUTION

- Bolus 250 mg: IV – 5 mL water for injection;
  IM – 1 mL 1% lignocaine hydrochloride
- Bolus 1 g: IV – 10 mL water for injection;
  IM – 3–5 mL 1% lignocaine hydrochloride
- Infusion: 2 g in 40 mL of calcium-free solution,
  e.g. sodium chloride 0.9%, glucose 5%
- Incompatible with calcium-containing solutions,
  e.g. Hartmann's, Ringer's

ROUTE

- IV, IM

RATE OF ADMINISTRATION

- Bolus: over 2–4 min
- Infusion: over at least 30 min

COMMENTS

- Doses of 50 mg/kg or over should be given by slow IV infusion
- For IM injection doses greater than 1 g should be divided and injected at more than one site

Other information

- Calcium ceftriaxone has appeared as a precipitate in urine or been mistaken for gallstones in patients receiving higher than recommended doses
- Monitor levels in dialysis patients
- For severe renal impairment the maximum daily dose recommended = 2 g
- Contains 3.6 mmol sodium per gram of ceftriaxone
- In severe renal impairment accompanied by hepatic insufficiency, the plasma concentration of ceftriaxone should be determined at regular intervals and the dosage adjusted

Cefuroxime (oral)

Clinical use

Antibacterial agent

Dose in normal renal function

125–500 mg every 12 hrs
Gonorrhoea:
single dose of 1 g

Pharmacokinetics

Molecular weight (daltons)	510.5
% Protein binding	35–50
% Excreted unchanged in urine	90
Volume of distribution (L/kg)	0.13–1.8
Half-life – normal/ESRF (hrs)	1.2/17

Dose in renal impairment GFR (mL/min)

20–50	Dose as in normal renal function
10–20	Dose as in normal renal function
<10	Dose as in normal renal function

Dose in patients undergoing renal replacement therapies

CAPD	Unknown dialysability. Dose as in normal renal function
HD	Unknown dialysability. Dose as in normal renal function
CAV/VVHD	Unknown dialysability. Dose as in normal renal function

Important drug interactions

CYCLOSPORIN

–

POTENTIALLY HAZARDOUS INTERACTIONS WITH OTHER DRUGS

–

Administration

RECONSTITUTION

–

ROUTE

• Oral

RATE OF ADMINISTRATION

–

COMMENTS

• Take with or after food

Other information

–

Cefuroxime (parenteral)

Clinical use

Antibacterial agent

Dose in normal renal function

750 mg–1.5 g every 6–8 hrs
(total dose 3–6 g daily)

Pharmacokinetics

Molecular weight (daltons)	446.4
% Protein binding	33
% Excreted unchanged in urine	90
Volume of distribution (L/kg)	0.13–1.8
Half-life – normal/ESRF (hrs)	1.2/17

Dose in renal impairment GFR (mL/min)

20–50	750 mg–1.5 g every 8 hrs
10–20	750 mg–1.5 g every 8–12 hrs
<10	750 mg–1.5 g every 24 hrs

Dose in patients undergoing renal replacement therapies

CAPD	Unknown dialysability. Dose as in GFR = <10 mL/min
HD	Unknown dialysability. Dose as in GFR = <10 mL/min
CAV/VVHD	Unknown dialysability. Dose as in GFR = 10–20 mL/min

Important drug interactions

CYCLOSPORIN

–

POTENTIALLY HAZARDOUS INTERACTIONS WITH OTHER DRUGS

–

Administration

RECONSTITUTION

• IM: 1 mL of water for injection to each 250 mg
• IV bolus: 2 mL of water for injection to each 250 mg, but 15 mL of water for injection to 1.5 g
• IV infusion: 1.5 g in 50 mL of water for injection

ROUTE

• IM, IV

RATE OF ADMINISTRATION

• IV bolus: over 3–5 min
• IV infusion: over 30 min

COMMENTS

• Do not mix in syringe with aminoglycoside antibiotics
• Injection may also be reconstituted with sodium chloride 0.9%, glucose 5%, glucose saline or Hartmann's solution
• Cefuroxime and metronidazole can be mixed (see manufacturer's guidelines)

Other information

• At high doses, care in patients receiving concurrent treatment with potent diuretics such as frusemide and aminoglycosides as combination can adversely affect renal function
• Each 750-mg vial ≡ 1.8 mmol sodium

Celiprolol

Clinical use

Beta-adrenoreceptor blocker used for mild to moderate hypertension

Dose in normal renal function

200 mg daily (maximum 400 mg daily)

Pharmacokinetics

Molecular weight (daltons)	416
% Protein binding	–
% Excreted unchanged in urine	10
Volume of distribution (L/kg)	–
Half-life – normal/ESRF (hrs)	4–5/5

Dose in renal impairment GFR (mL/min)

20–50	Dose as in normal renal function
10–20	Dose as in normal renal function
<10	150–300 mg daily

Dose in patients undergoing renal replacement therapies

CAPD	Unknown dialysability. Dose as in GFR = <10 mL/min
HD	Unknown dialysability. Dose as in GFR = <10 mL/min
CAV/VVHD	Unknown dialysability. Dose as in normal renal function

Important drug interactions

CYCLOSPORIN

–

POTENTIALLY HAZARDOUS INTERACTIONS WITH OTHER DRUGS

- Anaesthetics: enhanced hypotensive effect
- Anti-arrhythmics: increased risk of myocardial depression and bradycardia; with amiodarone increased risk of bradycardia and AV block
- Calcium-channel blockers: increased risk of bradycardia and AV block with diltiazem; severe hypotension and heart failure occasionally with nifedipine; asystole, severe hypotension and heart failure with verapamil
- Sympathomimetics: risk of severe hypertension
- Antihypertensives: enhanced hypotensive effects. Increased risk of withdrawal hypertension with clonidine. Increased risk of first-dose hypotensive effect with post-synaptic alpha-blockers

Administration

RECONSTITUTION

–

ROUTE

- Oral

RATE OF ADMINISTRATION

–

COMMENT

- Take ½–1 hr before food

Other information

- Manufacturer states that it is not recommended for patients with GFR < 15 mL/min

Cephalexin

Clinical use

Antibacterial agent

Dose in normal renal function

1 g every 12 hrs (occasionally 1 g every 8 hrs or 3 g every 12 hrs). Maximum 6 g daily
Recurrent UTI prophylaxis:
125 mg at night

Pharmacokinetics

Molecular weight (daltons)	365.4
% Protein binding	20
% Excreted unchanged in urine	98
Volume of distribution (L/kg)	0.35
Half-life – normal/ESRF (hrs)	0.7/16

Dose in renal impairment GFR (mL/min)

20–50	Dose as in normal renal function
10–20	500 mg every 12 hrs
<10	250–500 mg every 12 hrs

Dose in patients undergoing renal replacement therapies

CAPD	Dialysed. Dose as in GFR = <10 mL/min
HD	Dialysed. Dose as in GFR = <10 mL/min
CAV/VVHD	Dialysed. Dose as in GFR = 10–20 mL/min

Important drug interactions

CYCLOSPORIN

–

POTENTIALLY HAZARDOUS INTERACTIONS WITH OTHER DRUGS

–

Administration

RECONSTITUTION

–

ROUTE

• Oral

RATE OF ADMINISTRATION

–

COMMENTS

–

Other information

• Use dose for normal renal function to treat urinary tract infection in end-stage renal failure
• High doses, together with the use of nephrotoxic drugs such as aminoglycosides or potent diuretics, may adversely affect renal function

Cephamandole

Clinical use

Antibacterial agent

Dose in normal renal function

500 mg–2 g every 4–8 hrs

Pharmacokinetics

Molecular weight (daltons)	462.5
% Protein binding	75
% Excreted unchanged in urine	50–100
Volume of distribution (L/kg)	0.16–0.25
Half-life – normal/ESRF (hrs)	1/6–11

Dose in renal impairment GFR (mL/min)

20–50	500 mg–2 g every 6 hrs
10–20	500 mg–2 g every 6–8 hrs
<10	500 mg–2 g every 12 hrs

Dose in patients undergoing renal replacement therapies

CAPD	Unknown dialysability. 500 mg–1 g every 12 hrs
HD	Unknown dialysability. 500 mg–1 g every 12 hrs
CAV/VVHD	Unknown dialysability. Dose as in GFR = 10–20 mL/min

Important drug interactions

CYCLOSPORIN

–

POTENTIALLY HAZARDOUS INTERACTIONS WITH OTHER DRUGS

• Anticoagulants: effects of warfarin and nicoumalone may be enhanced

Administration

RECONSTITUTION

• IM: each gram of cephamandole should be reconstituted with 3 mL of water for injection or sodium chloride 0.9%

• IV: each gram of cephamandole should be reconstituted with 10 mL of water for injection, glucose 5% or sodium chloride 0.9%

ROUTE

• IV or deep IM injection

RATE OF ADMINISTRATION

• IV bolus: 1 g over 3–5 min

COMMENTS

• For intermittent IV infusion: 100 mL of diluent should be added to 2 g of cephamandole. If water for injection is used, reconstitute with approximately 20 mL/g to avoid a hypotonic solution

• For continuous IV infusion: add reconstituted solution to appropriate infusion solution

• Give aminoglycoside at a separate site to cephamandole

Other information

• Nephrotoxicity has been reported following concomitant administration of aminoglycoside antibiotics and cephalosporins

• Kefadol contains 1.19 mmol/g sodium

Cephradine

Clinical use

Antibacterial agent

Dose in normal renal function

Oral:
250–500 mg every 6 hrs (or 500 mg–1 g every
12 hrs)
Injection:
2–4 g daily (in four divided doses). Maximum
8 g/day

Pharmacokinetics

Molecular weight (daltons)	349.4
% Protein binding	10
% Excreted unchanged in urine	100
Volume of distribution (L/kg)	0.25–0.46
Half-life – normal/ESRF (hrs)	0.7–1.3/6–15

Dose in renal impairment
GFR (mL/min)

20–50	Dose as in normal renal function
10–20	Dose as in normal renal function
<10	250 mg every 6 hrs

Dose in patients undergoing renal replacement therapies

CAPD	Dialysed. Dose as in GFR = <10 mL/min
HD	Dialysed. Dose as in GFR = <10 mL/min
CAV/VVHD	Unknown dialysability. Dose as in normal renal function

Important drug interactions

CYCLOSPORIN

–

POTENTIALLY HAZARDOUS INTERACTIONS WITH
OTHER DRUGS

–

Administration

RECONSTITUTION

• IM: 2 mL of water for injection or sodium
  chloride 0.9% to each 500 mg
• IV bolus: 5 mL of water for injection, sodium
  chloride 0.9% or glucose 5% to each 500 mg
• IV infusions: 10 mL of suitable diluent to 1-g vial,
  then add to infusion solution

ROUTE

• Oral, IM, IV

RATE OF ADMINISTRATION

• IV bolus: over 3–5 min

COMMENTS

–

Other information

–

Cetirizine

Clinical use

Antihistamine – symptomatic relief of allergy, such as hay fever and urticaria

Dose in normal renal function

10 mg daily

Pharmacokinetics

Molecular weight (daltons)	461.8
% Protein binding	93
% Excreted unchanged in urine	60–70
Volume of distribution (L/kg)	0.4–0.6
Half-life – normal/ESRF (hrs)	7–10/20

Dose in renal impairment GFR (mL/min)

20–50	Dose as in normal renal function
10–20	Dose as in normal renal function
<10	5 mg daily

Dose in patients undergoing renal replacement therapies

CAPD	Unknown dialysability. Dose as in GFR = <10 mL/min
HD	Not dialysed. Dose as in GFR = <10 mL/min
CAV/VVHD	Unknown dialysability. Dose as in normal renal function

Important drug interactions

CYCLOSPORIN

–

POTENTIALLY HAZARDOUS INTERACTIONS WITH OTHER DRUGS

• Concomitant use of astemizole and terfenadine not recommended (risk of hazardous arrhythmias)

Administration

RECONSTITUTION

–

ROUTE

• Oral

RATE OF ADMINISTRATION

–

COMMENTS

• Available as tablets and solution

Other information

• Manufacturer recommends halving the dose in renal impairment

Chloral hydrate

Clinical use

Insomnia (short-term use)

Dose in normal renal function

500 mg–1 g at night. Maximum 2 g/day

Pharmacokinetics

Molecular weight (daltons)	165.4
% Protein binding	70–80
% Excreted unchanged in urine	<5
Volume of distribution (L/kg)	0.6
Half-life – normal/ESRF (hrs)	7–14/–

Dose in renal impairment GFR (mL/min)

20–50	Dose as in normal renal function
10–20	500 mg at night
<10	Avoid

Dose in patients undergoing renal replacement therapies

CAPD	Unknown dialysability. Probably not. Avoid
HD	Unknown dialysability. Probably not. Avoid
CAV/VVHD	Unknown dialysability. Probably not. Dose as in GFR = 10–20 mL/min

Important drug interactions

CYCLOSPORIN

–

POTENTIALLY HAZARDOUS INTERACTIONS WITH OTHER DRUGS

• Anticoagulants: when chloral hydrate is added to or withdrawn from the drug regimen, or its dosage changed, careful monitoring of prothrombin time is required

Administration

RECONSTITUTION

–

ROUTE

• Oral – tablets/elixir

RATE OF ADMINISTRATION

–

COMMENTS

• Take with water (or milk) 15–30 min before bedtime

Other information

• Avoid in patients with marked hepatic or renal impairment, severe cardiac disease, marked gastritis and those susceptible to acute attacks of porphyria
• Chloral hydrate followed by intravenous frusemide may result in sweating, hot flushes and variable blood pressure, including hypertension

Chlorambucil

Clinical use

Antineoplastic agent used for Hodgkin's disease,
non-Hodgkin's lymphoma (NHL), chronic
lymphocytic leukemia (CLL), Waldenstrom's
macroglobulinaemia (WM), ovarian carcinoma (OC)
and advanced breast cancer (ABC)

Dose in normal renal function

Hodgkin's disease = 0.2 mg/kg/day (4–8 weeks)

NHL = 0.1–0.2 mg/kg/day (4–8 weeks)

CLL = initially 0.15 mg/kg/day, then 4 weeks after
first course ended 0.1 mg/kg/day

WM = initially 6–12 mg/day, reducing to
maintenance dose of 2–8 mg/day

OC = 0.2 mg/kg/day

ABC = 0.2 mg/kg/day for 6 weeks
(or 14–20 mg/day)

Pharmacokinetics

Molecular weight (daltons)	304.2
% Protein binding	99
% Excreted unchanged in urine	<1
Volume of distribution (L/kg)	0.86
Half-life – normal/ESRF (hrs)	1/–

Dose in renal impairment
GFR (mL/min)

20–50	Dose as in normal renal function
10–20	Dose as in normal renal function
<10	Dose as in normal renal function

Dose in patients undergoing renal replacement therapies

CAPD	Not dialysed. Dose as in normal renal function
HD	Not dialysed. Dose as in normal renal function
CAV/VVHD	Not dialysed. Dose as in normal renal function

Important drug interactions

CYCLOSPORIN

–

POTENTIALLY HAZARDOUS INTERACTIONS WITH
OTHER DRUGS

• Patients who receive phenylbutazone may require
  reduced doses of chlorambucil

Administration

RECONSTITUTION

–

ROUTE

• Oral

RATE OF ADMINISTRATION

–

COMMENTS

–

Other information

• Chlorambucil is extensively metabolised in the
  liver, principally to phenylacetic acid mustard,
  which is pharmacologically active

• Chlorambucil is excreted in the urine, almost
  exclusively as metabolites

Chloramphenicol

Clinical use

Antibacterial agent

Dose in normal renal function

Oral/IV:

50 mg/kg/day in divided doses every 6 hrs
(maximum 100 mg/kg/day)

Eye drops:

every 2 hrs initially, continue for 48 hrs after eye
appears normal

Eye ointment:

every 6–8 hrs or at night
(if using drops in the day)

Ear drops:

2–3 drops every 8–12 hrs

Pharmacokinetics

Molecular weight (daltons)	323.1
% Protein binding	45–60
% Excreted unchanged in urine	10
Volume of distribution (L/kg)	0.5–1.0
Half-life – normal/ESRF (hrs)	1.6–3.3/3–7

Dose in renal impairment
GFR (mL/min)

20–50	Dose as in normal renal function
10–20	Dose as in normal renal function
<10	Dose as in normal renal function

Dose in patients undergoing renal replacement therapies

CAPD	Not dialysed. Dose as in normal renal function
HD	Not dialysed. Dose as in normal renal function
CAV/VVHD	Not dialysed. Dose as in normal renal function

Important drug interactions

CYCLOSPORIN

–

POTENTIALLY HAZARDOUS INTERACTIONS WITH
OTHER DRUGS

• Anticoagulants: effect of warfarin and nicoumalone
enhanced

• Antidiabetics: effect of sulphonylureas enhanced

• Anti-epileptics: metabolism accelerated by
phenobarbitone (reduced plasma concentration of
chloramphenicol). Increased plasma concentration
of phenytoin (risk of toxicity)

Administration

RECONSTITUTION

• Chloromycetin: add 11.75 mL water for injection
to 300-mg vial – gives 25 mg/mL; add 11 mL water
for injection to 1.2-g vial – gives 100 mg/mL

• Kemicetine: 1-g vial – reconstitute with water for
injection, sodium chloride 0.9% or glucose 5%
1.7 mL = 400 mg/mL solution
3.2 mL = 250 mg/mL solution
4.2 mL = 200 mg/mL solution
9.2 mL = 100 mg/mL solution

ROUTE

• Oral, IV, IM (Kemicetine only), topical

RATE OF ADMINISTRATION

• IV: over at least 1 min

COMMENTS

–

Other information

• Manufacturers recommend monitoring serum
levels in patients with renal impairment –
micromedex therapeutic range 10–25
micrograms/mL

• Chloromycetin: 300-mg vial = 0.94 mmol sodium;
1.2-g vial = 3.75 mmol sodium

• Kemicetine: 1-g vial = 3.14 mmol sodium

Chlordiazepoxide

Clinical use

Anxiety (short-term use), alcohol withdrawal, muscle spasm

Dose in normal renal function

Anxiety:

30–100 mg daily in divided doses

Insomnia associated with anxiety, muscle spasm:
10–30 mg daily

Alcohol withdrawal:

25–100 mg repeated, if necessary, after 2–4 hrs

Pharmacokinetics

Molecular weight (daltons)	299.8
% Protein binding	94–97
% Excreted unchanged in urine	<5
Volume of distribution (L/kg)	0.3–0.5
Half-life – normal/ESRF (hrs)	5–30/unchanged

Dose in renal impairment GFR (mL/min)

20–50	Dose as in normal renal function
10–20	Dose as in normal renal function
<10	50% of normal dose

Dose in patients undergoing renal replacement therapies

CAPD	Not dialysed. Dose as in GFR = <10 mL/min
HD	Not dialysed. Dose as in GFR = <10 mL/min
CAV/VVHD	Unknown dialysability. Dose as in normal renal function

Important drug interactions

CYCLOSPORIN

–

POTENTIALLY HAZARDOUS INTERACTIONS WITH OTHER DRUGS

• Rifampicin may increase the metabolism of chlordiazepoxide

• Cimetidine inhibits metabolism of benzodiazepines

Administration

RECONSTITUTION

–

ROUTE

• Oral

RATE OF ADMINISTRATION

–

COMMENTS

• May be administered parenterally, by deep IM or slow IV, in doses similar to those stated for oral administration

Other information

• Active metabolite

Chlormethiazole

Clinical use

Alcohol withdrawal, sedation, restlessness and agitation

Dose in normal renal function

Alcohol withdrawal:

2–4 capsules stat, then day 1: 3 capsules 3 or 4 times daily; day 2: 2 capsules 3 or 4 times daily; day 3: 1 capsule 4 times daily. Reduce over a further 4–6 days. Give a total treatment of not more than 9 days

Insomnia:

1–2 capsules at night

Restlessness and agitation:

1 capsule 3 times daily

Pharmacokinetics

Molecular weight (daltons)	162
% Protein binding	65
% Excreted unchanged in urine	0.1–5
Volume of distribution (L/kg)	4–16
Half-life – normal/ESRF (hrs)	4–6/unchanged

Dose in renal impairment GFR (mL/min)

20–50	Dose as in normal renal function
10–20	Dose as in normal renal function
<10	Dose as in normal renal function

Dose in patients undergoing renal replacement therapies

CAPD	Unknown dialysability. Dose as in normal renal function
HD	Dialysed. Dose as in normal renal function
CAV/VVHD	Unknown dialysability. Dose as in normal renal function

Important drug interactions

CYCLOSPORIN

–

POTENTIALLY HAZARDOUS INTERACTIONS WITH OTHER DRUGS

• Cimetidine: inhibits metabolism of chlormethiazole

Administration

RECONSTITUTION

• Ready reconstituted 0.8% solution

ROUTE

• Oral, IV

RATE OF ADMINISTRATION

• IV infusion: start at 3–7.5 mL/min until shallow sleep is induced, then reduce to 0.5–1 mL/min to maintain shallow sleep and adequate spontaneous respiration. Rapid deep sedation under medical supervision only can be achieved by giving 40–100 mL over 3–5 min followed by the normal maintenance dose

COMMENTS

• Infusion should be stored in a refrigerator

Other information

• Chlormethiazole has a high hepatic extraction ratio
• Increased cerebral sensitivity in renal impairment
• Infusion causes electrolyte imbalance
• Manufacturer recommends caution should be exercised in patients with chronic renal disease

Chloroquine

Clinical use

1. Treatment of malaria
2. Prophylaxis and suppression of malaria
3. Treatment of amoebic hepatitis and abscess
4. Treatment of discoid and systemic lupus erythematosus
5. Treatment of rheumatoid arthritis

Dose in normal renal function

Oral:

1. 1 g chloroquine phosphate – in many cases followed by 500 mg 6–8 hrs later, then 500 mg/day for 2 days

2. 500 mg chloroquine phosphate once a week on the same day each week (start 1 week before exposure to risk and continue until 4 weeks after leaving the malarious area)

3. 1 g chloroquine phosphate daily for 2 days followed by 250 mg every 12 hrs for 2 or 3 weeks

4. 250 mg chloroquine phosphate every 12 hrs for 1–2 weeks followed by a maintenance dose of 250 mg daily

5. 250 mg chloroquine phosphate daily

Pharmacokinetics

Molecular weight (daltons)	319.9
% Protein binding	50–65
% Excreted unchanged in urine	40
Volume of distribution (L/kg)	large
Half-life – normal/ESRF	2–4days/5–50 days

Dose in renal impairment GFR (mL/min)

20–50	Dose as in normal renal function
10–20	Dose as in normal renal function
<10	50% of normal dose

Dose in patients undergoing renal replacement therapies

CAPD	Not dialysed. Dose as in GFR = <10 mL/min
HD	Not dialysed. Dose as in GFR = <10 mL/min
CAV/VVHD	Not dialysed. Dose as in normal renal function

Important drug interactions

CYCLOSPORIN

• Increases plasma cyclosporin concentration (increased risk of toxicity)

POTENTIALLY HAZARDOUS INTERACTIONS WITH OTHER DRUGS

• Chloroquine possibly increases the plasma concentration of digoxin

Administration

RECONSTITUTION

–

ROUTE

• Oral, IV, IM/SC in rare cases

RATE OF ADMINISTRATION

• IV infusion: administer dose of 10 mg/kg of chloroquine base in sodium chloride 0.9% by slow IV infusion over 8 hrs followed by three further 8-hr infusions containing 5 mg base/kg (total dose 25 mg base/kg over 32 hrs)

COMMENTS

• Oral: do not take indigestion remedies at the same time of day as this medicine

• Chloroquine sulphate inj. 5.45% w/v (equivalent to 40 mg chloroquine base/mL) is available

Other information

• Excretion is increased in alkaline urine

• Cautioned in patients with renal or hepatic disease

• Bone marrow suppression may occur with extended treatment

Chlorpheniramine

Clinical use

Antihistamine – used for relief of allergy, pruritus and treatment or prophylaxis of anaphylaxis

Dose in normal renal function

Oral:
4 mg 4–6 times a day (maximum 24 mg/day)
IV/IM/SC:
10–20 mg (maximum 40 mg/day)

Pharmacokinetics

Molecular weight (daltons)	391 (chlorpheniramine maleate)
% Protein binding	72
% Excreted unchanged in urine	20
Volume of distribution (L/kg)	6–12
Half-life – normal/ESRF (hrs)	14–24/–

Dose in renal impairment GFR (mL/min)

20–50	Dose as in normal renal function
10–20	4 mg 4 times a day
<10	4 mg 3–4 times a day

Dose in patients undergoing renal replacement therapies

CAPD	Unknown dialysability. Dose as in GFR = <10 mL/min
HD	Unknown dialysability. Dose as in GFR = <10 mL/min
CAV/VVHD	Unknown dialysability. Dose as in GFR = 10–20 mL/min

Important drug interactions

CYCLOSPORIN

–

POTENTIALLY HAZARDOUS INTERACTIONS WITH OTHER DRUGS

• Inhibits phenytoin metabolism and can lead to phenytoin toxicity

Administration

RECONSTITUTION

–

ROUTE

• Oral, IV

RATE OF ADMINISTRATION

• Bolus over 1 min

COMMENTS

• Injection reported to cause stinging or burning sensation at site of injection

Other information

• Tends to be more efficacious but more sedating than terfenadine in treatment of pruritus
• Increased cerebral sensitivity in patients with renal impairment

Chlorpromazine

Clinical use

Anti-emetic, anxiety and agitation, antipsychotic, hiccups

Dose in normal renal function

Anti-emetic:
oral: 10–25 mg every 4–6 hrs; IM: 25–50 mg every 3–4 hrs

Antipsychotic, anxiety and agitation:
oral: 25 mg every 8 hrs initially, increase as necessary (up to 1 g daily); IM: 25–50 mg every 6–8 hrs

Hiccups:
oral: 25–50 mg every 6–8 hrs; IM: 25–50 mg initially

Pharmacokinetics

Molecular weight (daltons)	319
% Protein binding	91–99
% Excreted unchanged in urine	<1
Volume of distribution (L/kg)	7.4
Half-life – normal/ESRF (hrs)	11–42/unchanged

Dose in renal impairment GFR (mL/min)

20–50	Dose as in normal renal function
10–20	Dose as in normal renal function
<10	Start with small dose

Dose in patients undergoing renal replacement therapies

CAPD	Not dialysed. Dose as in normal renal function. Start with small dose
HD	Not dialysed. Dose as in normal renal function. Start with small dose
CAV/VVHD	Unknown dialysability. Dose as in normal renal function

Important drug interactions

CYCLOSPORIN

–

POTENTIALLY HAZARDOUS INTERACTIONS WITH OTHER DRUGS

- Anaesthetics: enhanced hypotensive effect
- Antidepressants: increased plasma level of tricyclics
- Anticonvulsants: antagonises effect lowering anticonvulsant threshold
- ACE inhibitors: severe postural hypotension
- Adrenergic neurone blockers: antagonism of hypotensive effect

Administration

RECONSTITUTION

–

ROUTE

- Oral, deep IM

RATE OF ADMINISTRATION

–

COMMENTS

–

Other information

- Start with small doses in severe renal impairment due to increased cerebral sensitivity

Chlorpropamide

Clinical use

Diabetes mellitus, diabetes insipidus

Dose in normal renal function

Diabetes mellitus:

initially 250 mg daily (elderly patients 100–125 mg, but avoid). Maximum 500 mg daily

Diabetes insipidus:

initially 100 mg daily

Pharmacokinetics

Molecular weight (daltons)	276.7
% Protein binding	88–96
% Excreted unchanged in urine	47
Volume of distribution (L/kg)	0.09–0.27
Half-life – normal/ESRF (hrs)	24–48/50–200

Dose in renal impairment GFR (mL/min)

20–50	50% of normal dose
10–20	Avoid
<10	Avoid

Dose in patients undergoing renal replacement therapies

CAPD	Unknown dialysability. Avoid
HD	Unknown dialysability. Avoid
CAV/VVHD	Unknown dialysability. Avoid

Important drug interactions

CYCLOSPORIN

–

POTENTIALLY HAZARDOUS INTERACTIONS WITH OTHER DRUGS

- Analgesics: azapropazone, phenylbutazone and possibly other NSAIDs enhance the effects of the sulphonylureas
- Antibacterials: chloramphenicol, co-trimoxazole, 4-quinolones, sulphonamides and trimethoprim enhance the effect of sulphonylureas. Rifamycins reduce the effect of sulphonylureas
- Antifungals: fluconazole and miconazole increase plasma concentrations of sulphonylureas
- Antihistamines: depressed thrombocyte count with concomitant use of oral antidiabetics and ketotifen
- Uricosurics: sulphinpyrazone enhances effect of sulphonylureas

Administration

RECONSTITUTION

–

ROUTE

- Oral

RATE OF ADMINISTRATION

–

COMMENTS

- Take with breakfast

Other information

- Chlorpropamide can enhance antidiuretic hormone and very rarely cause hyponatraemia
- Contraindicated in patients with serious impairment of hepatic, renal or thyroid function – severe risk of metabolic acidosis
- Prolonged hypoglycaemia can occur in azotemic patients

Chlorthalidone

Clinical use

Thiazide-like diuretic – used for hypertension, oedema, diabetes insipidus

Dose in normal renal function

Hypertension:

25–50 mg daily

Oedema:

50 mg daily initially, or 100–200 mg on alternate days

Diabetes insipidus:

100 mg every 12 hrs initially, reducing to 50 mg daily where possible

Pharmacokinetics

Molecular weight (daltons)	338.8
% Protein binding	76–90
% Excreted unchanged in urine	50
Volume of distribution (L/kg)	3.9
Half-life – normal/ESRF (hrs)	44–80/–

Dose in renal impairment GFR (mL/min)

20–50	Dose as in normal renal function
10–20	Dose as in normal renal function
<10	Avoid

Dose in patients undergoing renal replacement therapies

CAPD	Unknown dialysability. Avoid
HD	Unknown dialysability. Avoid
CAV/VVHD	Unknown dialysability. Dose as in normal renal function

Important drug interactions

CYCLOSPORIN

–

POTENTIALLY HAZARDOUS INTERACTIONS WITH OTHER DRUGS

- ACE inhibitors: enhanced hypotensive effect
- Anti-arrhythmics: toxicity of amiodarone, disopyramide, flecainide and quinidine increased if hypokalaemia occurs. Action of lignocaine, mexiletine and tocainide antagonised by hypokalaemia
- Antihistamines: hypokalaemia increases risk of ventricular arrhythmias with astemizole and terfenadine
- Antihypertensives: enhanced hypotensive effect, increased risk of first-dose hypotensive effect of post-synaptic alpha-blockers such as prazosin
- Antimalarials: electrolyte disturbances increase risk of ventricular arrhythmias with halofantrine
- Cardiac glycosides: increased risk of toxicity if hypokalaemia occurs
- Lithium: lithium excretion reduced by thiazides – increased plasma lithium concentration and risk of toxicity
- Antidiabetics: dosage of insulin or oral antidiabetic agents may need adjusting

Administration

RECONSTITUTION

–

ROUTE

- Oral

RATE OF ADMINISTRATION

–

COMMENTS

- A single dose at breakfast time is preferable

Other information

- Can precipitate diabetes mellitus and gout, and can cause severe electrolyte disturbances and an increase in serum lipids

Cholestyramine

Clinical use

Hyperlipidaemias, pruritis associated with partial biliary obstruction and primary biliary cirrhosis, diarrhoeal disorders

Dose in normal renal function

Lipid reduction:
8–24 g daily (in single or up to 4 divided doses). Maximum 36 g daily
Pruritis:
4–8 g daily
Diarrhoeal disorders:
12–24 g daily. Maximum 36 g daily

Pharmacokinetics

Molecular weight (daltons)	–
% Protein binding	0
% Excreted unchanged in urine	0
Volume of distribution (L/kg)	Not absorbed
Half-life – normal/ESRF (hrs)	Not absorbed

Dose in renal impairment GFR (mL/min)

20–50	Dose as in normal renal function
10–20	Dose as in normal renal function
<10	Dose as in normal renal function

Dose in patients undergoing renal replacement therapies

CAPD	Not dialysed. Dose as in normal renal function
HD	Not dialysed. Dose as in normal renal function
CAV/VVHD	Not dialysed. Dose as in normal renal function

Important drug interactions

CYCLOSPORIN

–

POTENTIALLY HAZARDOUS INTERACTIONS WITH OTHER DRUGS

• Anticoagulants: effect of nicoumalone, phenindione and warfarin may be enhanced or reduced
• Valproate, cardiac glycosides, mycophenolate mofetil: absorption reduced

Administration

RECONSTITUTION

• Mix with water, or a suitable liquid such as fruit juice, and stir to a uniform consistency
• May also be mixed with skimmed milk, thin soups, apple sauce, etc.

ROUTE

• Oral

RATE OF ADMINISTRATION

–

COMMENTS

• Do not take in dry form
• Administer other drugs at least 1 hr before or 4–6 hrs after cholestyramine
• Prepare powder immediately prior to administration

Other information

• Hyperchloraemic acidosis occasionally reported on prolonged use of cholestyramine
• On chronic use, an increased bleeding tendency may occur associated with vitamin K deficiency

Cilastatin

Clinical use

With imipenem (as Primaxin), antibacterial agent

Dose in normal renal function

Of Primaxin (in terms of imipenem dose)

IV:

1–2 g/day in 3 to 4 equally divided doses. Maximum 50 mg/kg/day or not exceeding 4 g

IM:

0.5–1.5 g daily (once or twice daily)

Pharmacokinetics

Molecular weight (daltons)	380.4
% Protein binding	44
% Excreted unchanged in urine	60
Volume of distribution (L/kg)	0.22
Half-life – normal/ESRF (hrs)	1/12

Dose in renal impairment GFR (mL/min)

31–70	500 mg every 6–8 hrs
21–30	500 mg every 8–12 hrs
5–20	250–500 mg every 12 hrs
<5	Avoid unless haemodialysis commenced within 48 hrs

Dose in patients undergoing renal replacement therapies

CAPD	Unknown dialysability. 250 mg every 12 hrs
HD	Dialysed. Dose as in GFR = 5–20 mL/min
CAV/VVHD	Dialysed. Dose as in GFR = 5–20 mL/min

Important drug interactions

CYCLOSPORIN

• With Primaxin

POTENTIALLY HAZARDOUS INTERACTIONS WITH OTHER DRUGS

• With Primaxin: increased toxicity with ganciclovir (convulsions reported)

Administration

RECONSTITUTION

Of Primaxin:

• IV: for each 250 mg add 50 mL of diluent
• IM: for each 500 mg add 2 mL of 1% lignocaine

ROUTE

• IM, IV

RATE OF ADMINISTRATION

• 250 mg and 500 mg: infuse over 20–30 min
• 1000-mg dose: infuse over 40–60 min
• IM: give by deep intramuscular injection into a large muscle mass

COMMENTS

• Each vial of Primaxin contains imipenem and cilastatin in equal amounts
• The IV formulation should not be used intramuscularly
• In patients who develop nausea during infusion, slow down infusion rate
• Diluents: sodium chloride 0.9%; glucose 5% and sodium chloride 0.9%; glucose 5% and sodium chloride 0.225%
• Incompatible with lactate
• Do not mix or add to any other antibiotics
• IM: use immediately after reconstitution

Other information

On Primaxin:

• Cilastatin component unnecessary in renal failure
• Patients with CNS disorders and/or compromised renal function (accumulation of Primaxin may occur) have shown CNS side-effects, e.g. convulsions
• Primaxin: IM – 500-mg vial = 1.47 mmol sodium; IV – 250-mg vial = 0.86 mmol sodium, 500-mg vial = 1.72 mmol sodium

Cilazapril

Clinical use

Angiotensin-converting enzyme inhibitor used for hypertension and congestive heart disease

Dose in normal renal function

Essential hypertension:

1–2.5 mg daily. Maximum 5 mg daily

Renovascular hypertension:

0.25–0.5 mg daily initially. Adjust maintenance dose individually)

Cardiac failure:

0.5 mg daily initially

Pharmacokinetics

Molecular weight (daltons)	435.5
% Protein binding	–
% Excreted unchanged in urine	91
Volume of distribution (L/kg)	20
Half-life – normal/ESRF (hrs)	9/–

Dose in renal impairment
GFR (mL/min)

20–50	Initially 1 mg once daily (maximum 5 mg daily)
10–20	Initially 0.5 mg once daily (maximum 2.5 mg daily)
<10	0.25–0.5 mg once daily and adjust according to response

Dose in patients undergoing renal replacement therapies

CAPD	Unknown dialysability. Dose as in GFR = <10 mL/min
HD	Unknown dialysability. Dose as in GFR = <10 mL/min
CAV/VVHD	Unknown dialysability. Dose as in GFR = 10–20 mL/min

Important drug interactions

CYCLOSPORIN

• Decreased renal function

POTENTIALLY HAZARDOUS INTERACTIONS WITH OTHER DRUGS

• Increased risk of hyperkalaemia
• Anaesthetics: enhanced hypotensive effect
• NSAIDs: antagonism of hypotensive effect and increased risk of renal failure, hyperkalaemia
• Diuretics: enhanced hypotensive effect, hyperkalaemia with potassium-sparing diuretics
• Epoetin: increased risk of hyperkalaemia
• Lithium: ACE inhibitors reduce excretion of lithium (increased plasma lithium concentration)
• Potassium salts: hyperkalaemia

Administration

RECONSTITUTION

–

ROUTE

• Oral

RATE OF ADMINISTRATION

–

COMMENTS

• Take dose about the same time each day

Other information

• Data refer to active drug – cilazaprilat
• Symptomatic hypotension reported in patients with sodium or volume depletion, i.e. sickness, diarrhoea, on diuretics, low-sodium diet or post dialysis
• Renal failure has been reported in association with ACE inhibitors in patients with renal artery stenosis, post renal transplant, or those with congestive heart failure
• A high incidence of anaphylactoid reactions has been reported in patients dialysed with high-flux polyacrylonitrile membranes and treated concomitantly with an ACE inhibitor – this combination should therefore be avoided
• Hyperkalaemia and other side-effects are more common in patients with impaired renal function
• Close monitoring of renal function during therapy is necessary in those with renal insufficiency

Cimetidine

Clinical use

Gastric and duodenal ulcer treatment and prophylaxis, reflux oesophagitis, Zollinger-Ellison syndrome (unlicensed use: refractory uraemic pruritus)

Dose in normal renal function

Oral:

duodenal and gastric ulceration treatment: 800 mg at night or 400 mg twice daily. Rarely, up to 2.4 g daily

Prophylaxis:

400 mg at night or 400 mg twice daily

Reflux oesophagitis: 400 mg every 6 hrs

IM:

200 mg every 4–6 hrs. Maximum 2.4 g daily

IV bolus:

200 mg every 4–6 hrs

IV infusion:

400 mg every 4–6 hrs intermittent or 50–100 mg/hr continuous. Maximum 2.4 g daily

Pharmacokinetics

Molecular weight (daltons)	252
% Protein binding	20
% Excreted unchanged in urine	50–70
Volume of distribution (L/kg)	0.8–1.3
Half-life – normal/ESRF (hrs)	1.5–2/5

Dose in renal impairment GFR (mL/min)

20–50	Dose as in normal renal function
10–20	50% of normal dose
<10	25–50% of normal dose

Dose in patients undergoing renal replacement therapies

CAPD	Not dialysed. Dose as in GFR = <10 mL/min
HD	Not dialysed. Dose as in GFR = <10 mL/min
CAV/VVHD	Unknown dialysability. Dose as in GFR = 10–20 mL/min

Important drug interactions

CYCLOSPORIN

• Possibly increases cyclosporin levels

POTENTIALLY HAZARDOUS INTERACTIONS WITH OTHER DRUGS

• Anti-arrhythmics: increased plasma concentration of many anti-arrhythmics
• Anticoagulants: enhanced effect of nicoumalone and warfarin
• Anti-epileptics: inhibits metabolism of carbamazepine, phenytoin and valproate. Plasma levels increased
• Theophylline: inhibits metabolism. Plasma levels increased

Administration

RECONSTITUTION

–

ROUTE

• Oral, IM, IV

RATE OF ADMINISTRATION

• IV infusion: 400 mg in 100 mL sodium chloride 0.9% over 30–60 min
• IV bolus: 200 mg over at least 2 min. Dilute larger doses to 10 mL and give over 20 min
• Continuous IV infusion: 50–100 mg/hr

COMMENTS

• Avoid bolus if possible

Other information

• Inhibits tubular secretion of creatinine
• Uraemic patients are susceptible to mental confusion

Ciprofloxacin

Clinical use

Antibacterial agent

Dose in normal renal function

Oral:

250–750 mg every 12 hrs

IV:

100–400 mg every 12 hrs

Pharmacokinetics

Molecular weight (daltons)	331
% Protein binding	20–40
% Excreted unchanged in urine	50–70
Volume of distribution (L/kg)	2.5
Half-life – normal/ESRF (hrs)	3–6/6–9

Dose in renal impairment GFR (mL/min)

20–50	Dose as in normal renal function
10–20	50% of normal dose
<10	50% of normal dose

Dose in patients undergoing renal replacement therapies

CAPD	Dialysed. Oral: 250 mg every 8–12 hrs. IV: 100 mg every 12 hrs
HD	Dialysed. Oral: 250–500 mg every 12 hrs. IV: 100 mg every 12 hrs
CAV/VVHD	Dialysed. Oral: 500–750 mg every 12 hrs. IV: 200 mg every 12 hrs

Important drug interactions

CYCLOSPORIN

• Variable response. No interaction seen locally

• Some reports of increased nephrotoxicity

POTENTIALLY HAZARDOUS INTERACTIONS WITH OTHER DRUGS

• Analgesics: increased risk of convulsions with NSAIDs

• Anticoagulants: anticoagulant effect enhanced

• Theophylline: increased plasma levels of theophylline

Administration

RECONSTITUTION

–

ROUTE

• Oral, IV

RATE OF ADMINISTRATION

• Infusion: over 30–60 min

COMMENTS

• Swallow tablets whole, do not chew

• Do not take milk, iron preparations, indigestion remedies or phosphate binders at the same time as ciprofloxacin orally

Other information

• Intra-peritoneal ciprofloxacin in CAPD dose range 25–100 mg/L

• In CAPD peritonitis, oral ciprofloxacin up to 500 mg 4 times daily may be administered

• The bioavailability of the oral and IV forms are approximately equivalent

Cisapride

Clinical use

Dyspepsia, gastro-oesophageal reflux and other symptoms of impaired gastric motility

Dose in normal renal function

10 mg 3–4 times a day (once daily for maintenance therapy)

Pharmacokinetics

Molecular weight (daltons)	484
% Protein binding	98
% Excreted unchanged in urine	<1
Volume of distribution (L/kg)	2.4
Half-life – normal/ESRF (hrs)	7–10/–

Dose in renal impairment GFR (mL/min)

20–50	5 mg 3–4 times a day and titrate as necessary
10–20	5 mg 3–4 times a day and titrate as necessary
<10	5 mg 3–4 times a day and titrate as necessary

Dose in patients undergoing renal replacement therapies

CAPD	Unknown dialysability. Dose as in GFR = <10 mL/min
HD	Unknown dialysability. Dose as in GFR = <10 mL/min
CAV/VVHD	Unknown dialysability. Dose as in GFR = 10–20 mL/min

Important drug interactions

CYCLOSPORIN

• Higher and earlier peak cyclosporin level in blood/plasma

POTENTIALLY HAZARDOUS INTERACTIONS WITH OTHER DRUGS

• Antibacterials: clarithromycin and erythromycin can possibly inhibit metabolism (risk of ventricular arrhythmias)
• Antifungals: imidazoles inhibit metabolism (ventricular arrhythmias reported)
• Anticoagulants: effects enhanced

Administration

RECONSTITUTION

–

ROUTE

• Oral

RATE OF ADMINISTRATION

–

COMMENTS

• Preferably take 15–30 min before a meal

Other information

• Start with low dose and increase according to response providing patient can tolerate it
• Predominantly metabolised hepatically to inactive renally excreted metabolites

Cisplatin

Clinical use

Antineoplastic agent, used for testicular and metastatic ovarian tumours, also cervical tumours, lung carcinoma and bladder cancer

Dose in normal renal function

Single-agent therapy:

50–120 mg/m^2 as a single IV dose every 2–4 weeks or 15–20 mg/m^2 IV daily for 5 days every 3–4 weeks

Combination therapy:

20 mg/m^2 and upward, IV every 2–4 weeks

Pharmacokinetics

Molecular weight (daltons)	300
% Protein binding	90
% Excreted unchanged in urine	27–45
Volume of distribution (L/kg)	0.5
Half-life – normal/ESRF (hrs)	0.3–0.5/–

Dose in renal impairment GFR (mL/min)

20–50	See 'Other information'
10–20	See 'Other information'
<10	See 'Other information'

Dose in patients undergoing renal replacement therapies

CAPD	Unknown dialysability. Dose as in GFR = <10 mL/min
HD	Dialysed. Dose as in GFR = <10 mL/min
CAV/VVHD	Unknown dialysability. Dose as in GFR = 10–20 mL/min

Important drug interactions

CYCLOSPORIN

–

POTENTIALLY HAZARDOUS INTERACTIONS WITH OTHER DRUGS

• Antibacterials: aminoglycosides and capreomycin increase risk of nephrotoxicity and possibility of ototoxicity

Administration

RECONSTITUTION

• Lagap cisplatin: no reconstitution necessary
• Faulding/Pharmacia cisplatin: dissolve in water for injection to form a 1 mg/mL solution (use within 20 hrs, protect from light, store at room temperature)

ROUTE

• IV infusion

RATE OF ADMINISTRATION

• Over 6–8 hrs

COMMENTS

• Pre-treatment hydration with 1–2 L of fluid infused for 8–12 hrs prior to cisplatin dose is recommended in order to initiate diuresis. The drug is then well diluted in sodium chloride 0.9% or glucose saline solutions to ensure hydration and maintain urine output. Adequate hydration **must** be maintained during the following 24 hrs, with potassium and magnesium supplementation given as necessary
• Cisplatin solutions react with aluminium – do not use equipment containing aluminium

Other information

• Dose modification depends not only on the degree of renal dysfunction, but also on the intended dose and the therapeutic end-point. In general, any patient with a GFR < 70 mL/min should be highlighted as 'at risk' from cisplatin renal toxicity. Furthermore, dose modification will depend on the risk/benefit ratio for that patient. Consequently, the clinical decision may range from complete omission of cisplatin if palliation is intended, to treatment at full dose if cure is possible, with the damage to renal function being justified on the balance of the benefit to the patient of the chemotherapy. An alternative approach is consideration of a change to carboplatin, which can be dosed specifically according to GFR
• Ototoxicity, nephrotoxicity and myelosuppression reported. Check hearing, renal function and haematology before treatment and before each subsequent course (also during treatment)
• Hypomagnesaemia, hypocalcaemia and hyperuricaemia observed
• The addition of mannitol to the infusion may aid diuresis and protect the kidneys

Clarithromycin

Clinical use

Antibacterial agent; adjunct in treatment of
duodenal ulcers by eradication of H. pylori

Dose in normal renal function

Oral:
250–500 mg every 12 hrs
IV:
500 mg every 12 hrs

Pharmacokinetics

Molecular weight (daltons)	748
% Protein binding	70
% Excreted unchanged in urine	15
Volume of distribution (L/kg)	2–4
Half-life – normal/ESRF (hrs)	2.3–6/–

Dose in renal impairment GFR (mL/min)

20–50	Oral: 250–500 mg every 12 hrs IV: 500 mg every 12 hrs
10–20	Oral: 250–500 mg every 12–24 hrs IV: 250–500 mg every 12 hrs
<10	Oral: 250 mg every 12–24 hrs IV: 250 mg every 12 hrs

Dose in patients undergoing renal replacement therapies

CAPD	Unknown dialysability. Dose as in GFR = <10 mL/min
HD	Unknown dialysability. Dose as in GFR = <10 mL/min
CAV/VVHD	Unknown dialysability. Dose as in GFR = 10–20 mL/min

Important drug interactions

CYCLOSPORIN

• Increases plasma cyclosporin concentration
(although may take ~5 days after starting
clarithromycin before increase in cyclosporin
levels is seen)

POTENTIALLY HAZARDOUS INTERACTIONS WITH
OTHER DRUGS

• Anticoagulants: effect of nicoumalone and warfarin
is potentially enhanced
• Anticonvulsants: increased plasma carbamazepine
concentration
• Antihistamines: inhibits the metabolism of
terfenadine and astemizole (risk of hazardous
arrhythmias)
• Cisapride: possibly inhibits the metabolism of
cisapride (risk of ventricular arrhythmias)
• Theophylline: increased plasma theophylline
concentration

Administration

RECONSTITUTION

• Add 10 mL water for injection to vial (500 mg).
Add reconstituted product to 250 mL glucose 5%
or sodium chloride 0.9%. (Stable in 100 mL, but
more likely to cause phlebitis, pain and
inflammation at the injection site)

ROUTE

• IV infusion into one of the larger proximal veins.
Not to be administered by bolus or IM injection

RATE OF ADMINISTRATION

• Over 60 min

COMMENTS

–

Other information

Use with caution in renal or hepatic failure

Clindamycin

Clinical use

Antibacterial agent

Dose in normal renal function

Oral:

150–450 mg every 6 hrs. Endocarditis prophylaxis 600 mg 1 hr before procedure

IV/IM:

0.6–4.5 g daily in 2–4 divided doses. Prophylaxis 300 mg 15 min before then 150 mg 6 hrs later

Pharmacokinetics

Molecular weight (daltons)	479.5 as hydrochloride in capsules; 505 as phosphate in injection
% Protein binding	60–95
% Excreted unchanged in urine	10–13
Volume of distribution (L/kg)	0.6–1.2
Half-life – normal/ESRF (hrs)	2–4/3–5

Dose in renal impairment GFR (mL/min)

20–50	Dose as in normal renal function
10–20	Dose as in normal renal function
<10	Dose as in normal renal function

Dose in patients undergoing renal replacement therapies

CAPD	Not dialysed. Dose as in normal renal function
HD	Not dialysed. Dose as in normal renal function
CAV/VVHD	Not dialysed. Dose as in normal renal function

Important drug interactions

CYCLOSPORIN

–

POTENTIALLY HAZARDOUS INTERACTIONS WITH OTHER DRUGS

• Muscle relaxants: enhanced neuromuscular blockade
• Erythromycin: antagonism demonstrated in vitro, manufacturer recommends that the two drugs should not be administered concurrently

Administration

RECONSTITUTION

• Dilute prior to IV administration. Each 300 mg in at least 50 mL of diluent. Compatible diluents: sodium chloride 0.9% or glucose 5%

ROUTE

• IV infusion, IM

RATE OF ADMINISTRATION

• Each 300 mg in 50 mL over 10 min

COMMENTS

• Administration of more than 1200 mg in a single 1-hr infusion is not recommended
• Single IM injections of greater than 600 mg are not recommended

Other information

• Capsules should be swallowed whole with a glass of water (200 ml)
• Pseudomembranous colitis may occur
• Periodic kidney and liver function tests should be carried out during prolonged therapy
• Dosage may require reduction in patients with severe renal impairment due to prolonged half-life

Clodronate sodium

Clinical use

Bisphosphonate for: (1) management of osteolytic lesions, hypercalcaemia and bone pain associated with skeletal metastases in patients with breast cancer or multiple myeloma; (2) maintenance of acceptable serum Ca^{2+} levels in patients with hypercalcaemia of malignancy

Dose in normal renal function

• Loron/Bonefos: 1600–3200 mg daily
• Loron 520: 1040–2080 mg daily

Pharmacokinetics

Molecular weight (daltons)	360.9
% Protein binding	36
% Excreted unchanged in urine	70–90
Volume of distribution (L/kg)	0.25
Half-life – normal/ESRF (hrs)	13/increased

Dose in renal impairment GFR (mL/min)

20–50	Dose as in normal renal function
10–20	50% of normal dose
<10	25% of normal dose

Dose in patients undergoing renal replacement therapies

CAPD	Unknown dialysability. Dose as in GFR = <10 mL/min
HD	Unknown dialysability. Dose as in GFR = <10 mL/min
CAV/VVHD	Unknown dialysability. Dose as in GFR = 10–20 mL/min

Important drug interactions

CYCLOSPORIN

–

POTENTIALLY HAZARDOUS INTERACTIONS WITH OTHER DRUGS

–

Administration

RECONSTITUTION

• Single infusion: 1500 mg sodium clodronate to 500 mL sodium chloride 0.9% or glucose 5%
• Multiple infusions : 300 mg sodium clodronate to 500 mL sodium chloride 0.9% or glucose 5%

ROUTE

• Oral, IV infusion

RATE OF ADMINISTRATION

• Single infusion: 1500 mg over 4 hrs
• Multiple infusions: 300 mg over at least 2 hrs

COMMENTS

• Multiple infusions should be repeated on successive days until normocalcaemia is achieved, or to a maximum of 7 days
• Whichever method of infusion is employed, most patients will achieve normocalcaemia within 5 days

Other information

• Renal failure has been associated with IV use of bisphosphonates. Smaller doses (up to 300 mg daily) over 2–3 hrs are less likely to be associated with renal impairment than high doses by short IV infusion
• Reversible elevations of creatinine have been reported. Renal function should be monitored during treatment
• Orally: avoid food for 1 hr before and after treatment, particularly calcium-containing products; also avoid iron, mineral supplements and antacids

Clomipramine

Clinical use

Depressive illness, phobic and obsessional states; adjunctive treatment of cataplexy associated with narcolepsy

Dose in normal renal function

10–250 mg daily

Pharmacokinetics

Molecular weight (daltons)	351.3
% Protein binding	97
% Excreted unchanged in urine	–
Volume of distribution (L/kg)	12
Half-life – normal/ESRF (hrs)	19–37/–

Dose in renal impairment GFR (mL/min)

20–50	Dose as in normal renal function
10–20	Not known. Start at lower doses and monitor effect
<10	Not known. Start at lower doses and monitor effect

Dose in patients undergoing renal replacement therapies

CAPD	Not dialysed. Dose as in GFR = <10 mL/min
HD	Not dialysed. Dose as in GFR = <10 mL/min
CAV/VVHD	Not dialysed. Dose as in GFR = 10–20 mL/min

Important drug interactions

CYCLOSPORIN

–

Potentially hazardous interactions with other drugs

- Anti-arrhythmics: increased risk of ventricular arrhythmias with drugs which prolong QT interval
- MAOIs: CNS excitation and hypertension: tricyclics should not be started until 2 weeks after stopping MAOI; MAOI should not be started until at least 1 week after tricyclic has stopped
- Anti-epileptics: convulsive threshold can be lowered
- Antihistamines: increased risk of ventricular arrhythmias with astemizole and terfenadine
- Sympathomimetics: hypertension and arrhythmias reported

Administration

RECONSTITUTION

- IV infusion: initially 25–50 mg in 200–500 mL of sodium chloride 0.9% or glucose 5%. If satisfactory response, increase dose, but volume of infusion fluid may be reduced to a minimum of 125 mL

ROUTE

- IV, IM

RATE OF ADMINISTRATION

- Initially, infuse over 1.5–3 hrs. If there is a satisfactory response, infusion duration may be decreased to a minimum of 45 min

COMMENTS

- IM injection: 25 mg increasing to a maximum of 150 mg daily
- Monitor blood pressure during the infusion as hypotension may occur

Other information

- Normal doses have been used in dialysis patients long term, but caution is needed as parent drug and active metabolites may accumulate

Clonazepam

Clinical use

Benzodiazepine – anticonvulsant, anxiolytic

Dose in normal renal function

1–8 mg daily

Pharmacokinetics

Molecular weight (daltons)	315.7
% Protein binding	47–86
% Excreted unchanged in urine	<1
Volume of distribution (L/kg)	1.5–4.5
Half-life – normal/ESRF (hrs)	18–45/–

Dose in renal impairment GFR (mL/min)

20–50	Dose as in normal renal function
10–20	Dose as in normal renal function
<10	Dose as in normal renal function

Dose in patients undergoing renal replacement therapies

CAPD	Unknown dialysability. Dose as in normal renal function
HD	Unknown dialysability. Dose as in normal renal function
CAV/VVHD	Unknown dialysability. Dose as in normal renal function

Important drug interactions

CYCLOSPORIN

–

POTENTIALLY HAZARDOUS INTERACTIONS WITH OTHER DRUGS

–

Administration

RECONSTITUTION

• IV bolus: add the contents of the diluent ampoule (1 mL water for injection) to the contents of the clonazepam ampoule (1 mg in 1 mL solvent)
• IV infusion: up to 3 mg (3 amps) added to 250 mL sodium chloride 0.9%, glucose 5% or glucose/sodium chloride 0.9%

ROUTE

• IV bolus or infusion

RATE OF ADMINISTRATION

• IV bolus: 1 mg over approximately 30 sec

COMMENTS

• IV infusion of clonazepam is potentially hazardous (especially if prolonged), calling for close and constant observation and best carried out in specialist centres with ICU facilities. Risks include apnoea, hypotension and deep unconsciousness

Other information

• In long-term administration, active metabolites may accumulate and lower doses should be used
• Clonazepam is one of several agents which are used in restless leg syndrome, and has also been tried in the management of intractable hiccup where chlorpromazine has failed

Clonidine

Clinical use

All grades of essential and secondary hypertension

Dose in normal renal function

0.05–0.1 mg 3 times a day, increasing gradually to 1.8 mg or more

Pharmacokinetics

Molecular weight (daltons)	266
% Protein binding	20–40
% Excreted unchanged in urine	45
Volume of distribution (L/kg)	3–6
Half-life – normal/ESRF (hrs)	6–23/39–42

Dose in renal impairment GFR (mL/min)

20–50	Dose as in normal renal function
10–20	Dose as in normal renal function
<10	Dose as in normal renal function

Dose in patients undergoing renal replacement therapies

CAPD	Unknown dialysability. Dose as in normal renal function
HD	Unknown dialysability. Dose as in normal renal function
CAV/VVHD	Unknown dialysability. Dose as in normal renal function

Important drug interactions

CYCLOSPORIN

–

POTENTIALLY HAZARDOUS INTERACTIONS WITH OTHER DRUGS

• Central nervous system depressants
• Beta-adrenoreceptor antagonists
• Antipsychotics (haloperidol and chlorpromazine)

Administration

RECONSTITUTION

–

ROUTE

• Oral

RATE OF ADMINISTRATION

–

COMMENTS

–

Other information

• Use in renal impairment: clonidine plasma concentrations for a given dose are 2–3 times higher in patients with severe renal impairment. However, blood pressure control appears to be satisfactory and adverse effects are not increased
• Clearance of clonidine by haemodialysis is not sufficient to require an additional post-dialysis dose
• Clonidine withdrawal: rebound hypertension occurs if the drug is abruptly withdrawn
• Tricyclic antidepressants may decrease efficacy

Co-amoxiclav (amoxycillin/clavulanic acid)

Clinical use

Antibacterial agent

Dose in normal renal function

For treatment of infections:

IV – 1.2 g every 8 hrs (increasing to every 6 hrs in severe infection); oral – 375 mg 3 times daily (maximum 625 mg 3 times daily)

Pharmacokinetics

Molecular weight (daltons)	amoxycillin: 365.4; clavulanic acid: 199.2
% Protein binding	amoxycillin: 18; clavulanic acid: 22
% Excreted unchanged in urine	amoxycillin: 78–94; clavulanic acid: 29–57
Volume of distribution (L/kg)	amoxycillin: 0.21; clavulanic acid: 0.21
Half-life – normal/ESRF (hrs)	amoxycillin: 1.4–2.0; clavulanic acid: 0.8–1.0

Dose in renal impairment GFR (mL/min)

20–50	Dose as in normal renal function
10–20	IV: 1.2 g stat followed by 600 mg IV every 12 hrs Oral: 375 mg or 625 mg two–three daily
<10	IV: 1.2 g stat followed by 600 mg IV every 24 hrs Oral: 375 mg two–three daily

Dose in patients undergoing renal replacement therapies

CAPD	Dialysed. Dose as in GFR = <10 mL/min
HD	Dialysed. Dose as in GFR = <10 mL/min
CAV/VVHD	Dialysed. Dose as in GFR = 10–20 mL/min

Important drug interactions

CYCLOSPORIN

–

POTENTIALLY HAZARDOUS INTERACTIONS WITH OTHER DRUGS

• Anticoagulants: effects of nicoumalone and warfarin are potentially enhanced
• Oral contraceptives: potentially reduced efficacy
• Methotrexate: reduced excretion thereby increasing risk of toxicity

Administration

RECONSTITUTION

• IV: 600 mg with 10 mL water for injection; 1.2 g with 20 mL water for injection

ROUTE

• Oral, IV. Not for IM injection

RATE OF ADMINISTRATION

• IV bolus: over 3–4 min
• Infusion: infuse over 30–40 min in 100 mL sodium chloride 0.9%

COMMENTS

• IV preparation is less stable in infusion solutions containing glucose, dextran or bicarbonate. May be injected into drip tubing over period of 3–4 min
• Do not mix with aminoglycosides

Other information

• CSM has advised that cholestatic jaundice may occur if treatment exceeds a period of 14 days or up to 6 weeks after treatment has been stopped. The incidence of cholestatic jaundice occurring with co-amoxiclav is higher in males than in females and particularly prevalent in men over the age of 65 years
• The probability of co-amoxiclav-associated cholestatic jaundice is 6 times higher than with amoxycillin
• Each 1.2-g vial contains: sodium 3.1 mmol, potassium 1 mmol

Co-codamol (paracetamol/codeine phosphate)

Clinical use

Analgesia

Dose in normal renal function

1–2 tablets up to 4 times a day

Pharmacokinetics

Molecular weight (daltons)	paracetamol: 151; codeine: 372 (codeine phosphate mw = 406)
% Protein binding	paracetamol: 20–30; codeine: 7
% Excreted unchanged in urine	paracetamol: 3; codeine: <5
Volume of distribution (L/kg)	paracetamol: 1.0–2.0; codeine: 3–4
Half-life – normal/ESRF (hrs)	paracetamol: 1.9–2.5/unchanged; codeine: 2.5–3.5/–

Dose in renal impairment GFR (mL/min)

20–50	Dose as in normal renal function
10–20	75% of normal dose
<10	50% of normal dose

Dose in patients undergoing renal replacement therapies

CAPD	Unknown dialysability. Dose as in GFR = <10 mL/min
HD	Unknown dialysability. Dose as in GFR = <10 mL/min
CAV/VVHD	Unknown dialysability. Dose as in GFR = 10–20 mL/min

Important drug interactions

CYCLOSPORIN

–

POTENTIALLY HAZARDOUS INTERACTIONS WITH OTHER DRUGS

–

Administration

RECONSTITUTION

–

ROUTE

• Oral

RATE OF ADMINISTRATION

–

COMMENTS

• Available in two strengths: (1) 8/500 – 8 mg codeine phosphate/500 mg paracetamol; (2) 30/500 – 30 mg codeine phosphate/500 mg paracetamol

• 30/500 formulation: may cause drowsiness due to increased cerebral sensitivity in patients with renal failure

Other information

• Effervescent formulations of Solpadol and Tylex (30/500) should be avoided in renal impairment. They contain 18.6 mmol sodium per tablet and 13.6 mmol sodium per tablet, respectively

• Caution is recommended when giving paracetamol to patients with renal impairment. Plasma concentrations of the glucuronide and sulphate conjugates of paracetamol are increased in patients with moderate renal impairment and in patients on dialysis. Paracetamol itself may be regenerated from these metabolites

• In renal impairment, opioid analgesics may produce a prolonged effect with increased cerebral sensitivity

Codeine phosphate

Clinical use

Analgesic, anti-diarrhoeal, cough suppressant

Dose in normal renal function

30–60 mg up to 4 times a day

Pharmacokinetics

Molecular weight (daltons)	codeine: 372; codeine phosphate: 406
% Protein binding	7
% Excreted unchanged in urine	<5
Volume of distribution (L/kg)	3–4
Half-life – normal/ESRF (hrs)	2.5–3.5/–

Dose in renal impairment GFR (mL/min)

20–50	Dose as in normal renal function
10–20	75% of normal dose
<10	50% of normal dose

Dose in patients undergoing renal replacement therapies

CAPD	Unknown dialysability. Dose as in GFR = <10 mL/min
HD	Unknown dialysability. Dose as in GFR = <10 mL/min
CAV/VVHD	Unknown dialysability. Dose as in GFR = 10–20 mL/min

Important drug interactions

CYCLOSPORIN

–

POTENTIALLY HAZARDOUS INTERACTIONS WITH OTHER DRUGS

–

Administration

RECONSTITUTION

• 60 mg/mL

ROUTE

• IV

RATE OF ADMINISTRATION

• IV bolus

COMMENTS

–

Other information

• Increased risk of drowsiness due to increased cerebral sensitivity in patients with renal failure
• Increased risk of constipation – care required in patients on CAPD

Co-dydramol (paracetamol/dihydrocodeine)

Clinical use

Analgesia

Dose in normal renal function

1–2 tablets up to 4 times a day

Pharmacokinetics

Molecular weight (daltons)	paracetamol: 151; dihydrocodeine: 452
% Protein binding	paracetamol: 20–30; dihydrocodeine: –
% Excreted unchanged in urine	paracetamol: 3; dihydrocodeine: –
Volume of distribution (L/kg)	paracetamol: 1.0–2.0; dihydrocodeine: 1.1
Half-life – normal/ESRF (hrs)	paracetamol: 1.9–2.5/unchanged; dihydrocodeine: 3.4–4.5/6+

Dose in renal impairment GFR (mL/min)

20–50	1–2 tablets every 4 hrs
10–20	75% of dose every 6 hrs
<10	50% of dose every 6–8 hrs

Dose in patients undergoing renal replacement therapies

CAPD	Not dialysed. Dose as in GFR = <10 mL/min
HD	Not dialysed. Dose as in GFR = <10 mL/min
CAV/VVHD	Unknown dialysability. Dose as in GFR = 10–20 mL/min

Important drug interactions

CYCLOSPORIN

–

POTENTIALLY HAZARDOUS INTERACTIONS WITH OTHER DRUGS

–

Administration

RECONSTITUTION

–

ROUTE

• Oral

RATE OF ADMINISTRATION

–

COMMENTS

–

Other information

• Active metabolites of dihydrocodeine accumulate in renal impairment (drowsiness/lightheadedness/constipation). Increased cerebral sensitivity in patients with renal failure

Colchicine

Clinical use

Acute gout. Short-term prophylaxis during initial therapy with allopurinol and uricosuric drugs

Dose in normal renal function

Acute:

1 mg then 0.5 mg every 2–3 hrs until pain relieved or vomiting/diarrhoea occurs. Maximum of 10 mg per course

Short-term prophylaxis:

500 micrograms 2–3 times a day

Pharmacokinetics

Molecular weight (daltons)	399
% Protein binding	30–50
% Excreted unchanged in urine	5–20
Volume of distribution (L/kg)	1–2
Half-life – normal/ESRF (hrs)	19/40

Dose in renal impairment GFR (mL/min)

20–50	Dose as in normal renal function
10–20	Dose as in normal renal function
<10	50% of normal dose

Dose in patients undergoing renal replacement therapies

CAPD	Unknown dialysability. Dose as in GFR = <10 mL/min
HD	Not dialysed. Dose as in GFR = <10 mL/min
CAV/VVHD	Unknown dialysability. Dose as in GFR = 10–20 mL/min

Important drug interactions

CYCLOSPORIN

• Risk of myopathy or rhabdomyolysis, also increased blood cyclosporin concentrations and nephrotoxicity

POTENTIALLY HAZARDOUS INTERACTIONS WITH OTHER DRUGS

–

Administration

RECONSTITUTION

–

ROUTE

• Oral

RATE OF ADMINISTRATION

–

COMMENTS

–

Other information

• If nausea, vomiting or diarrhoea occur, stop therapy
• In ESRD colchicine can be administered concurrently with allopurinol, but seek specialist advice

Colestipol

Clinical use

Hyperlipidaemias, particularly type IIa

Dose in normal renal function

5 g once or twice daily, increased if necessary at intervals of 1–2 months to a maximum of 30 g daily

Pharmacokinetics

Molecular weight (daltons)	–
% Protein binding	0
% Excreted unchanged in urine	0
Volume of distribution (L/kg)	Not absorbed
Half-life – normal/ESRF (hrs)	Not absorbed

Dose in renal impairment GFR (mL/min)

20–50	Dose as in normal renal function
10–20	Dose as in normal renal function
<10	Dose as in normal renal function

Dose in patients undergoing renal replacement therapies

CAPD	Not dialysed. Dose as in normal renal function
HD	Not dialysed. Dose as in normal renal function
CAV/VVHD	Not dialysed. Dose as in normal renal function

Important drug interactions

CYCLOSPORIN

• No reports of an interaction. However, cyclosporin levels should be carefully monitored if colestipol and cyclosporin are prescribed concurrently, as colestipol may interfere with cyclosporin absorption

POTENTIALLY HAZARDOUS INTERACTIONS WITH OTHER DRUGS

• Anticoagulants: may enhance or reduce effects of nicoumalone, phenindione and warfarin

Administration

RECONSTITUTION

–

ROUTE

• Oral

RATE OF ADMINISTRATION

–

COMMENTS

• Other drugs should be taken at least 1 hr before or 4–6 hrs after colestipol to reduce possible interference with absorption
• Colestipol granules may be administered as a suspension in water or a flavoured vehicle
• Colestipol orange contains 32.5 mg aspartame (18.2 mg phenylalanine) per sachet

Other information

• Colestipol may interfere with the absorption of fat-soluble vitamins

Co-proxamol (paracetamol/dextropropoxyphene)

Clinical use

Analgesia

Dose in normal renal function

1–2 tablets, 3 or 4 times daily. Maximum 8 tablets daily

Pharmacokinetics

Molecular weight (daltons)	paracetamol: 151; dextropropoxyphene HCl: 376
% Protein binding	paracetamol: 20–30; dextropropoxyphene HCl: 80
% Excreted unchanged in urine	paracetamol: 3; dextropropoxyphene HCl: 1
Volume of distribution (L/kg)	paracetamol: 1.0–2.0; dextropropoxyphene HCl: ~16
Half-life – normal/ESRF (hrs)	paracetamol: 1.9–2.5/unchanged; dextropropoxyphene HCl: 6–12/–

Dose in renal impairment GFR (mL/min)

20–50	Dose as in normal renal function
10–20	75% of normal dose
<10	50% of normal dose

Dose in patients undergoing renal replacement therapies

CAPD	Unknown dialysability. Dose as in GFR = <10 mL/min
HD	Unknown dialysability. Dose as in GFR = <10 mL/min
CAV/VVHD	Unknown dialysability. Dose as in GFR = 10–20 mL/min

Important drug interactions

CYCLOSPORIN

–

POTENTIALLY HAZARDOUS INTERACTIONS WITH OTHER DRUGS

–

Administration

RECONSTITUTION

–

ROUTE

• Oral

RATE OF ADMINISTRATION

–

COMMENTS

• May cause drowsiness and increased cerebral sensitivity in patients with renal failure

Other information

• Caution is recommended when giving paracetamol to patients with renal impairment. Plasma concentrations of the glucuronide and sulphate conjugates of paracetamol are increased in patients with moderate renal impairment and in patients on dialysis

• In renal impairment, opioid analgesics may produce a prolonged effect with increased cerebral sensitivity

• The elimination of the drug is prolonged and plasma concentrations are increased so that adjustment of the dose may be necessary

Cortisone acetate

Clinical use

Glucocorticoid replacement in adrenocortical insufficiency

Dose in normal renal function

25–37.5 mg daily in divided doses

Pharmacokinetics

Molecular weight (daltons)	402.5
% Protein binding	90–95
% Excreted unchanged in urine	0
Volume of distribution (L/kg)	0.3
Half-life – normal/ESRF (hrs)	0.5–2/3.5

Dose in renal impairment GFR (mL/min)

20–50	Dose as in normal renal function
10–20	Dose as in normal renal function
<10	Dose as in normal renal function

Dose in patients undergoing renal replacement therapies

CAPD	Unknown dialysability. Dose as in normal renal function
HD	Unknown dialysability. Dose as in normal renal function
CAV/VVHD	Unknown dialysability. Dose as in normal renal function

Important drug interactions

CYCLOSPORIN

–

POTENTIALLY HAZARDOUS INTERACTIONS WITH OTHER DRUGS

- Rifamycins accelerate metabolism of corticosteroids
- Anti-epileptics: carbamazepine, phenobarbitone, phenytoin and primidone accelerate metabolism of corticosteroids
- Increased risk of hypokalaemia with amphotericin

Administration

RECONSTITUTION

–

ROUTE

- Oral

RATE OF ADMINISTRATION

–

COMMENTS

–

Other information

- Treatment of adrenocortical insufficiency with hydrocortisone is now generally preferred since cortisone itself is inactive and must be converted by the liver to hydrocortisone, its active metabolite, and hence, in some liver disorders, its bioavailability is less reliable
- Mineralocorticoid activity is usually supplemented by fludrocortisone acetate by mouth
- Cortisone acetate has been used in the treatment of many allergic and inflammatory disorders, but prednisolone or other synthetic glucocorticoids are generally preferred because of their reduced sodium-retaining properties

Co-trimoxazole (trimethoprim/ sulphamethoxazole)

Clinical use

Antibacterial agent for treatment and prophylaxis of pneumocystis carinii pneumonitis (PCP)

Dose in normal renal function

IV:

60 mg/kg of co-trimoxazole twice a day

Oral:

60 mg/kg of co-trimoxazole twice a day

Oral prophylaxis:

960 mg daily

Pharmacokinetics

Molecular weight (daltons)	sulphamethoxazole: 253; trimethoprim: 290
% Protein binding	sulphamethoxazole: 50; trimethoprim: 30–70
% Excreted unchanged in urine	sulphamethoxazole: 70; trimethoprim: 40–70
Volume of distribution (L/kg)	sulphamethoxazole: 0.28–0.38 (altered in uraemia); trimethoprim: 1–2.2
Half-life – normal/ESRF (hrs)	sulphamethoxazole: 10/20–50; trimethoprim: 9–13/20–49

Dose in renal impairment GFR (mL/min)

20–50	Dose as in normal renal function
10–20	60 mg/kg twice a day for 3 days, then 30 mg/kg twice a day
<10	60mg/kg once a day or 30 mg/kg twice daily. (This should only be given if haemodialysis facilities are available)

Dose in patients undergoing renal replacement therapies

CAPD	Not dialysed. Dose as in GFR = <10 mL/min
HD	Dialysed. Dose as in GFR = <10 mL/min
CAV/VVHD	Dialysed. Dose as in GFR = 10–20 mL/min

Important drug interactions

CYCLOSPORIN

• Increased risk of nephrotoxicity. No significant changes in cyclosporin levels

POTENTIALLY HAZARDOUS INTERACTIONS WITH OTHER DRUGS

• Anticoagulants: effect of warfarin enhanced

• Antidiabetics: effect of sulphonylureas enhanced

• Anti-epileptics: antifolate effect and plasma concentration of phenytoin increased

Administration

RECONSTITUTION

–

ROUTE

• IV

RATE OF ADMINISTRATION

• Over 30 min – 1½ hrs centrally (or 2–3 hrs for high doses) (unlicensed)

COMMENTS

• For an IV infusion dilute 5 mL co-trimoxazole strong solution with 125 mL sodium chloride 0.9% or glucose 5% and infuse over 1½ hrs Alternatively, dilute 5 mL to 75 mL glucose 5% and administer over 1 hr. Can infuse undiluted solution via central line (unlicensed)

Other information

• After 2–3 days plasma samples collected 12 hrs post-dose should have levels of sulphamethoxazole not higher than 150 micrograms/mL. If higher, stop treatment until levels fall below 120 micrograms/mL

• Plasma levels of trimethoprim should be 5 micrograms/mL or higher for optimum efficacy

• Folic acid supplementation may be necessary during chronic therapy

• Monthly blood counts advisable

Cyclizine

Clinical use

Nausea, vomiting, vertigo, motion sickness, labyrinthine disorders

Dose in normal renal function

Oral/IV/IM: 50 mg up to 3 times daily

Pharmacokinetics

Molecular weight (daltons)	266
% Protein binding	–
% Excreted unchanged in urine	<1
Volume of distribution (L/kg)	–
Half-life – normal/ESRF (hrs)	20/–

Dose in renal impairment GFR (mL/min)

20–50	Dose as in normal renal function
10–20	Dose as in normal renal function
<10	Dose as in normal renal function

Dose in patients undergoing renal replacement therapies

CAPD	Unknown dialysability. Dose as in normal renal function
HD	Unknown dialysability. Dose as in normal renal function
CAV/VVHD	Unknown dialysability. Dose as in normal renal function

Important drug interactions

CYCLOSPORIN

–

POTENTIALLY HAZARDOUS INTERACTIONS WITH OTHER DRUGS

• Other antihistamines: concomitant use of astemizole or terfenadine not recommended – increased risk of hazardous arrhythmias

Administration

RECONSTITUTION

–

ROUTE

• Oral, IV

RATE OF ADMINISTRATION

• Slow IV

COMMENTS

• Increased cerebral sensitivity in patients with renal failure

Other information

–

Cyclophosphamide

Clinical use

Antineoplastic agent for: (1) immunosuppression of autoimmune diseases; (2) treatment of malignant disease

Dose in normal renal function

Oral (for autoimmune disease):
1–2.5 mg/kg/day
IV:
usually 0.5–1 g/m² repeated at intervals, e.g. monthly (pulse therapy)

Pharmacokinetics

Molecular weight (daltons)	279
% Protein binding	parent drug: 13; alkylating metabolites: 50–60
% Excreted unchanged in urine	10–15
Volume of distribution (L/kg)	0.62
Half-life – normal/ESRF (hrs)	4–7.5/10

Dose in renal impairment GFR (mL/min)

20–50	Dose as in normal renal function
10–20	75–100% of normal dose
<10	50–75% of normal dose

Dose in patients undergoing renal replacement therapies

CAPD	Dialysed. Dose as in GFR = <10 mL/min. Following dose do not perform CAPD exchange for 12 hrs
HD	Dialysed. Dose as in GFR = <10 mL/min. Dose at minimum of 12 hrs before HD session
CAV/VVHD	Dialysed. Dose as in GFR = 10–20 mL/min

Important drug interactions

CYCLOSPORIN

–

POTENTIALLY HAZARDOUS INTERACTIONS WITH OTHER DRUGS

–

Administration

RECONSTITUTION

• Add 5 mL water for injection to each 100 mg

ROUTE

• Oral, IV

RATE OF ADMINISTRATION

• Directly into vein over 1–2 min or directly into tubing of fast-running IV infusion with patient supine

COMMENTS

• IV route occasionally used for pulse therapy. Can be administered as an IV infusion

Other information

• Patients receiving chronic indefinite therapy may be at increased risk of developing urothelial carcinoma

• If patient is anuric and on dialysis, neither the cyclophosphamide nor its metabolites nor mesna should appear in the urinary tract. The use of mesna may therefore be unnecessary, although this would be a clinical decision

• If the patient is still passing urine, mesna should be given to prevent urothelial toxicity

Cycloserine

Clinical use

Antibacterial agent used for treatment of active pulmonary or extra-pulmonary tuberculosis

Dose in normal renal function

Initially 250 mg every 12 hrs for 2 weeks, increased according to blood concentration and response to maximum 500 mg every 12 hrs

Pharmacokinetics

Molecular weight (daltons)	102
% Protein binding	<20
% Excreted unchanged in urine	60–70
Volume of distribution (L/kg)	0.11–0.26
Half-life – normal/ESRF (hrs)	10/–

Dose in renal impairment GFR (mL/min)

20–50	250–500 mg every 12–24 hrs. Monitor blood levels weekly
10–20	250–500 mg every 12–24 hrs. Monitor blood levels weekly
<10	250 mg every 24 hrs. Monitor blood levels weekly

Dose in patients undergoing renal replacement therapies

CAPD	Unknown dialysability. Dose as in GFR = <10 mL/min
HD	Dialysed. Dose as in GFR = <10 mL/min
CAV/VVHD	Likely to be dialysed. Dose as in GFR = 10–20 mL/min

Important drug interactions

CYCLOSPORIN

–

POTENTIALLY HAZARDOUS INTERACTIONS WITH OTHER DRUGS

• Increased plasma concentration of phenytoin – risk of toxicity

Administration

RECONSTITUTION

–

ROUTE

• Oral

RATE OF ADMINISTRATION

–

COMMENTS

• May cause drowsiness and increased cerebral sensitivity in patients with renal impairment
• Blood concentration monitoring is required, especially in renal impairment, if dose exceeds 500 mg daily or if there are signs of toxicity. Blood concentration should not exceed 30 mg/L
• Contraindicated in severe renal insufficiency

Other information

• Can cause CNS toxicity
• Pyridoxine has been used in an attempt to treat or prevent neurological reactions, but its value is unproven

Cyclosporin

Clinical use

Immunosuppressant – used for prophylaxis of
kidney transplant rejection

Dose in normal renal function

Oral:

2–15 mg/kg/day based on levels (see local protocol)

IV:

One-third to one-half of oral dose
(see local protocol)

Pharmacokinetics

Molecular weight (daltons)	1203
% Protein binding	96–99
% Excreted unchanged in urine	<1
Volume of distribution (L/kg)	3.5–7.4
Half-life – normal/ESRF (hrs)	3–16/unchanged

Dose in renal impairment
GFR (mL/min)

20–50	Dose as in normal renal function
10–20	Dose as in normal renal function
<10	Dose as in normal renal function

Dose in patients undergoing renal replacement therapies

CAPD	Not dialysed. Dose as in normal renal function. Adjust according to levels
HD	Not dialysed. Dose as in normal renal function. Adjust according to levels
CAV/VVHD	Not dialysed. Dose as in normal renal function. Adjust according to levels

Important drug interactions

CYCLOSPORIN

–

POTENTIALLY HAZARDOUS INTERACTIONS WITH
OTHER DRUGS

- Increased risk of hyperkalaemia with ACE
  inhibitors, potassium-sparing diuretics
- Increased risk of nephrotoxicity with NSAIDs,
  aminoglycosides, cotrimoxazole, trimethoprim,
  4-quinolones, amphotericin, colchicine, melphalan
- Increased plasma cyclosporin levels with
  amiodarone, propafenone, doxycycline,
  erythromycin, clarithromycin, itraconazole,
  ketoconazole, miconazole, fluconazole,
  chloroquine, diltiazem, nicardipine, nifedipine,
  verapamil, high-dose methylprednisolone, danazol,
  progestogens, cimetidine
- Decreased plasma cyclosporin levels with
  rifampicin, IV trimethoprim, IV sulphadimidine,
  carbamazepine, phenobarbitone, phenytoin,
  griseofulvin, octreotide
- Increased risk of neurotoxicity with doxorubicin
- Increased toxicity with methotrexate
- Increased risk of myopathy with HMG CoA
  reductase inhibitors
- Increased half-life with tacrolimus

Administration

RECONSTITUTION

- Dilute dose 1:20 to 1:100 with sodium chloride
  0.9% or glucose 5%

ROUTE

- Oral, IV peripherally or centrally

RATE OF ADMINISTRATION

- Over 2 hrs peripherally or 1 hr centrally

COMMENTS

–

Other information

- Dose and monitor blood levels in accordance
  with local protocol

Cyproterone acetate

Clinical use

Control of libido in severe hypersexuality and sexual deviation in adult males; (2) management of patients with prostatic cancer (LHRH 'flare', palliative treatment, hot flushes)

Dose in normal renal function

Control of hypersexuality:
50 mg twice daily

Prostatic cancer:
200–300 mg/day

Pharmacokinetics

Molecular weight (daltons)	417
% Protein binding	–
% Excreted unchanged in urine	<1
Volume of distribution (L/kg)	10–30
Half-life – normal/ESRF (hrs)	38/–

Dose in renal impairment GFR (mL/min)

20–50	Dose as in normal renal function
10–20	Dose as in normal renal function
<10	Dose as in normal renal function

Dose in patients undergoing renal replacement therapies

CAPD	Unknown dialysability. Dose as in normal renal function
HD	Unknown dialysability. Dose as in normal renal function
CAV/VVHD	Unknown dialysability. Dose as in normal renal function

Important drug interactions

CYCLOSPORIN

–

POTENTIALLY HAZARDOUS INTERACTIONS WITH OTHER DRUGS

–

Administration

RECONSTITUTION

–

ROUTE

• Oral

RATE OF ADMINISTRATION

–

COMMENTS

• May cause drowsiness and increased CNS sensitivity in patients with renal impairment

Other information

• The CSM has advised that, in view of the hepatotoxicity associated with long-term doses of 300 mg daily, the use of cyproterone acetate in prostatic cancer should be restricted to short courses to cover testosterone flare associated with gonadorelin analogues, treatment of hot flushes after orchidectomy or gonadorelin analogues and for patients who have not responded to (or are intolerant of) other treatments

• Direct hepatic toxicity including jaundice, hepatitis and hepatic failure have been reported. Liver function tests should be performed before treatment and whenever symptoms suggestive of hepatotoxicity occur

Cytarabine

Clinical use

Antineoplastic agent, used for acute leukaemias

Dose in normal renal function

'High-dose infusional therapy':
$1-3$ g/m^2 every 12 hrs for up to 6 days
'Low-dose (conventional) therapy':
100 mg/m^2

Pharmacokinetics

Molecular weight (daltons)	243
% Protein binding	13
% Excreted unchanged in urine	6
Volume of distribution (L/kg)	2.6
Half-life – normal/ESRF (hrs)	0.5–3/unchanged

Dose in renal impairment GFR (mL/min)

20–50	100% of conventional low-dose regime. For high dose, see 'Other information'
10–20	100% of conventional low-dose regime. For high dose, see 'Other information'
<10	100% of conventional low-dose regime. For high dose, see 'Other information'

Dose in patients undergoing renal replacement therapies

CAPD	Unknown dialysability. Dose as in GFR = <10 mL/min
HD	Unknown dialysability. Dose as in GFR = <10 mL/min
CAV/VVHD	Unknown dialysability. Dose as in GFR = <10 mL/min

Important drug interactions

CYCLOSPORIN

–

POTENTIALLY HAZARDOUS INTERACTIONS WITH OTHER DRUGS

–

Administration

RECONSTITUTION

• Reconstitute/dilute with water for injection BP, glucose 5% or sodium chloride 0.9%

ROUTE

• Cytarabine injection (Faulding) only: IV inf, IV inj, IM, SC (200 mg/mL available for intrathecal use)
• Cytosar®: IV inf, IV inj, SC

RATE OF ADMINISTRATION

• IV inj: rapid
• IV inf: infuse over 1–24 hrs (1 hr is adequate for high dose)

COMMENTS

• Cytarabine inj (Faulding): administered intrathecally for leukaemic meningitis in doses up to 10–30 mg/m^2 3 times a week
• As a rule, patients have been seen to tolerate higher doses when given by rapid IV injection as compared with slow infusion. This difference is due to the rapid metabolism of cytarabine and the consequent short duration of action of the high dose

Other information

• Elevated baseline serum creatinine (>1.2 mg/dL) was an independent risk factor for the development of neurotoxicity during treatment with high-dose cytarabine. Furthermore, retrospective analysis implicates impaired renal function as an independent risk factor for high-dose cytarabine-induced cerebral and cerebellar toxicity. The incidence of neurotoxicity was 86–100% following administration of high-dose cytarabine to patients with Clcr <40 mL/min and 60–76% following administration to patients with Clcr <60 mL/min. In contrast, when patients with Clcr >60 mL/min received high-dose cytarabine, the incidence of neurotoxicity was found to be 8%, which correlates with the overall incidence of this adverse effect. Accordingly, it has been suggested that high-dose cytarabine should be used with caution in patients with impaired renal function. For Clcr of 30–45 mL/min, 50% of normal cytarabine dose should be prescribed, and for Clcr of 45–60 mL/min, 60% of normal cytarabine dose (high-dose regime) should be prescribed. High-dose cytarabine should be avoided for Clcr = 30 mL/min or less

Cytomegalovirus (CMV) human immunoglobulin (unlicensed product)

Clinical use

Prophylaxis for renal transplant recipients at risk of primary cytomegalovirus (CMV) disease. Treatment of CMV disease (usually with ganciclovir)

Dose in normal renal function

See local protocols

Pharmacokinetics

Molecular weight (daltons)	150
% Protein binding	N/A
% Excreted unchanged in urine	0
Volume of distribution (L/kg)	1
Half-life – normal/ESRF (hrs)	50

Dose in renal impairment GFR (mL/min)

20–50	Dose as in normal renal function
10–20	Dose as in normal renal function
<10	Dose as in normal renal function

Dose in patients undergoing renal replacement therapies

CAPD	Not dialysed. Dose as in normal renal function
HD	Not dialysed. Dose as in normal renal function
CAV/VVHD	Not dialysed. Dose as in normal renal function

Important drug interactions

CYCLOSPORIN

• No effect on efficacy of CMV immunoglobulin

POTENTIALLY HAZARDOUS INTERACTIONS WITH OTHER DRUGS

–

Administration

RECONSTITUTION

–

ROUTE

• IV peripherally or centrally

RATE OF ADMINISTRATION

–

COMMENTS

• Follow guidelines supplied by manufacturer

Other information

• Can give 10 mg IV chlorpheniramine 1 hr before administration
• Monitor for anaphylaxis, have adrenaline available
• Do not mix with any other drugs or infusion fluids

Dalteparin sodium (LMWH)

Clinical use

(1) Peri- and post-operative surgical thromboprophylaxis; (2) prevention of thrombus formation in extracorporeal circulation during HD; (3) treatment of DVT

Dose in normal renal function

Dose according to risk of thrombosis

Moderate risk:

2500 iu (antifactor Xa) SC 1–2 hrs prior to surgery, thereafter 2500 iu SC daily for 5 days

High risk:

2500 iu (antifactor Xa) SC 1–2 hrs prior to surgery, 2500 iu 12 hrs later, thereafter 5000 iu SC daily for 5 days

Pharmacokinetics

Molecular weight (daltons)	Average MW = 4000–6000
% Protein binding	–
% Excreted unchanged in urine	–
Volume of distribution (L/kg)	0.06–0.13
Half-life – normal/ESRF (hrs)	3.8

Dose in renal impairment GFR (mL/min)

20–50	Dose as in normal renal function
10–20	Dose as in normal renal function
<10	Dose as in normal renal function

Dose in patients undergoing renal replacement therapies

CAPD	Not dialysed. Dose as in normal renal function
HD	Not dialysed. Dose as in normal renal function
CAV/VVHD	Not dialysed. Dose as in normal renal function

Important drug interactions

CYCLOSPORIN

–

POTENTIALLY HAZARDOUS INTERACTIONS WITH OTHER DRUGS

• Anticoagulant/antiplatelet agents, e.g. aspirin, dextran, warfarin, may enhance effects of dalteparin
• Increased risk of haemorrhage with ketorolac
• Nitrates: glyceryl trinitrate infusion increases excretion

Administration

RECONSTITUTION

• Dalteparin solution for injection (ampoules) is compatible with sodium chloride 0.9% and glucose 5%

ROUTE

• SC injection into abdominal wall (pre-filled syringes)
• IV bolus/infusion (ampoules)

RATE OF ADMINISTRATION

–

COMMENTS

–

Other information

• Dalteparin is also indicated for prevention of clotting in the extracorporeal circulation during haemodialysis or haemofiltration. Dose for >4-hr session: IV bolus of 35 iu (antifactor Xa) per kg body weight, followed by infusion of 13 iu/kg/hr. Dose for <4-hr session: as above or single IV bolus injection of 5000 iu
• Antifactor Xa levels should be regularly monitored in new patients on haemodialysis during the first weeks; later less frequent monitoring is generally required. Consult the manufacturer's literature
• Patients undergoing acute HD have a narrower therapeutic dose range and should be monitored frequently
• Bleeding may be provoked, especially at high doses corresponding to antifactor Xa levels greater than 1.5 iu/mL
• The prolongation of the APTT induced by dalteparin is fully neutralised by protamine, but the anti-Xa activity is only neutralised to about 25–50%
• 1 mg of protamine inhibits the effect of 100 iu (antifactor Xa) of dalteparin
• The half-life is prolonged in uraemic patients as dalteparin sodium is eliminated primarily through the kidneys. However, it is not known how this affects current dosage guidelines

Daunorubicin

Clinical use

Antineoplastic agent, used for acute leukaemias

Dose in normal renal function

30–45 mg/m^2, or as for local protocol

Pharmacokinetics

Molecular weight (daltons)	564
% Protein binding	–
% Excreted unchanged in urine	25–30 (over 7 days)
Volume of distribution (L/kg)	–
Half-life – normal/ESRF (hrs)	18–27/–

Dose in renal impairment GFR (mL/min)

20–50	Dose as in normal renal function
10–20	Dose as in normal renal function
<10	Dose as in normal renal function

Dose in patients undergoing renal replacement therapies

CAPD	Unknown dialysability. Dose as in normal renal function
HD	Unknown dialysability. Dose as in normal renal function
CAV/VVHD	Unknown dialysability. Dose as in normal renal function

Important drug interactions

CYCLOSPORIN

–

POTENTIALLY HAZARDOUS INTERACTIONS WITH OTHER DRUGS

–

Administration

RECONSTITUTION

• Reconstitute 20-mg vial with 4 mL water for injection giving a concentration of 5 mg/mL. Dilute calculated dose of daunorubicin further in sodium chloride 0.9% to give a final concentration of 1 mg/mL

ROUTE

• IV

RATE OF ADMINISTRATION

• 1 mg/mL solution should be infused over 20 min into the tubing or a side-arm of a rapidly flowing IV infusion of sodium chloride 0.9%

COMMENTS

• Do not administer IM or SC – extremely irritating to tissues

Other information

• Daunorubicin is potentially cardiotoxic
• Monitor blood uric acid and urea levels
• Daunorubicin is extensively metabolised. The liver clears 40–50% of drug, largely into bile
• Manufacturer's literature suggests that in patients with a serum creatinine of 105–265 micromol/L, the dose should be reduced to 75% of normal, and if the creatinine is >265 micromol/L, the dose should be 50% of normal
• A liposomal formulation of daunorubicin is now available (DaunoXome®)

Desferrioxamine

Clinical use

Chelating agent used in the treatment of acute iron poisoning and chronic iron or aluminium overload

Dose in normal renal function

20–40 mg/kg/day. Exact dosages should be determined for each individual

Pharmacokinetics

Molecular weight (daltons)	657
% Protein binding	–
% Excreted unchanged in urine	30–35
Volume of distribution (L/kg)	2–2.5
Half-life – normal/ESRF (hrs)	6/–

Dose in renal impairment GFR (mL/min)

20–50	Dose as in normal renal function
10–20	Dose as in normal renal function
<10	50% of normal dose

Dose in patients undergoing renal replacement therapies

CAPD	Treatment of aluminium overload: 1 g once or twice each week prior to final exchange of the day by slow IV infusion, IM, SC or IP
HD	Treatment of aluminium overload: 1 g once each week administered during the last hour of dialysis as a slow IV infusion
CAV/VVHD	Dose schedule unknown. Metal chelates will be removed by dialysis

Important drug interactions

CYCLOSPORIN

–

POTENTIALLY HAZARDOUS INTERACTIONS WITH OTHER DRUGS

• Avoid prochlorperazine and methotrimeprazine (prolonged unconsciousness)

Administration

RECONSTITUTION

• Dissolve contents of one vial (500 mg) in 5 mL of water for injection = 10% solution. If for IV administration, the 10% solution can be diluted with sodium chloride 0.9%, glucose 5% or glucose/sodium chloride

ROUTE

• IV, SC (bolus or continuous infusion), IM, IP (CAPD, CCPD), PO (acute iron poisoning)

RATE OF ADMINISTRATION

• IV (acute overdose): max 15 mg/kg/hr. Reduce after 4–6 hrs so that total dose does not exceed 80 mg/kg/24 hrs

• SC: infuse over 8–12 hrs. Local irritation may occur

COMMENTS

• The urine in patients treated with desferrioxamine for severe iron intoxication may appear orange/red

• SC infusion is about 90% as effective as IV administration, which is now the route of choice in transfusion-related iron overload

• For oral administration, 5–10 mg should be dissolved in 50–100 mL water

• IM injection is less effective than SC

Other information

• Studies suggest that during HD only a small amount of plasma desferrioxamine transfers across the dialysis membrane

• Contraindicated in patients with severe renal disease, except those on dialysis

• Desferrioxamine may predispose to development of infection with Yersinia species

• In haemodialysis patients treated with desferrioxamine post-dialysis session, the half-life has been found to be extended to 19 hrs between dialysis sessions

• In treatment of acute iron poisoning, effectiveness of treatment is dependent on an adequate urine output. If oliguria or anuria develop, PD or HD may be necessary

Desmopressin (DDAVP)

Clinical use

Post-biopsy bleeding (unlicensed indication);
pre-biopsy prophylaxis (unlicensed indication)

Dose in normal renal function

Males: 16 micrograms; females: 12 micrograms;
or 300–400 nanograms/kg

Pharmacokinetics

Molecular weight (daltons)	1070
% Protein binding	0
% Excreted unchanged in urine	N/A
Volume of distribution (L/kg)	–
Half-life – normal/ESRF (hrs)	6–24/–

Dose in renal impairment GFR (mL/min)

20–50	Dose as in normal renal function
10–20	Dose as in normal renal function
<10	Dose as in normal renal function

Dose in patients undergoing renal replacement therapies

CAPD	Dialysis unlikely. Dose as in normal renal function
HD	Dialysis unlikely. Dose as in normal renal function
CAV/VVHD	Dialysis unlikely. Dose as in normal renal function

Important drug interactions

CYCLOSPORIN

–

POTENTIALLY HAZARDOUS INTERACTIONS WITH OTHER DRUGS

–

Administration

RECONSTITUTION

• Dilute dose to 50 mL with sodium chloride 0.9%

ROUTE

• IV peripherally

RATE OF ADMINISTRATION

• Over 30 min

COMMENTS

• Do not inject at a faster rate – greater risk of tachyphylaxis

Other information

• Emergency treatment of more generalised bleeding unresponsive to normal treatments: 0.1–0.5 micrograms/kg 4 times a day + IV premarin 0.6 mg/kg/day for up to 5 days
• DDAVP works as a haemostatic by stimulating Factor 8 production
• Onset of action less than 1 hr. Duration of effect 4–8 hrs

Dexamethasone

Clinical use

Corticosteroid, used in cerebral oedema.
Anti-emetic (unlicensed indication)

Dose in normal renal function

10–20 mg IV followed by 4–6 mg IV or IM every 6 hrs

Pharmacokinetics

Molecular weight (daltons)	393
% Protein binding	70
% Excreted unchanged in urine	8
Volume of distribution (L/kg)	0.6–1
Half-life – normal/ESRF (hrs)	3/–

Dose in renal impairment GFR (mL/min)

20–50	Dose as in normal renal function
10–20	Dose as in normal renal function
<10	Dose as in normal renal function

Dose in patients undergoing renal replacement therapies

CAPD	Dialysis unlikely. Dose as in normal renal function
HD	Dialysis unlikely. Dose as in normal renal function
CAV/VVHD	Dialysis unlikely. Dose as in normal renal function

Important drug interactions

CYCLOSPORIN

–

POTENTIALLY HAZARDOUS INTERACTIONS WITH OTHER DRUGS

• Rifampicin: accelerates dexamethasone metabolism
• Anti-epileptics: accelerate dexamethasone metabolism

Administration

RECONSTITUTION

–

ROUTE

• Oral, IV, IM

RATE OF ADMINISTRATION

• IV slowly over not less than 5 min. If there is underlying cardiac pathology, infusion over 20–30 min advised

COMMENTS

–

Other information

• Dexamethasone sodium phosphate 5 mg ≡ dexamethasone 4 mg
• Injection solution can be administered orally or via nasogastric tube
• Tablets will disperse in water

Diamorphine

Clinical use

Opiate analgesic – used for control of severe pain, and for pain relief in myocardial infarction

Dose in normal renal function

SC/IM:
5–10 mg 4-hourly increasing dose as necessary
IV:
2.5–5 mg (elderly patients – reduce dose by half)

Pharmacokinetics

Molecular weight (daltons)	424
% Protein binding	40
% Excreted unchanged in urine	<10
Volume of distribution (L/kg)	40–50
Half-life – normal/ESRF	1.7–3.5 min/–

Dose in renal impairment GFR (mL/min)

20–50	Dose as in normal renal function
10–20	Use small doses, e.g. 2.5 mg SC/IM approx 6-hourly and titrate to response
<10	Use small doses, e.g. 2.5 mg SC/IM approx 8-hourly and titrate to response

Dose in patients undergoing renal replacement therapies

CAPD	Not dialysed. Dose as in GFR = <10 mL/min
HD	Dialysed. Dose as in GFR = <10 mL/min
CAV/VVHD	Unknown dialysability. Dose as in GFR = 10–20 mL/min

Important drug interactions

CYCLOSPORIN

–

POTENTIALLY HAZARDOUS INTERACTIONS WITH OTHER DRUGS

–

Administration

RECONSTITUTION

• 1 mL water for injection or sodium chloride 0.9% (less may be used, e.g. for SC injection use 0.1 mL for 10 mg)

ROUTE

• IV, IM, SC

RATE OF ADMINISTRATION

• IV: 1 mg/min

COMMENTS

• Monitor BP and respiratory rates

Other information

• Increased cerebral sensitivity in renal impairment which can result in excessive sedation and serious respiratory depression necessitating ventilation
• More potent than morphine
• Extreme caution required with regular dosing – accumulation of active metabolites may occur
• Naloxone for effect reversal must be readily available if required

Diazepam

Clinical use

Benzodiazepine – used for peri-operative sedation (IV), also anxiolytic and muscle relaxant

Dose in normal renal function

Pre-med:

0.1–0.2 mg/kg IV

Anxiety:

2 mg 3 times a day, increasing if necessary to 15–30 mg daily in divided doses

Pharmacokinetics

Molecular weight (daltons)	285
% Protein binding	94–99
% Excreted unchanged in urine	<1
Volume of distribution (L/kg)	1.1–1.8
Half-life – normal/ESRF (hrs)	20–90/unchanged

Dose in renal impairment GFR (mL/min)

20–50	Dose as in normal renal function
10–20	Use small doses and titrate to response
<10	Use small doses and titrate to response

Dose in patients undergoing renal replacement therapies

CAPD	Not dialysed. Dose as in GFR = <10 mL/min
HD	Not dialysed. Dose as in GFR = <10 mL/min
CAV/VVHD	Unknown dialysability. Dose as in GFR = 10–20 mL/min

Important drug interactions

CYCLOSPORIN

–

POTENTIALLY HAZARDOUS INTERACTIONS WITH OTHER DRUGS

• Isoniazid inhibits metabolism of diazepam
• Rifampicin enhances metabolism of diazepam

Administration

RECONSTITUTION

–

ROUTE

• IV injection peripherally

RATE OF ADMINISTRATION

• 5 mg (1 mL)/min

COMMENTS

–

Other information

• Active metabolites are renally excreted and therefore accumulate in renal impairment
• Increased cerebral sensitivity in renal impairment which may result in excessive sedation and encephalopathy
• Always have flumazenil available to reverse effect
• Protein binding decreased in ESRD
• Vd increased in ESRD
• IV emulsion formulation (Diazemuls) less likely to cause thrombophlebitis

Diclofenac

Clinical use

NSAID and analgesic

Dose in normal renal function

75–150 mg daily in divided doses

Pharmacokinetics

Molecular weight (daltons)	318
% Protein binding	99
% Excreted unchanged in urine	<1
Volume of distribution (L/kg)	0.12–0.17
Half-life – normal/ESRF (hrs)	1–2/unchanged

Dose in renal impairment GFR (mL/min)

20–50	Dose as in normal renal function
10–20	Dose as in normal renal function, but avoid if possible
<10	Dose as in normal renal function, but only use if ESRD on dialysis

Dose in patients undergoing renal replacement therapies

CAPD	Not dialysed. Dose as in normal renal function
HD	Not dialysed. Dose as in normal renal function
CAV/VVHD	Not dialysed. Dose as in normal renal function

Important drug interactions

CYCLOSPORIN

• Increased risk of nephrotoxicity

POTENTIALLY HAZARDOUS INTERACTIONS WITH OTHER DRUGS

• Lithium: excretion decreased
• Cytotoxic agents: reduced excretion of methotrexate
• Anticoagulants: effects of nicoumalone and warfarin enhanced
• Antidiabetic agents: effects of sulphonylureas enhanced
• Anti-epileptic agents: effects of phenytoin enhanced
• ACE inhibitors: antagonism of hypotensive effect; increased risk of renal damage and hyperkalaemia

Administration

RECONSTITUTION

–

ROUTE

• Oral

RATE OF ADMINISTRATION

–

COMMENTS

–

Other information

• Diclofenac should be used with caution in uraemic patients predisposed to gastrointestinal bleeding or uraemic coagulopathies
• Inhibition of renal prostaglandin synthesis by NSAIDs may interfere with renal function, especially in the presence of existing renal disease. Avoid if possible; if not, check serum creatinine 48–72 hrs after starting NSAID. If raised, discontinue NSAID therapy
• Use normal doses in patients with ESRD on dialysis
• Use with great caution in renal transplant recipients – it can reduce intra-renal autocoid synthesis

Diflunisal

Clinical use

NSAID and analgesic

Dose in normal renal function

250–500 mg twice daily

Pharmacokinetics

Molecular weight (daltons)	250
% Protein binding	99
% Excreted unchanged in urine	<3
Volume of distribution (L/kg)	0.1
Half-life – normal/ESRF (hrs)	5–20/62

Dose in renal impairment GFR (mL/min)

20–50	Dose as in normal renal function
10–20	50% of normal dose, but avoid if possible
<10	50% of normal dose, but only use if ESRD on dialysis

Dose in patients undergoing renal replacement therapies

CAPD	Not dialysed. Dose as in normal renal function
HD	Not dialysed. Dose as in normal renal function
CAV/VVHD	Not dialysed. Dose as in normal renal function

Important drug interactions

CYCLOSPORIN

• Increased risk of nephrotoxicity

POTENTIALLY HAZARDOUS INTERACTIONS WITH OTHER DRUGS

• Lithium: decreased excretion
• Cytotoxic agents: decreased excretion of methotrexate
• Anticoagulants: effects of nicoumalone and warfarin enhanced
• Antidiabetic agents: effects of sulphonylureas enhanced
• Anti-epileptic agents: effects of phenytoin enhanced
• ACE inhibitors: antagonism of hypotensive effect; increased risk of renal damage and hyperkalaemia

Administration

RECONSTITUTION

–

ROUTE

• Oral

RATE OF ADMINISTRATION

–

COMMENTS

–

Other information

• Diflunisal should be used with caution in uraemic patients predisposed to gastrointestinal bleeding or uraemic coagulopathies
• Inhibition of renal prostaglandin synthesis by NSAIDs may interfere with renal function, especially in the presence of existing renal disease
• Avoid use of NSAIDs if possible; if not, check serum creatinine 48–72 hrs after starting NSAID. If raised, discontinue NSAID therapy
• Use normal doses in patients with ESRD on dialysis
• Use with great caution in renal transplant recipients – it can reduce intra-renal autocoid synthesis

Digitoxin

Clinical use

Heart failure, supraventricular arrhythmias

Dose in normal renal function

Maintenance dose 100 micrograms alternate days; may be increased to 200 micrograms daily if necessary

Pharmacokinetics

Molecular weight (daltons)	765
% Protein binding	>90
% Excreted unchanged in urine	20–25
Volume of distribution (L/kg)	0.6
Half-life – normal/ESRF (hrs)	144–200/210

Dose in renal impairment GFR (mL/min)

20–50	Dose as in normal renal function
10–20	Dose as in normal renal function
<10	Give 50–75% of normal dose

Dose in patients undergoing renal replacement therapies

CAPD	Not dialysed. Dose as in GFR = <10 mL/min
HD	Not dialysed. Dose as in GFR = <10 mL/min
CAV/VVHD	Unknown dialysability. Dose as in GFR = 10–20 mL/min

Important drug interactions

CYCLOSPORIN

–

POTENTIALLY HAZARDOUS INTERACTIONS WITH OTHER DRUGS

- Anti-arrhythmics: amiodarone increases digitoxin levels
- Antifungals: increased toxicity if hypokalaemia occurs with amphotericin; plasma levels of digitoxin increased by itraconazole
- Calcium-channel blockers: increased digitoxin levels
- Diuretics: increased digitoxin toxicity if hypokalaemia occurs
- Antimalarials: quinine, hydroxychloroquine and chloroquine increase plasma levels of digitoxin

Administration

RECONSTITUTION

–

ROUTE

- Oral

RATE OF ADMINISTRATION

–

COMMENTS

–

Other information

- Volume of distribution is decreased by uraemia
- Digitoxin is largely metabolised in the liver where 8–10% is converted to digoxin. More digitoxin is converted to digoxin in severe renal impairment

Digoxin

Clinical use

Atrial fibrillation, cardiac failure

Dose in normal renal function

Digitalisation: 1–1.5 mg in divided doses over 24 hrs followed by 62.5–500 micrograms daily adjusted according to response

Pharmacokinetics

Molecular weight (daltons)	781
% Protein binding	20–30
% Excreted unchanged in urine	76–85; IV: 50–70
Volume of distribution (L/kg)	5–8
Half-life – normal/ESRF (hrs)	30–40/84–104

Dose in renal impairment GFR (mL/min)

	Digitalisation using 750 micrograms–1 mg. Interval between normal or reduced doses may need to be lengthened
20–50	125–250 micrograms per day
10–20	125–250 micrograms per day. Monitor levels
<10	Dose commonly 62.5 micrograms 3 times a week after HD, or 62.5 micrograms daily. Monitor levels

Dose in patients undergoing renal replacement therapies

CAPD	Not dialysed. Dose as in GFR = <10 mL/min
HD	Not dialysed. Dose as in GFR = <10 mL/min
CAV/VVHD	Unknown dialysability. Dose as in GFR = 10–20 mL/min

Important drug interactions

CYCLOSPORIN

• Raised digoxin serum/blood levels

POTENTIALLY HAZARDOUS INTERACTIONS WITH OTHER DRUGS

• Anti-arrhythmics: amiodarone, propafenone and quinidine increase digoxin plasma level (half maintenance dose of digoxin)

• Quinine: increases plasma concentration of digoxin (half maintenance dose)

• Calcium-channel blockers: increase digoxin plasma levels

• Diuretics: increase toxicity if hypokalaemia occurs; effects enhanced by spironolactone

• Concurrent erythromycin or omeprazole administration decreases digoxin clearance

• Antifungals: increased toxicity if hypokalaemia occurs with amphotericin; plasma concentration of digoxin increased by itraconazole

• Antimalarials: quinine, hydroxychloroquine and chloroquine raise plasma concentrations of digoxin; increased risk of bradycardia with mefloquine

Administration

RECONSTITUTION

• IV administration, dilute dose to 50 mL with sodium chloride 0.9%

ROUTE

• Oral, IV

RATE OF ADMINISTRATION

• IV: infuse over 30 min–2 hrs

COMMENTS

• IV dosing may be used for very rapid control (infused over 1–2 hrs)

Other information

• If possible, take blood sample prior to commencing therapy for determination of digoxin immunoreactive-like substance

• Complex kinetics in renal impairment. Vd and total body clearance reduced in ESRD

• Steady-state plasma monitoring advisable. Normal range 0.8–2 nanograms/mL

• Hypokalaemia, hypomagnesaemia, marked hypercalcaemia and hypothyroidism increase toxicity

• Increases uraemic gastrointestinal symptoms

• Concomitant administration of phosphate binders reduces gastrointestinal absorption by up to 25%

Dihydrocodeine

Clinical use

Analgesia

Dose in normal renal function

Oral:
30 mg every 4–6 hrs
SC/IM:
up to 50 mg every 4–6 hrs

Pharmacokinetics

Molecular weight (daltons)	452
% Protein binding	–
% Excreted unchanged in urine	–
Volume of distribution (L/kg)	1.1
Half-life – normal/ESRF (hrs)	3.4–4.5/>6

Dose in renal impairment GFR (mL/min)

20–50	Dose as in normal renal function
10–20	Avoid or use small doses and titrate to response
<10	Avoid or use small doses and titrate to response

Dose in patients undergoing renal replacement therapies

CAPD	Unknown dialysability. Dose as in GFR = <10 mL/min
HD	Unknown dialysability. Dose as in GFR = <10 mL/min
CAV/VVHD	Unknown dialysability. Dose as in GFR = 10–20 mL/min

Important drug interactions

CYCLOSPORIN

–

POTENTIALLY HAZARDOUS INTERACTIONS WITH OTHER DRUGS

–

Administration

RECONSTITUTION

–

ROUTE

• Oral, IM/SC

RATE OF ADMINISTRATION

–

COMMENTS

–

Other information

• Increased and prolonged effect in renal impairment, enhancing respiratory depression and constipation
• Increased CNS sensitivity in renal impairment
• Accumulation of active metabolites can occur. Caution is needed
• Effects can be reversed by naloxone
• Oral liquid formulation contains ethanol. Caution is needed if patient is on metronidazole

Diltiazem

Clinical use

Calcium-channel blocker, used for prophylaxis and treatment of angina and hypertension

Dose in normal renal function

Angina:

60–120 mg 3 times daily

Hypertension:

180–480 mg daily

Pharmacokinetics

Molecular weight (daltons)	451
% Protein binding	98
% Excreted unchanged in urine	<10
Volume of distribution (L/kg)	3–5
Half-life – normal/ESRF (hrs)	2/3.5

Dose in renal impairment GFR (mL/min)

20–50	Dose as in normal renal function
10–20	Dose as in normal renal function
<10	Dose as in normal renal function

Dose in patients undergoing renal replacement therapies

CAPD	Not dialysed. Dose as in normal renal function
HD	Not dialysed. Dose as in normal renal function
CAV/VVHD	Unknown dialysability. Dose as in normal renal function

Important drug interactions

CYCLOSPORIN

• Increases cyclosporin plasma concentrations

POTENTIALLY HAZARDOUS INTERACTIONS WITH OTHER DRUGS

• Increased risk of bradycardia and AV block and myocardial depression if prescribed with amiodarone
• Metabolism increased by rifampicin
• Enhances effect of carbamazepine and increases plasma levels of phenytoin
• Risk of bradycardia and AV block if co-prescribed with beta-blockers
• Increased plasma concentration of digoxin
• Enhances effect of theophylline

Administration

RECONSTITUTION

–

ROUTE

• Oral

RATE OF ADMINISTRATION

–

COMMENTS

–

Other information

• Active metabolites
• Monitor heart rate early on in therapy. If it falls below 50 beats/min, do not increase dose
• Maintain patient on same brand

Dipyridamole

Clinical use

Antiplatelet agent

Dose in normal renal function

100–200 mg 3 times daily

Pharmacokinetics

Molecular weight (daltons)	505
% Protein binding	99
% Excreted unchanged in urine	–
Volume of distribution (L/kg)	2.4
Half-life – normal/ESRF (hrs)	12/–

Dose in renal impairment GFR (mL/min)

20–50	Dose as in normal renal function
10–20	Dose as in normal renal function
<10	Dose as in normal renal function

Dose in patients undergoing renal replacement therapies

CAPD	Not dialysed. Dose as in normal renal function
HD	Not dialysed. Dose as in normal renal function
CAV/VVHD	Not dialysed. Dose as in normal renal function

Important drug interactions

CYCLOSPORIN

–

POTENTIALLY HAZARDOUS INTERACTIONS WITH OTHER DRUGS

• Effects of adenosine enhanced and extended
• Anticoagulants: enhanced effect

Administration

RECONSTITUTION

–

ROUTE

• Oral

RATE OF ADMINISTRATION

–

COMMENTS

–

Other information

–

Disopyramide

Clinical use

Ventricular and supraventricular arrhythmias

Dose in normal renal function

100–200 mg 4 times daily

Pharmacokinetics

Molecular weight (daltons)	340
% Protein binding	40–80
% Excreted unchanged in urine	35–65
Volume of distribution (L/kg)	0.8–2.6
Half-life – normal/ESRF (hrs)	5–8/10–18

Dose in renal impairment GFR (mL/min)

20–50	100 mg every 8 hrs or 150 mg every 12 hrs
10–20	100 mg every 12 hrs
<10	150 mg every 24 hrs (monitor levels)

Dose in patients undergoing renal replacement therapies

CAPD	Not dialysed. Dose as in GFR = <10 mL/min
HD	Not dialysed. Dose as in GFR = <10 mL/min
CAV/VVHD	Unknown dialysability. Dose as in GFR = 10–20 mL/min

Important drug interactions

CYCLOSPORIN

–

POTENTIALLY HAZARDOUS INTERACTIONS WITH OTHER DRUGS

- Amiodarone increases risk of ventricular arrhythmias
- Increased myocardial depression with any anti-arrhythmic
- Plasma levels reduced by rifampicin and phenytoin, and increased by erythromycin
- Increased risk of ventricular arrhythmias with astemizole and terfenadine

Administration

RECONSTITUTION

–

ROUTE

- Oral, IV

RATE OF ADMINISTRATION

- Not >3 mL/min

COMMENTS

- May be given by IV infusion peripherally at rate of 0.4 mg/kg/hr

Other information

- Use with caution in patients with impaired renal function
- Do not give renally impaired patients sustained-release preparations
- Optimum therapeutic plasma level 2–5 mg/L
- Haemoperfusion can be used in cases of severe poisoning

Dobutamine

Clinical use

Inotropic agent

Dose in normal renal function

2.5–10 micrograms/kg/min up to 40 micrograms/kg/min according to response

Pharmacokinetics

Molecular weight (daltons)	301.4
% Protein binding	–
% Excreted unchanged in urine	<10
Volume of distribution (L/kg)	0.25
Half-life – normal/ESRF	2 min/–

Dose in renal impairment GFR (mL/min)

20–50	Dose as in normal renal function
10–20	Dose as in normal renal function
<10	Dose as in normal renal function

Dose in patients undergoing renal replacement therapies

CAPD	Not dialysed. Dose as in normal renal function
HD	Not dialysed. Dose as in normal renal function
CAV/VVHD	Not dialysed. Dose as in normal renal function

Important drug interactions

CYCLOSPORIN

–

POTENTIALLY HAZARDOUS INTERACTIONS WITH OTHER DRUGS

• Antagonised by beta-blockers

Administration

RECONSTITUTION

• Dilute to at least 50 mL with sodium chloride 0.9% or glucose 5%

ROUTE

• Continuous IV infusion centrally via CRIP (or peripherally via a large vein)

RATE OF ADMINISTRATION

• Varies with dose

COMMENTS

• 250 mg may be diluted in as little as 50 mL diluent

Other information

• Cardiac and BP monitoring advised
• Sodium bicarbonate rapidly inactivates dobutamine
• Solution may turn pink, but potency is unaffected by this
• Can cause hypokalaemia

Domperidone

Clinical use

Acute nausea and vomiting (including that caused by levodopa and bromocriptine); functional dyspepsia

Dose in normal renal function

Nausea and vomiting:
adults 10–20 mg orally at 4–8-hourly intervals

Pharmacokinetics

Molecular weight (daltons)	426
% Protein binding	>90
% Excreted unchanged in urine	<1
Volume of distribution (L/kg)	5.7
Half-life – normal/ESRF (hrs)	7.5/–

Dose in renal impairment GFR (mL/min)

20–50	Dose as in normal renal function
10–20	Dose as in normal renal function
<10	Dose as in normal renal function

Dose in patients undergoing renal replacement therapies

CAPD	Unknown dialysability. Dose as in normal renal function
HD	Unknown dialysability. Dose as in normal renal function
CAV/VVHD	Unknown dialysability. Dose as in normal renal function

Important drug interactions

CYCLOSPORIN

–

POTENTIALLY HAZARDOUS INTERACTIONS WITH OTHER DRUGS

–

Administration

RECONSTITUTION

–

ROUTE

• Oral, PR

RATE OF ADMINISTRATION

–

COMMENTS

• Treatment of acute nausea and vomiting: maximum period of treatment is 12 weeks
• Treatment of functional dyspepsia: administer before food; maximum period of treatment is 12 weeks

Other information

• Domperidone has the advantage over metoclopramide and the phenothiazines of being less likely to cause central effects such as sedation and dystonic reactions, as it does not readily cross the blood–brain barrier

Dopamine

Clinical use

Increases renal blood perfusion at low 'renal' dose. At higher dose, has inotropic effect and eventually is vasoconstricting

Dose in normal renal function

Renal dose:

2–5 micrograms/kg/min

Inotropic dose:

5–10 micrograms/kg/min

Vasoconstricting dose:

>10 micrograms/kg/min

NB: Individual patient sensitivity may affect these ranges

Pharmacokinetics

Molecular weight (daltons)	190
% Protein binding	–
% Excreted unchanged in urine	–
Volume of distribution (L/kg)	–
Half-life – normal/ESRF	2 min/–

Dose in renal impairment GFR (mL/min)

20–50	Dose as in normal renal function
10–20	Dose as in normal renal function
<10	Dose as in normal renal function

Dose in patients undergoing renal replacement therapies

CAPD	Not dialysed. Dose as in normal renal function
HD	Not dialysed. Dose as in normal renal function
CAV/VVHD	Not dialysed. Dose as in normal renal function

Important drug interactions

CYCLOSPORIN

• May reduce risk of cyclosporin nephrotoxicity

POTENTIALLY HAZARDOUS INTERACTIONS WITH OTHER DRUGS

• Antidepressants: hypertensive crisis with MAOIs

Administration

RECONSTITUTION

• Add 200 mg to 250 mL sodium chloride 0.9% or glucose 5%, then renal dose (mL/hr) = 0.1875 x patient's weight in kg, i.e. for 60-kg patient, dose is 11.25 mL/hr of this solution

ROUTE

• IV peripherally into large vein (centrally for inotropic dose). Central route always preferable

RATE OF ADMINISTRATION

• Via CRIP as indicated above

COMMENTS

• Minimum dilution 200 mg in 50 mL
• Not compatible with sodium bicarbonate – rapid deactivation of dopamine

Other information

• Causes renal vasoconstriction at inotropic dose
• Cardiac and BP monitoring advised
• Very severe tissue damage caused by extravasation
• 'Renal effects' consist of a mixture of renal/ splanchnic vasodilation, a direct tubular (diuretic) effect and improved perfusion secondary to an increase in cardiac output

Dopexamine

Clinical use

Inotropic support in heart failure associated with cardiac surgery

Dose in normal renal function

IV infusion:

0.5 micrograms/kg/min and may be increased to 1 microgram/kg/min and then in increments (0.5–1 micrograms/kg/min) up to 6 micrograms/kg/min at not less than 15-min intervals

Pharmacokinetics

Molecular weight (daltons)	429
% Protein binding	–
% Excreted unchanged in urine	10
Volume of distribution (L/kg)	0.45
Half-life – normal/ESRF	Mean 7 min/–

Dose in renal impairment GFR (mL/min)

20–50	Dose as in normal renal function and adjust to response
10–20	Dose as in normal renal function and adjust to response
<10	Dose as in normal renal function and adjust to response

Dose in patients undergoing renal replacement therapies

CAPD	Unknown dialysability. Dose as in normal renal function
HD	Unknown dialysability. Dose as in normal renal function
CAV/VVHD	Unknown dialysability. Dose as in normal renal function

Important drug interactions

CYCLOSPORIN

–

POTENTIALLY HAZARDOUS INTERACTIONS WITH OTHER DRUGS

• Antidepressants: risk of hypertensive crisis with MAOIs
• Beta-blockers: risk of severe hypertension
• Other sympathomimetics: risk of severe hypertension

Administration

RECONSTITUTION

• IV infusion of 400 or 800 micrograms/mL in glucose 5% or sodium chloride 0.9%
• Peripheral administration: concentration of infusion solution must not exceed 1 mg/mL
• Central administration: concentration not >4 mg/mL

ROUTE

• By intravenous infusion into a central or large peripheral vein

RATE OF ADMINISTRATION

• See dosage instructions

COMMENTS

• During the administration of dopexamine the rate of administration and duration of therapy should be adjusted according to the patient's response as determined by heart rate and rhythm, blood pressure, urine flow and measurement of cardiac output

Other information

• The duration of therapy is dependent on the patient's overall response to treatment
• Avoid abrupt withdrawal

Dothiepin

Clinical use

Tricyclic antidepressant

Dose in normal renal function

50–225 mg daily

Pharmacokinetics

Molecular weight (daltons)	332
% Protein binding	–
% Excreted unchanged in urine	56 (mainly as metabolites)
Volume of distribution (L/kg)	11–78
Half-life – normal/ESRF (hrs)	14–24/–

Dose in renal impairment GFR (mL/min)

20–50	Dose as in normal renal function
10–20	Start with small dose, i.e. 25 mg at night
<10	Start with small dose, i.e. 25 mg at night

Dose in patients undergoing renal replacement therapies

CAPD	Not dialysed. Dose as in GFR = <10 mL/min
HD	Not dialysed. Dose as in GFR = <10 mL/min
CAV/VVHD	Unknown dialysability. Dose as in GFR = 10–20 mL/min

Important drug interactions

CYCLOSPORIN

–

POTENTIALLY HAZARDOUS INTERACTIONS WITH OTHER DRUGS

• MAOIs: CNS excitation and hypertension
• SSRIs: may increase dothiepin blood levels
• Anti-epileptics: antagonism – reduced convulsive threshold
• Antihistamines: increased antimuscarinic and sedative effects. Increased risk of arrhythmias with terfenadine and astemizole
• Adrenaline/noradrenaline: hypertension and arrhythmias

Administration

RECONSTITUTION

–

ROUTE

• Oral

RATE OF ADMINISTRATION

–

COMMENTS

–

Other information

• Metabolites are active and partly renally excreted
• Metabolites accumulate and cause excessive sedation
• 25–50 mg usually effective without too much sedation

Doxapram

Clinical use

Post-operative respiratory depression; acute respiratory failure

Dose in normal renal function

Post-operative respiratory depression:

IV injection 0.5–1.5 mg/kg repeated at hourly intervals or IV infusion 2–5 mg/min adjusted according to response

Pharmacokinetics

Molecular weight (daltons)	433
% Protein binding	–
% Excreted unchanged in urine	<5
Volume of distribution (L/kg)	0.58–2.74
Half-life – normal/ESRF (hrs)	2.4–4.1/–

Dose in renal impairment GFR (mL/min)

20–50	Dose as in normal renal function
10–20	Dose as in normal renal function
<10	Dose as in normal renal function

Dose in patients undergoing renal replacement therapies

CAPD	Unknown dialysability. Dose as in normal renal function
HD	Unknown dialysability. Dose as in normal renal function
CAV/VVHD	Unknown dialysability. Dose as in normal renal function

Important drug interactions

CYCLOSPORIN

–

POTENTIALLY HAZARDOUS INTERACTIONS WITH OTHER DRUGS

–

Administration

RECONSTITUTION

–

ROUTE

• IV bolus, IV infusion

RATE OF ADMINISTRATION

• IV injection: over at least 30 sec

• IV infusion post-operative: 2–3 mg/min, adjust according to response

• IV infusion acute respiratory failure: 1.5–4 mg/min, adjust according to response

COMMENTS

• Doxapram has a narrow margin of safety; the minimum effective dosage should be used and maximum recommended dosages should not be exceeded

Other information

• Unlike naloxone, doxapram does not reverse the other effects of opioid analgesics (i.e. analgesia)

Doxazosin

Clinical use

Alpha-adrenoreceptor blocker, used for
hypertension and benign prostatic hyperplasia

Dose in normal renal function

Hypertension:

1 mg daily, increased after 1–2 weeks to 2 mg daily,
and thereafter to 4 mg daily, if necessary; maximum
16 mg daily

Pharmacokinetics

Molecular weight (daltons)	548
% Protein binding	98
% Excreted unchanged in urine	<5
Volume of distribution (L/kg)	1–1.7
Half-life – normal/ESRF (hrs)	9.5–12.5/13

Dose in renal impairment
GFR (mL/min)

20–50	Dose as in normal renal function
10–20	Dose as in normal renal function
<10	Dose as in normal renal function

Dose in patients undergoing renal replacement therapies

CAPD	Not dialysed. Dose as in normal renal function
HD	Not dialysed. Dose as in normal renal function
CAV/VVHD	Not dialysed. Dose as in normal renal function

Important drug interactions

CYCLOSPORIN

–

POTENTIALLY HAZARDOUS INTERACTIONS WITH
OTHER DRUGS

- Anaesthetics: enhanced hypotensive effect
- Antidepressants: enhanced hypotensive effect
- Beta-blockers: increased first-dose hypotensive effect
- Calcium-channel blockers: enhanced hypotensive effect
- Diuretics: increased first-dose hypotensive effect

Administration

RECONSTITUTION

–

ROUTE

- Oral

RATE OF ADMINISTRATION

–

COMMENTS

–

Other information

- At steady state, the half-life is calculated at 22 hrs (elimination $t^{1/2}$) providing 24 hrs duration of action

Doxepin

Clinical use

Tricyclic antidepressant

Dose in normal renal function

Initially 75 mg daily, increased as necessary to maximum of 300 mg daily in 3 divided doses

Pharmacokinetics

Molecular weight (daltons)	316
% Protein binding	95
% Excreted unchanged in urine	<1
Volume of distribution (L/kg)	20
Half-life – normal/ESRF (hrs)	8–25/10–30

Dose in renal impairment GFR (mL/min)

20–50	Dose as in normal renal function
10–20	Dose as in normal renal function
<10	Dose as in normal renal function

Dose in patients undergoing renal replacement therapies

CAPD	Not dialysed. Dose as in normal renal function
HD	Not dialysed. Dose as in normal renal function
CAV/VVHD	Not dialysed. Dose as in normal renal function

Important drug interactions

CYCLOSPORIN

–

POTENTIALLY HAZARDOUS INTERACTIONS WITH OTHER DRUGS

• Alcohol: enhanced effect
• Other antidepressants: risk of enhanced CNS effects and excitation with MAOIs
• Antihistamines: enhanced antimuscarinic and sedative effects. Increased risk of ventricular arrhythmias with astemizole and terfenadine
• Antimalarials: increased risk of ventricular arrhythmias with halofantrine
• Sympathomimetics: increased risk of hypertension and ventricular arrhythmias
• Anti-arrhythmics: increased risk of ventricular arrhythmias with drugs which prolong the QT interval, e.g. amiodarone, disopyramide, procainamide, quinidine
• Anti-epileptics: effects antagonised (convulsive threshold lowered)
• Antihypertensives: enhanced hypotensive effect
• Beta-blockers: risk of ventricular arrhythmias with sotalol

Administration

RECONSTITUTION

–

ROUTE

• Oral

RATE OF ADMINISTRATION

–

COMMENTS

–

Other information

–

Doxorubicin

Clinical use

Antineoplastic agent – used for acute leukaemias, lymphomas, sarcomas and malignant neoplasms of bladder, breast, lung, ovary, stomach and thyroid

Dose in normal renal function

60–75 mg/m^2 every 3 weeks when doxorubicin is used alone, or see local protocol

Pharmacokinetics

Molecular weight (daltons)	580
% Protein binding	80–85
% Excreted unchanged in urine	<15
Volume of distribution (L/kg)	21.5
Half-life – normal/ESRF (hrs)	35/unchanged

Dose in renal impairment GFR (mL/min)

20–50	Dose as in normal renal function
10–20	Dose as in normal renal function
<10	Dose as in normal renal function

Dose in patients undergoing renal replacement therapies

CAPD	Unknown dialysability. Dose as in normal renal function
HD	Unknown dialysability. Dose as in normal renal function
CAV/VVHD	Unknown dialysability. Dose as in normal renal function

Important drug interactions

CYCLOSPORIN

• Increased risk of neurotoxicity

POTENTIALLY HAZARDOUS INTERACTIONS WITH OTHER DRUGS

–

Administration

RECONSTITUTION

• Reconstitute with water for injection or sodium chloride 0.9%

ROUTE

• IV, intra-arterial, intravesical (bladder instillation)

RATE OF ADMINISTRATION

• IV: give via the tubing of a fast-running intravenous infusion of sodium chloride 0.9% or glucose 5%, taking 2–3 min over the injection

COMMENTS

• For bladder instillation the concentration of doxorubicin in the bladder should be 50 mg per 50 mL. To avoid undue dilution in urine, the patient should be instructed not to drink any fluid in the 12 hrs prior to instillation. This should limit urine production to approximately 50 mL/hr

Other information

• A cumulative dose of 450–550 mg/m^2 should only be exceeded with extreme caution. Above this level, the risk of irreversible congestive cardiac failure increases greatly

• Patients with impaired hepatic function have prolonged and elevated plasma concentrations of both the drug and its metabolites. Dose reduction is required

Doxycycline

Clinical use

Antibacterial agent and prophylaxis/treatment of malaria

Dose in normal renal function

200 mg on day 1, then 100 mg daily;
severe infections 200 mg daily

Pharmacokinetics

Molecular weight (daltons)	463
% Protein binding	80–93
% Excreted unchanged in urine	33–45
Volume of distribution (L/kg)	0.75
Half-life – normal/ESRF (hrs)	15–24/18–25

Dose in renal impairment GFR (mL/min)

20–50	Dose as in normal renal function
10–20	Dose as in normal renal function
<10	Dose as in normal renal function

Dose in patients undergoing renal replacement therapies

CAPD	Unknown dialysability. Dose as in normal renal function
HD	Insignificant dialysability. Dose as in normal renal function
CAV/VVHD	Unknown dialysability. Dose as in normal renal function

Important drug interactions

CYCLOSPORIN

• Possibly increases plasma cyclosporin concentration

POTENTIALLY HAZARDOUS INTERACTIONS WITH OTHER DRUGS

–

Administration

RECONSTITUTION

–

ROUTE

• Oral

RATE OF ADMINISTRATION

–

COMMENTS

• Do not take iron preparations, indigestion remedies or phosphate binders at the same time of day as doxycycline

Other information

–

Enalapril maleate

Clinical use

Angiotensin-converting enzyme inhibitor, used for hypertension and congestive heart failure

Dose in normal renal function

2.5–40 mg daily

Pharmacokinetics

Molecular weight (daltons)	493
% Protein binding	30–60
% Excreted unchanged in urine	43
Volume of distribution (L/kg)	1.7 ± 0.7
Half-life – normal/ESRF (hrs)	11–24/34–60

Dose in renal impairment
GFR (mL/min)

20–50	Dose as in normal renal function
10–20	Start with 2.5 mg per day then dose according to response
<10	Start with 2.5 mg per day then dose according to response

Dose in patients undergoing renal replacement therapies

CAPD	Dialysed. Dose as in GFR = <10 mL/min
HD	Dialysed. Dose as in GFR = <10 mL/min
CAV/VVHD	Unknown dialysability. Dose as in GFR = 10–20 mL/min

Important drug interactions

CYCLOSPORIN

• Increased risk of hyperkalaemia

POTENTIALLY HAZARDOUS INTERACTIONS WITH OTHER DRUGS

• Epoetin: increased risk of hyperkalaemia

• Lithium levels may be increased
• NSAIDs: antagonism of hypotensive effect; increased risk of hyperkalaemia and renal damage
• Diuretics: enhanced hypotensive effect; increased risk of hyperkalaemia with potassium-sparing diuretics
• Potassium supplements: increased risk of hyperkalaemia
• Anaesthetics: enhanced hypotensive effects

Administration

RECONSTITUTION

–

ROUTE

• Oral

RATE OF ADMINISTRATION

–

COMMENTS

–

Other information

• Side-effects, e.g. hyperkalaemia, metabolic acidosis, are more common in patients with impaired renal function
• Close monitoring of renal function during therapy is necessary in those with renal insufficiency
• Renal failure has been reported in association with ACE inhibitors in patients with renal artery stenosis, post-renal transplant and severe congestive heart failure
• A high incidence of anaphylactoid reactions has been reported in patients dialysed with high-flux polyacrylonitrile membranes and treated concomitantly with an ACE inhibitor – this combination should therefore be avoided
• ACE inhibitor cough may be helped by sodium cromoglycate inhalers
• Enalapril maleate is a pro-drug that requires hepatic conversion to enalaprilat, with a long half-life, and as such is not suitable for use as an ACE inhibitor test-dose agent
• Enalaprilat injection is available on a 'named patient' basis

Enoxoparin

Clinical use

Low-molecular-weight heparin – used for prophylaxis of thromboembolic disorders of venous origin, treatment of deep vein thrombosis, and anticoagulation of the extracorporeal circulation during haemodialysis

Dose in normal renal function

Prophylaxis DVT:

low-risk surgery – 20 mg SC once daily, 2 hrs before surgery, thereafter for 7–10 days; high-risk surgery – 40 mg SC once daily, 12 hrs before surgery, thereafter for 7–10 days

Treatment DVT:

1 mg/kg (100 iu/kg) SC every 12 hrs

Pharmacokinetics

Molecular weight (daltons)	mean = 4500
% Protein binding	–
% Excreted unchanged in urine	–
Volume of distribution (L/kg)	7
Half-life – normal/ESRF (hrs)	4–5/–

Dose in renal impairment GFR (mL/min)

20–50	Dose as in normal renal function
10–20	Dose as in normal renal function
<10	Dose as in normal renal function

Dose in patients undergoing renal replacement therapies

CAPD	Not dialysed. Dose as in normal renal function
HD	Not dialysed. Dose as in normal renal function
CAV/VVHD	Not dialysed. Dose as in normal renal function

Important drug interactions

CYCLOSPORIN

–

POTENTIALLY HAZARDOUS INTERACTIONS WITH OTHER DRUGS

• Use with care in patients receiving oral anticoagulants, platelet aggregation inhibitors, NSAIDs, aspirin or dextran

Administration

RECONSTITUTION

–

ROUTE

• Deep SC injection

RATE OF ADMINISTRATION

–

COMMENTS

–

Other information

• In extracorporeal circulation during haemodialysis, 1 mg/kg (100 iu/kg) enoxoparin is introduced into the arterial line of the circuit at the beginning of the session. The effect of this dose is usually sufficient for a 4-hr session, although if fibrin rings are found, a further dose of 500–1000 micrograms/kg (50–100 iu/kg) may be given. For patients with a high risk of haemorrhage, the dose should be reduced to 500 micrograms/kg for double vascular access or 750 micrograms/kg for single vascular access

• The dose of protamine to neutralise the effect of enoxoparin should equal the dose of enoxoparin: 100 anti-heparin units of protamine should neutralise the anti-factor IIa activity generated by 1 mg (100 iu) of enoxoparin

• Rhône-Poulenc Rorer advise monitoring of the anti-factor Xa activity, whatever the severity of the renal impairment, when treatment doses are being employed. They also advise monitoring patients if prolonged treatment using prophylactic doses is given

Epoetin alpha (Eprex)

Clinical use

Management of anaemia associated with renal impairment before and on dialysis

Dose in normal renal function

Correction phase:

to raise haemoglobin to target level, 50 u/kg 3 times weekly SC. Increase according to response by 25 u/kg 3 times weekly at intervals of 4 weeks. Rise in haemoglobin should not exceed 2 g/100 mL/month (optimum rise in haemoglobin up to 1 g/100 mL/month to avoid hypertension). Target haemoglobin usually 10–12 g/100 mL

Maintenance phase:

adjust dose to maintain required haemoglobin level. The usual dose needed is 100–300 u/kg weekly in 2–3 divided doses

Pharmacokinetics

Molecular weight (daltons)	34 000
% Protein binding	–
% Excreted unchanged in urine	–
Volume of distribution (L/kg)	0.03–0.05
Half-life – normal/ESRF (hrs)	IV: 4/unchanged SC: ≅ 24/ unchanged

Dose in renal impairment
GFR (mL/min)

20–50	Dose as in normal renal function
10–20	Dose as in normal renal function
<10	Dose as in normal renal function

Dose in patients undergoing renal replacement therapies

CAPD	Not dialysed. Dose as in normal renal function
HD	Not dialysed. Dose as in normal renal function
CAV/VVHD	Not dialysed. Dose as in normal renal function

Important drug interactions

CYCLOSPORIN

–

POTENTIALLY HAZARDOUS INTERACTIONS WITH OTHER DRUGS

• Hyperkalaemia with ACE inhibitors

Administration

RECONSTITUTION

• Ready reconstituted

ROUTE

• SC (maximum 1 mL per injection site), IV

RATE OF ADMINISTRATION

–

COMMENTS

• May also be given IV over 2 min, but higher doses are normally needed to produce required response. (Does not represent cost-effective use)
• May be given intra-peritoneally, but larger doses are needed

Other information

• Pretreatment checks and appropriate correction/ treatment are needed for iron, folate and B12 deficiency, infection, inflammation or aluminium toxicity to produce optimum response to therapy
• Concomitant iron therapy (200–300 mg elemental oral iron) needed daily. IV iron may be needed for patients with very low serum ferritins (<100 nanograms/mL)
• Contains 2.5 mg/mL human serum albumin
• May increase heparin requirement during HD

Epoetin beta (Recormon)

Clinical use

Management of anaemia associated with renal impairment before and on dialysis

Dose in normal renal function

Correction phase:

to raise haemoglobin to target level, 20 u/kg SC 3 times weekly for 4 weeks increasing, according to response, in steps of 20 u/kg 3 times weekly at monthly intervals. Maximum dose 720 u/kg weekly. Target haemoglobin usually 10–12 g/100 mL

Maintenance dose:

to maintain haemoglobin at target level. Half correction phase dose, then adjust according to response at intervals of 1–2 weeks

Pharmacokinetics

Molecular weight (daltons)	34 000
% Protein binding	–
% Excreted unchanged in urine	–
Volume of distribution (L/kg)	0.03–0.05
Half-life – normal/ESRF (hrs)	IV: 4–12/ unchanged; SC: 13–28/unchanged

Dose in renal impairment
GFR (mL/min)

20–50	Dose as in normal renal function
10–20	Dose as in normal renal function
<10	Dose as in normal renal function

Dose in patients undergoing renal replacement therapies

CAPD	Not dialysed. Dose as in normal renal function
HD	Not dialysed. Dose as in normal renal function
CAV/VVHD	Not dialysed. Dose as in normal renal function

Important drug interactions

CYCLOSPORIN

–

POTENTIALLY HAZARDOUS INTERACTIONS WITH OTHER DRUGS

• Risk of hyperkalaemia with ACE inhibitors

Administration

RECONSTITUTION

• Reconstitute using diluent provided

ROUTE

• SC, IV

RATE OF ADMINISTRATION

–

COMMENTS

• May also be given IV over 2 min, but higher doses are needed to produce required response. (Does not represent cost-effective use)

Other information

• Pretreatment checks and appropriate correction/ treatment are needed for iron, folate and B12 deficiencies, infection, inflammation or aluminium toxicity to produce optimum response to therapy

• Concomitant iron therapy (200–300 mg elemental oral iron) needed daily. IV iron may be needed for patients with very low serum ferritins (<100 nanograms/mL)

• Does not contain human serum albumin, so is therefore suitable for Jehovah's Witnesses

• May increase heparin requirement during HD

Epoprostenol (Prostacyclin)

Clinical use

Vasodilator and inhibits platelet aggregation without prolonging bleeding time. Alternative to heparin to facilitate dialysis in patients with uraemic coagulopathy or disseminated intravascular coagulation. Also used in the treatment of peripheral vascular disease and pulmonary hypertension

Dose in normal renal function

2.5–10 nanograms/kg/min. If used in DIC, sepsis, peripheral cyanosis or microangiopathies, dose used is 5–20 nanograms/kg/min

Pharmacokinetics

Molecular weight (daltons)	353
% Protein binding	–
% Excreted unchanged in urine	–
Volume of distribution (L/kg)	–
Half-life – normal/ESRF	2–3 min/–

Dose in renal impairment GFR (mL/min)

20–50	Dose as in normal renal function
10–20	Dose as in normal renal function
<10	Dose as in normal renal function

Dose in patients undergoing renal replacement therapies

CAPD	Unknown dialysability. Dose as in normal renal function
HD	Unknown dialysability. Dose as in normal renal function
CAV/VVHD	Unknown dialysability. Dose as in normal renal function

Important drug interactions

CYCLOSPORIN

–

POTENTIALLY HAZARDOUS INTERACTIONS WITH OTHER DRUGS

• Increased hypotensive effect with 'acetate' dialysis

Administration

RECONSTITUTION

• 500-microgram vial with diluent provided gives solution of 10 000 nanograms/mL. Can be diluted further

ROUTE

• IV or into blood supplying dialyser

RATE OF ADMINISTRATION

• Via CRIP

COMMENTS

• Complicated dosing schedule – check calculations carefully
• Infusion rate may be calculated by the following formula:

$$\text{Dose rate} = \frac{\text{dosage (ng/kg/min)} \times \text{body weight (kg)} \times 60}{\text{concentration of infusion (ng/mL)}}$$
$$\text{(mL/hr)} \qquad \text{(usually 10 000)}$$

Other information

• Monitor BP and heart rate. Reduce dose if patient becomes hypotensive. Cardiovascular effects cease 30 min after stopping the infusion
• Some patients may exhibit allergic reaction to buffer solution used to reconstitute epoprostenol
• Solution retains 90% potency for 12 hrs after dilution
• The concentrated solution should be filtered using the filter provided in the pack

Erythromycin

Clinical use

Antibacterial agent

Dose in normal renal function

IV:

mild to moderate infection – 25 mg/kg/day; severe infection or immunocompromised patients –
50 mg/kg/day (maximum of 4 g per day for adults)
Oral:
250–500 mg every 6 hrs or 0.5–1 g every 12 hrs

Pharmokinetics

Molecular weight (daltons)	734
% Protein binding	60–95
% Excreted unchanged in urine	15
Volume of distribution (L/kg)	0.78 (increases in ESRF)
Half-life – normal/ESRF (hrs)	1.4/5–6

Dose in renal impairment GFR (mL/min)

20–50	Dose as in normal renal function
10–20	Dose as in normal renal function
<10	50–75% of normal dose, maximum 1.5 g daily

Dose in patients undergoing renal replacement therapies

CAPD	Unknown dialysability. Dose as in GFR = <10 mL/min
HD	Not dialysed. Dose as in GFR = <10 mL/min
CAV/VVHD	Unknown dialysability. Dose as in normal renal function

Important drug interactions

CYCLOSPORIN

• Markedly elevated cyclosporin blood levels – decreased levels on withdrawing drug. Monitor blood levels of cyclosporin carefully and adjust dose promptly as necessary

POTENTIALLY HAZARDOUS INTERACTIONS WITH OTHER DRUGS

• Increased blood levels of anticoagulants (e.g. warfarin), astemizole, carbamazepine, digoxin, disopyramide, terfenadine, theophylline/ aminophylline, phenytoin
• Risk of arrhythmias with astemizole, terfenadine

Administration

RECONSTITUTION

• 1 g with 20 mL water for injection, then dilute resultant solution further, e.g. 1 g in 100 mL (i.e. 10 mg/mL). [Some units use 50 mL with sodium chloride 0.9% (20 mg/mL)]

ROUTE

• Centrally

RATE OF ADMINISTRATION

• 1 hr using constant-rate infusion pump

COMMENTS

–

Other information

• May also give ⅓ of daily dose by infusion over 8 hrs peripherally at concentration of 1 g/250 mL (4 mg/mL). Repeat 8-hourly, i.e. continuously
• Increased risk of ototoxicity in renally impaired
• Avoid peaks produced by oral twice daily dosing, i.e. dose four times daily
• Monitor closely for thrombophlebitic reactions at site of infusion

Ethambutol

Clinical use

Antibacterial agent

Dose in normal renal function

15 mg/kg/day

Pharmacokinetics

Molecular weight (daltons)	204
% Protein binding	10–30
% Excreted unchanged in urine	75–90
Volume of distribution (L/kg)	3.9
Half-life – normal/ESRF (hrs)	4/7–15

Dose in renal impairment GFR (mL/min)

20–50	Dose as in normal renal function
10–20	24–36 hrs or 7.5–15 mg/kg/day
<10	48 hrs or 5–7.5 mg/kg/day

Dose in patients undergoing renal replacement therapies

CAPD	Dialysed. Dose as in GFR = 10–20 mL/min
HD	Dialysed. Dose as in GFR = <10 mL/min or on dialysis days give 25 mg/kg post-dialysis
CAV/VVHD	Dialysed. Dose as in GFR = 10–20 mL/min

Important drug interactions

CYCLOSPORIN

–

POTENTIALLY HAZARDOUS INTERACTIONS WITH OTHER DRUGS

–

Administration

RECONSTITUTION

–

ROUTE

• Oral

RATE OF ADMINISTRATION

–

COMMENTS

–

Other information

- Monitor plasma levels. Dosages should be individually determined and adjusted according to measured levels and renal replacement therapy
- Baseline visual acuity tests should be performed prior to initiating ethambutol
- Daily dosing is preferred by some specialists to aid compliance and ensure maximum therapeutic effect

Ethosuximide

Clinical use

Epilepsy

Dose in normal renal function

500–1500 mg daily in divided doses

Pharmacokinetics

Molecular weight (daltons)	141
% Protein binding	10
% Excreted unchanged in urine	17–40
Volume of distribution (L/kg)	0.7
Half-life – normal/ESRF (hrs)	35–55/unchanged

Dose in renal impairment GFR (mL/min)

20–50	Dose as in normal renal function
10–20	Dose as in normal renal function
<10	Dose as in normal renal function

Dose in patients undergoing renal replacement therapies

CAPD	Dialysed. Dose as in normal renal function
HD	Dialysed. Dose as in normal renal function
CAV/VVHD	Unknown dialysability. Dose as in normal renal function

Important drug interactions

CYCLOSPORIN

–

POTENTIALLY HAZARDOUS INTERACTIONS WITH OTHER DRUGS

- Isoniazid increases plasma concentrations
- Antidepressants and antipsychotics lower convulsive threshold
- Other anti-epileptics: concomitant administration may enhance toxicity

Administration

RECONSTITUTION

–

ROUTE

- Oral

RATE OF ADMINISTRATION

–

COMMENTS

–

Other information

–

Etidronate disodium

Clinical use

Bisphosphonate – used for Paget's disease of bone, hypercalcaemia of malignancy and treatment of vertebral osteoporosis (Didronel PMO)

Dose in normal renal function

Paget's disease and hypercalcaemia:

5–20 mg/kg daily

Vertebral osteoporosis:

400 mg daily for 14 days followed by 76 days of calcium carbonate 1.25 g (= 500 mg calcium)

Pharmacokinetics

Molecular weight (daltons)	250
% Protein binding	Depends on calcium concentration and pH
% Excreted unchanged in urine	40–60
Volume of distribution (L/kg)	0.3–1.3
Half-life – normal/ESRF (hrs)	2–6/–

Dose in renal impairment GFR (mL/min)

20–50	Maximum dose = 5 mg/kg/day
10–20	Avoid (but may use Didronel PMO for osteoporosis)
<10	Avoid (but may use Didronel PMO for osteoporosis)

Dose in patients undergoing renal replacement therapies

CAPD	Unknown dialysability. Dose as in GFR = <10 mL/min
HD	Unknown dialysability. Dose as in GFR = <10 mL/min
CAV/VVHD	Unknown dialysability. Dose as in GFR = 10–20 mL/min

Important drug interactions

CYCLOSPORIN

–

POTENTIALLY HAZARDOUS INTERACTIONS WITH OTHER DRUGS

• See 'Comments'

Administration

RECONSTITUTION

–

ROUTE

• Oral (Didronel IV no longer available in the UK)

RATE OF ADMINISTRATION

–

COMMENTS

• Take on an empty stomach. It is recommended that patients take the therapy with water at the midpoint of a 4-hr fast (i.e. 2 hrs before and 2 hrs after food)

• Do not give iron and mineral supplements, antacids or phosphate binders within 2 hrs of an etidronate dose

• Oral bioavailability is very low. Only about 4% of dose is absorbed

Other information

• Hypercalcaemia may cause or exacerbate impaired renal function

• The renal clearance of etidronate is 1.2 mL/min/kg, while the total body clearance is 2.2 mL/min/kg. Elimination is likely to be reduced in patients with renal impairment and elderly patients with reduced renal function, necessitating caution. Uptake of etidronate by bone represents non-renal clearance

• Occasional mild to moderate abnormalities in renal function (increased BUN and serum creatinine) have been observed when etidronate was given IV, as directed, to patients with hypercalcaemia of malignancy. These changes were reversible or remained stable without worsening after completion of the course of IV etidronate. In some patients with pre-existing renal impairment or in those who had received nephrotoxic drugs, further depression of renal function was seen. Appropriate monitoring of renal function is essential during treatment

Etodolac

Clinical use

NSAID, used for rheumatoid arthritis and osteoarthritis

Dose in normal renal function

200 mg or 300 mg twice daily, or 400 mg or 600 mg once daily; maximum 600 mg daily

Pharmacokinetics

Molecular weight (daltons)	287
% Protein binding	>99
% Excreted unchanged in urine	<5
Volume of distribution (L/kg)	0.4
Half-life – normal/ESRF (hrs)	5–7/unchanged

Dose in renal impairment GFR (mL/min)

20–50	Dose as in normal renal function, but avoid if possible
10–20	Dose as in normal renal function, but avoid if possible
<10	Dose as in normal renal function, but only use if ESRD on dialysis

Dose in patients undergoing renal replacement therapies

CAPD	Not dialysed. Dose as in normal renal function
HD	Not dialysed. Dose as in normal renal function
CAV/VVHD	Unlikely to be dialysed. Use lowest possible dose

Important drug interactions

CYCLOSPORIN

• Increased risk of nephrotoxicity

POTENTIALLY HAZARDOUS INTERACTIONS WITH OTHER DRUGS

• ACE inhibitors: antagonism of hypotensive effect
• Other NSAIDs: increased side-effects
• Sulphonylureas: effect possibly enhanced
• Methotrexate: reduced excretion
• Lithium: reduced excretion

Administration

RECONSTITUTION

–

ROUTE

• Oral

RATE OF ADMINISTRATION

–

COMMENTS

• Take with or after food

Other information

• Inhibition of renal prostaglandin synthesis by NSAIDs may interfere with renal function, especially in the presence of existing renal disease. Avoid if possible; if not, check serum creatinine 48–72 hrs after starting NSAID. If increased, discontinue therapy

• In patients with renal, cardiac or hepatic impairment, especially those taking diuretics, caution is required since the use of NSAIDs may result in deterioration of renal function. The dose should be kept as low as possible and renal function should be monitored

• Use normal doses in patients with ESRD on dialysis

• Use with caution in renal transplant recipients – etodolac can reduce intra-renal autocoid synthesis

• Accumulation of etodolac is unlikely in ARF, CRF or dialysis patients as it is metabolised in the liver

Etomidate

Clinical use

Intravenous induction of anaesthesia

Dose in normal renal function

0.3 mg/kg
High-risk patients:
0.1 mg/kg/min until anaesthetised (about 3 min)

Pharmacokinetics

Molecular weight (daltons)	244
% Protein binding	75
% Excreted unchanged in urine	2
Volume of distribution (L/kg)	2–4.5
Half-life – normal/ESRF (hrs)	4–5/unchanged

Dose in renal impairment
GFR (mL/min)

20–50	Dose as in normal renal function
10–20	Dose as in normal renal function
<10	Dose as in normal renal function

Dose in patients undergoing renal replacement therapies

CAPD	Unknown dialysability. Dose as in normal renal function
HD	Unknown dialysability. Dose as in normal renal function
CAV/VVHD	Unknown dialysability. Dose as in normal renal function

Important drug interactions

CYCLOSPORIN

–

POTENTIALLY HAZARDOUS INTERACTIONS WITH OTHER DRUGS

• Enhanced hypotensive effect with ACE inhibitors, antihypertensives, antipsychotics, beta-blockers, calcium-channel blockers
• Increased risk of arrhythmias with dopaminergics and sympathomimetics

Administration

RECONSTITUTION

• May be diluted with saline or glucose 5%. Incompatible with compound sodium lactate infusion BP (Hartmann's solution)

ROUTE

• Intravenous injection only

RATE OF ADMINISTRATION

• Slow

COMMENTS

–

Other information

• In cases of adrenocortical gland dysfunction and during very long surgical procedures, a prophylactic cortisol supplement may be required (e.g. 50–100 mg hydrocortisone)

Etoposide

Clinical use

Antineoplastic agent

Dose in normal renal function

IV:

60–120 mg/m^2 daily according to local protocol

Oral:

twice the relevant IV dose should be given daily according to local protocol

Pharmacokinetics

Molecular weight (daltons)	589
% Protein binding	74–94
% Excreted unchanged in urine	20–60
Volume of distribution (L/kg)	0.17–0.5
Half-life – normal/ESRF (hrs)	4–8/19

Dose in renal impairment GFR (mL/min)

20–50	See 'Other information'
10–20	See 'Other information'
<10	See 'Other information'

Dose in patients undergoing renal replacement therapies

CAPD	Unknown dialysability. Dose as in GFR = <10 mL/min
HD	Dialysed. Dose as in GFR = <10 mL/min
CAV/VVHD	Unknown dialysability. Dose as in GFR = 10–20 mL/min

Important drug interactions

CYCLOSPORIN

• 50% reduction in etoposide clearance

POTENTIALLY HAZARDOUS INTERACTIONS WITH OTHER DRUGS

–

Administration

RECONSTITUTION

• Dilute with sodium chloride 0.9% to give a solution concentration of not more than 0.25 mg/mL of etoposide

ROUTE

• Oral or IV. Must not be given by intra-cavitary injection

RATE OF ADMINISTRATION

• IV infusion: not less than 30 min

COMMENTS

–

Other information

• Avoid skin contact

• It has been suggested that patients with serum creatinine >130 micromol/L require a 30% dose reduction. This dose adjustment was calculated to result in equivalent total dose exposure in patients with reduced renal function. Furthermore, patients with raised bilirubin and/or decreased albumin may have an increase in free etoposide and hence greater myelosuppression

• Reaches a high concentration in kidney; possible accumulation in renal impairment

Famciclovir

Clinical use

Antiviral agent

Dose in normal renal function

Zoster:

250 mg 3 times a day or 750 mg once daily for 7 days

First genital herpes infection:

250 mg 3 times a day for 5 days

Acute recurrent genital herpes:

125 mg twice a day for 5 days

Pharmacokinetics

Of penciclovir (active metabolite)

Molecular weight (daltons)	253
% Protein binding	<20
% Excreted unchanged in urine	43–75
Volume of distribution (L/kg)	1.5
Half-life – normal/ESRF (hrs)	1.6–2.9/3.8–25

Dose in renal impairment GFR (mL/min)

30–59	Zoster and first-episode genital herpes: 250 mg twice a day. Recurrent genital herpes: dose as in normal renal function
10–29	Zoster and first-episode genital herpes: 250 mg daily. Recurrent genital herpes: 125 mg daily
<10	Zoster and first-episode genital herpes: 250 mg on alternate days. Recurrent genital herpes: 125 mg on alternate days

Dose in patients undergoing renal replacement therapies

CAPD	Moderate dialysability likely. Dose as in GFR = <10 mL/min
HD	Dialysed. Dose as in GFR = <10 mL/min post-dialysis on dialysis days
CAV/VVHD	Dialysability likely. Dose as in GFR = 10–29 mL/min

Important drug interactions

CYCLOSPORIN

–

POTENTIALLY HAZARDOUS INTERACTIONS WITH OTHER DRUGS

• Probenecid: decreased excretion of famciclovir
• Increased famciclovir levels reported with mycophenolate mofetil

Administration

RECONSTITUTION

–

ROUTE

• Oral

RATE OF ADMINISTRATION

–

COMMENTS

–

Other information

• Famciclovir is well absorbed after oral administration and is deacetylated and oxidised rapidly to form the potent and selective antiviral compound penciclovir

Famotidine

Clinical use

H_2-blocker, used for conditions associated with hyperacidity

Dose in normal renal function

20–800 mg daily (varies according to indication)

Pharmacokinetics

Molecular weight (daltons)	337
% Protein binding	15–22
% Excreted unchanged in urine	65–80
Volume of distribution (L/kg)	0.8–1.4
Half-life – normal/ESRF (hrs)	2.5–4/12–19

Dose in renal impairment GFR (mL/min)

20–50	Dose as in normal renal function
10–20	50% of normal dose
<10	20 mg at night (maximum)

Dose in patients undergoing renal replacement therapies

CAPD	Insignificant dialysability. Dose as in GFR = <10 mL/min
HD	Insignificant dialysability. Dose as in GFR = <10 mL/min
CAV/VVHD	Insignificant dialysability. Dose as in GFR = 10–20 mL/min

Important drug interactions

CYCLOSPORIN

–

POTENTIALLY HAZARDOUS INTERACTIONS WITH OTHER DRUGS

–

Administration

RECONSTITUTION

–

ROUTE

• Oral

RATE OF ADMINISTRATION

–

COMMENTS

–

Other information

–

Felodipine

Clinical use

Calcium-channel blocker, used for management of hypertension and angina

Dose in normal renal function

5–10 mg once daily

Pharmacokinetics

Molecular weight (daltons)	384
% Protein binding	99
% Excreted unchanged in urine	<1
Volume of distribution (L/kg)	9–10
Half-life – normal/ESRF (hrs)	10–14/21–24

Dose in renal impairment GFR (mL/min)

20–50	Dose as in normal renal function
10–20	Dose as in normal renal function
<10	Dose as in normal renal function

Dose in patients undergoing renal replacement therapies

CAPD	Not dialysed. Dose as in normal renal function
HD	Not dialysed. Dose as in normal renal function
CAV/VVHD	Not dialysed. Dose as in normal renal function

Important drug interactions

CYCLOSPORIN

–

POTENTIALLY HAZARDOUS INTERACTIONS WITH OTHER DRUGS

• Drugs that interfere with the cytochrome P450 enzyme system may affect plasma concentrations of felodipine: cimetidine, erythromycin, phenytoin, carbamazepine, phenobarbitone

• Grapefruit juice should not be taken together with felodipine

Administration

RECONSTITUTION

–

ROUTE

• Oral

RATE OF ADMINISTRATION

–

COMMENTS

–

Other information

–

Fenofibrate

Clinical use

Treatment of hyperlipidaemias

Dose in normal renal function

Initial dose is 300 mg daily. Adjust according to response within range 200–400 mg daily

Pharmacokinetics

Molecular weight (daltons)	361
% Protein binding	99
% Excreted unchanged in urine	30–60
Volume of distribution (L/kg)	0.89
Half-life – normal/ESRF (hrs)	20/140–360

Dose in renal impairment GFR (mL/min)

20–60	200 mg daily
10–20	100 mg daily
<10	Avoid

Dose in patients undergoing renal replacement therapies

CAPD	Unlikely to be dialysed. Avoid
HD	Unlikely to be dialysed. Avoid
CAV/VVHD	Unlikely to be dialysed. Dose as in GFR = 10–20 mL/min

Important drug interactions

CYCLOSPORIN

- Cyclosporin levels appear to be unaffected. However, it is recommended that concomitant therapy should be avoided because of the possibility of elevated serum creatinine levels

POTENTIALLY HAZARDOUS INTERACTIONS WITH OTHER DRUGS

- In patients taking anticoagulants, the dose of anticoagulant should be reduced by $\frac{1}{3}$ when treatment with fenofibrate is started, and then adjusted gradually if necessary

Administration

RECONSTITUTION

–

ROUTE

- Oral

RATE OF ADMINISTRATION

–

COMMENTS

–

Other information

- A few studies have noted that the use of second-generation fibrates in transplant recipients is hampered by frequent rises in serum creatinine

Fenoprofen

Clinical use

NSAID, used for osteoarthritis, rheumatoid arthritis
and ankylosing spondylitis

Dose in normal renal function

300–600 mg 4 times a day

Pharmacokinetics

Molecular weight (daltons)	559
% Protein binding	>99
% Excreted unchanged in urine	2–5
Volume of distribution (L/kg)	0.10
Half-life – normal/ESRF (hrs)	2–3/unchanged

Dose in renal impairment GFR (mL/min)

20–50	Start with low dose, but avoid if possible
10–20	Start with low dose, but avoid if possible
<10	Start with low dose, but only use if ESRD on dialysis

Dose in patients undergoing renal replacement therapies

CAPD	Unlikely to be dialysed. Start with low doses and increase according to response
HD	Unlikely to be dialysed. Start with low doses and increase according to response
CAV/VVHD	Unlikely to be dialysed. Dose as in GFR = 10–20 mL/min

Important drug interactions

CYCLOSPORIN

• Increased risk of nephrotoxicity

POTENTIALLY HAZARDOUS INTERACTIONS WITH
OTHER DRUGS

• ACE inhibitors: increased risk of hyperkalaemia.
  Reduced hypotensive effect
• Anticoagulants: possible enhancement of effects of
  warfarin and nicoumalone
• Sulphonylureas: effects possibly enhanced
• Methotrexate: excretion reduced
• Lithium: excretion reduced
• Anti-epileptics: effects of phenytoin enhanced

Administration

RECONSTITUTION

–

ROUTE

• Oral

RATE OF ADMINISTRATION

–

COMMENTS

–

Other information

• Contraindicated in patients with history of
  significantly impaired renal function
• Inhibition of renal prostaglandin synthesis by
  NSAIDs may interfere with renal function,
  especially in the presence of existing renal disease.
  Avoid use if possible. If not, check serum creatinine
  48–72 hrs after starting NSAID; if it has increased,
  discontinue therapy
• Possibility of decreased platelet aggregation
• Can use normal doses in patients with ESRD on
  dialysis
• Use with caution in renal transplant recipients –
  can reduce intra-renal autocoid synthesis
• Associated with nephrotic syndrome, interstitial
  nephritis, hyperkalaemia, sodium retention

Fentanyl

Clinical use

Narcotic analgesic for short surgical procedures or use in ventilated patients

Dose in normal renal function

Consult relevant data sheet

Pharmacokinetics

Molecular weight (daltons)	529
% Protein binding	79–87
% Excreted unchanged in urine	6–8
Volume of distribution (L/kg)	2–5
Half-life – normal/ESRF (hrs)	2–7/unchanged

Dose in renal impairment GFR (mL/min)

20–50	Dose as in normal renal function. Titrate according to response
10–20	75% of normal dose. Titrate according to response
<10	50% of normal dose. Titrate according to response

Dose in patients undergoing renal replacement therapies

CAPD	Not dialysed. Dose as in GFR = <10 mL/min
HD	Not dialysed. Dose as in GFR = <10 mL/min
CAV/VVHD	Not dialysed. Dose as in GFR = 10–20 mL/min

Important drug interactions

CYCLOSPORIN

–

POTENTIALLY HAZARDOUS INTERACTIONS WITH OTHER DRUGS

- MAOIs: concurrent administration with MAOIs, or within 2 weeks of their discontinuation, is contraindicated
- Non-selective CNS depressants may enhance or prolong respiratory depression
- Non-vagolytic muscle relaxants: bradycardia/ asystole can occur
- Droperidol: increased risk of hypotension

Administration

RECONSTITUTION

- Compatible with sodium chloride 0.9% and glucose 5%

ROUTE

- IV, IM (pre-med), topical (chronic pain)

RATE OF ADMINISTRATION

–

COMMENTS

–

Other information

- For short surgical procedures the degree of renal impairment is irrelevant
- For other indications, renal impairment may have a moderate effect on the elimination of the drug. However, as fentanyl is titrated to response, the usual method of administration remains valid

Ferrous gluconate

Clinical use

Iron deficiency anaemia. Prophylaxis and treatment of iron deficiency before and during epoetin therapy

Dose in normal renal function

Prophylaxis:

300 mg twice daily

Therapeutic:

300–600 mg 2–3 times daily

Pharmacokinetics

Molecular weight (daltons)	482
% Protein binding	–
% Excreted unchanged in urine	–
Volume of distribution (L/kg)	–
Half-life – normal/ESRF (hrs)	–

Dose in renal impairment GFR (mL/min)

20–50	Dose as in normal renal function
10–20	Dose as in normal renal function
<10	Dose as in normal renal function

Dose in patients undergoing renal replacement therapies

CAPD	Not dialysed. Dose as in normal renal function
HD	Not dialysed. Dose as in normal renal function
CAV/VVHD	Not dialysed. Dose as in normal renal function

Important drug interactions

CYCLOSPORIN

–

POTENTIALLY HAZARDOUS INTERACTIONS WITH OTHER DRUGS

• Reduced absorption of 4-quinolones

Administration

RECONSTITUTION

–

ROUTE

• Oral

RATE OF ADMINISTRATION

–

COMMENTS

–

Other information

• One 300-mg ferrous gluconate tablet contains 35 mg elemental iron. Best taken before food to aid absorption

• Phosphate-binding agents, e.g. calcium carbonate or magnesium carbonate, reduce absorption of iron from the gut

• Monitor serum iron, transferrin saturation and ferritin levels (in line with local policy)

Ferrous sulphate

Clinical use

Iron deficiency anaemia. Prophylaxis and treatment
of iron deficiency before and during epoetin
therapy

Dose in normal renal function

Prophylaxis:
200 mg daily
Therapeutic:
200 mg 2–3 times daily

Pharmacokinetics

Molecular weight (daltons)	278
% Protein binding	–
% Excreted unchanged in urine	–
Volume of distribution (L/kg)	–
Half-life – normal/ESRF (hrs)	–

Dose in renal impairment GFR (mL/min)

20–50	Dose as in normal renal function
10–20	Dose as in normal renal function
<10	Dose as in normal renal function

Dose in patients undergoing renal replacement therapies

CAPD	Not dialysed. Dose as in normal renal function
HD	Not dialysed. Dose as in normal renal function
CAV/VVHD	Not dialysed. Dose as in normal renal function

Important drug interactions

CYCLOSPORIN

–

POTENTIALLY HAZARDOUS INTERACTIONS WITH
OTHER DRUGS

• Decreases absorption of 4-quinolones

Administration

RECONSTITUTION

–

ROUTE

• Oral

RATE OF ADMINISTRATION

–

COMMENTS

–

Other information

• One 200-mg ferrous sulphate tablet contains
  65 mg elemental iron
• Absorption of iron may be enhanced with
  concurrent administration of ascorbic acid
• Phosphate-binding agents, e.g. calcium carbonate
  or magnesium carbonate, reduce absorption of
  iron from the gut
• Monitor serum iron, transferrin saturation and
  ferritin levels (in line with local policy)

Filgrastim

Clinical use

Recombinant human granulocyte–colony stimulating factor (rhG-CSF), used for treatment of neutropenia

Dose in normal renal function

0.5–1.2 MU/kg/day according to indication and patient response

Pharmacokinetics

Molecular weight (daltons)	18 799
% Protein binding	Very high
% Excreted unchanged in urine	0
Volume of distribution (L/kg)	0.15
Half-life – normal/ESRF (hrs)	3.5/–

Dose in renal impairment GFR (mL/min)

20–50	Dose as in normal renal function and titrate dose to response
10–20	Dose as in normal renal function and titrate dose to response
<10	Dose as in normal renal function and titrate dose to response

Dose in patients undergoing renal replacement therapies

CAPD	Not dialysed. Dose as in GFR = <10 mL/min
HD	Not dialysed. Dose as in GFR = <10 mL/min
CAV/VVHD	Not dialysed. Dose as in GFR = 10–20 mL/min

Important drug interactions

CYCLOSPORIN

–

POTENTIALLY HAZARDOUS INTERACTIONS WITH OTHER DRUGS

–

Administration

RECONSTITUTION

• IV: dilute with glucose 5% *only*. Minimum concentration 0.2 MU/mL. Add human serum albumen if concentration is less than 1.5 MU/mL
• SC: continuous infusion – dilute with 20 mL of glucose 5%

ROUTE

• IV, SC

RATE OF ADMINISTRATION

• IV: over 30 min or continuous IV infusion over 24 hrs
• SC: can give as continuous SC infusion over 24 hrs

COMMENTS

• Dilute Neupogen may be adsorbed to glass and plastic materials. Follow recommendations for dilution

Other informaiton

• One very small study (2–3 patients) concluded that body clearance of filgrastim was not affected by degree of renal impairment

Finasteride

Clinical use

Benign prostatic hypertrophy

Dose in normal renal function

5 mg daily

Pharmacokinetics

Molecular weight (daltons)	373
% Protein binding	≈93
% Excreted unchanged in urine	<0.05
Volume of distribution (L/kg)	1.07
Half-life – normal/ESRF (hrs)	6/–

Dose in renal impairment GFR (mL/min)

20–50	Dose as in normal renal function
10–20	Dose as in normal renal function
<10	Dose as in normal renal function

Dose in patients undergoing renal replacement therapies

CAPD	Unlikely to be dialysed. Dose as in normal renal function
HD	Unlikely to be dialysed. Dose as in normal renal function
CAV/VVHD	Unlikely to be dialysed. Dose as in normal renal function

Important drug interactions

CYCLOSPORIN

–

POTENTIALLY HAZARDOUS INTERACTIONS WITH OTHER DRUGS

–

Administration

RECONSTITUTION

–

ROUTE

• Oral

RATE OF ADMINISTRATION

–

COMMENTS

–

Other information

• Data sheet states that no dosage adjustment is required in renally impaired patients whose creatinine clearance is as low as 9 mL/min. No studies have been done in patients with creatinine clearance of less than 9 mL/min

Flecainide

Clinical use

Class Ic anti-arrhythmic agent used for the treatment of ventricular arrhythmias and tachycardias

Dose in normal renal function

Supraventricular arrhythmias:

100–300 mg daily in 2 divided doses

Ventricular arrhythmias:

200–400 mg daily in 2 divided doses

IV bolus:

2 mg/kg over not less than 10 min

IV infusion:

2 mg/kg over 30 min; then

first hour, 1.5 mg/kg/hr; subsequently, 0.1–0.25 mg/kg/hr; maximum 600 mg in 24 hrs

Pharmacokinetics

Molecular weight (daltons)	474
% Protein binding	52
% Excreted unchanged in urine	25
Volume of distribution (L/kg)	8.4–9.5
Half-life – normal/ESRF (hrs)	7–23/9–58

Dose in renal impairment GFR (mL/min)

20–50	See 'Other information'
10–20	See 'Other information'
<10	See 'Other information'

Dose in patients undergoing renal replacement therapies

CAPD	≈ 1% dialysed. Dose as in GFR = <10 mL/min
HD	≈ 1% dialysed. Dose as in GFR = <10 mL/min.
CAV/VVHD	Minimal removal. Dose as in GFR = 10–20 mL/min

Important drug interactions

CYCLOSPORIN

–

Potentially hazardous interactions with other drugs

- Other anti-arrhythmics: amiodarone increases plasma flecainide levels; increased risk of ventricular arrhythmias.
- Increased myocardial depression with any anti-arrhythmic
- Antidepressants: fluoxetine increases plasma flecainide levels; increased risk of ventricular arrhythmias with fluoxetine and tricyclics
- Antihistamines: increased risk of ventricular arrhythmias with astemizole and terfenadine
- Antimalarials: quinine increases plasma levels of flecainide; increased risk of arrhythmias with halofantrine
- Beta-blockers: increased myocardial depression and bradycardia
- Calcium-channel blockers: increased myocardial depression and asystole with verapamil
- Diuretics: cardiac toxicity is increased if hypokalaemia occurs

Administration

RECONSTITUTION

- Infusion: dilute with 5% glucose infusion. If chloride-containing solutions are used the injection should be added to a volume of not less than 500 mL, otherwise a precipitate will form

ROUTE

- Oral, IV bolus, IV infusion

RATE OF ADMINISTRATION

- See 'Other information'

COMMENTS

- Plasma levels of 200–1000 nanogram/mL may be needed to obtain the maximum therapeutic effect. Plasma levels above 700–1000 nanogram/mL are associated with increased likelihood of adverse experiences

Other information

- Product information recommends reducing dosing recommendations for IV infusion by half in patients with severe renal impairment, defined as being a creatinine clearance of less than 35 mL/min

- Product information recommends for patients with severe renal impairment as defined above that the maximum initial dosage should be 100 mg daily (or 50 mg twice daily), with frequent plasma level monitoring strongly recommended

- Electrolyte disturbances should be corrected before using flecainide
- Plasma levels quoted in product information are trough levels. Sample prior to dose

Flucloxacillin

Clinical use

Antibacterial agent

Dose in normal renal function

Oral:
250–500 mg every 6 hrs
IV/IM:
250 mg–2 g every 6 hrs

Pharmacokinetics

Molecular weight (daltons)	453
% Protein binding	95
% Excreted unchanged in urine	60–90
Volume of distribution (L/kg)	0–13 (altered in hypoalbuminaemia and uraemia)
Half-life – normal/ESRF (hrs)	0.8–1.0/3.0

Dose in renal impairment GFR (mL/min)

20–50	Dose as in normal renal function
10–20	Dose as in normal renal function
<10	Dose as in normal renal function up to a total daily dose of 4 g

Dose in patients undergoing renal replacement therapies

CAPD	Not dialysable. Dose as in GFR = <10 mL/min
HD	Not dialysable. Dose as in GFR = <10 mL/min
CAV/VVHD	Not dialysable. Dose as in normal renal function

Important drug interactions

CYCLOSPORIN

–

POTENTIALLY HAZARDOUS INTERACTIONS WITH OTHER DRUGS

• Reduces excretion of methotrexate

Administration

RECONSTITUTION

• IV: 250 mg and 500 mg in 5 mL water for injection; 1 g in 15 mL water for injection
• IM: 1.5 mL water for injection to 250 mg; 2 mL water for injection to 500 mg

ROUTE

• IV peripherally

RATE OF ADMINISTRATION

• 3–4 min

COMMENTS

–

Other information

• Monitor urine for protein at high doses
• Sodium content of injection 2.0 mmol/g
• Monitor liver function tests in hypoalbuminaemic patients receiving high doses of flucloxacillin (e.g. CAPD patients)

Fluconazole

Clinical use

Antifungal agent

Dose in normal renal function

50–400 mg daily

Pharmacokinetics

Molecular weight (daltons)	306
% Protein binding	12
% Excreted unchanged in urine	70
Volume of distribution (L/kg)	0.7
Half-life – normal/ESRF (hrs)	22/98

Dose in renal impairment GFR (mL/min)

>50	Dose as in normal renal function
20–50	Dose as in normal renal function
10–20	Dose as in normal renal function
<10	50% of normal dose

Dose in patients undergoing renal replacement therapies

CAPD	Dialysed. Dose as in GFR = <10 mL/min
HD	Dialysed. Dose as in GFR = <10 mL/min. Give post-dialysis.
CAV/VVHD	Dialysed. Dose as in normal renal function

Important drug interactions

CYCLOSPORIN

• Increases blood/serum cyclosporin levels

POTENTIALLY HAZARDOUS INTERACTIONS WITH OTHER DRUGS

• Potentiates effect of warfarin
• Increases phenytoin levels and effect
• Increases theophylline levels

Administration

RECONSTITUTION

• IV preparation supplied as solution

ROUTE

• Oral, IV

RATE OF ADMINISTRATION

• IV: 5–10 mL/min peripherally

COMMENTS

• Oral ≡ IV dose. Very high bioavailability

Other information

• Has been used as an adjunct to IV amphotericin and IP flucytosine in CAPD peritonitis
• No dose adjustment is required for single-dose therapy
• Recurrent yeast peritonitis: flucytosine 2000 mg orally stat, then 1000 mg daily in addition to fluconazole 150 mg IP or 200 mg orally on alternate days. Remove Tench-koff after 4–7 days if no response
• 3 hrs haemodialysis reduces blood levels by 50%

Flucytosine

Clinical use

Antifungal agent

Dose in normal renal function

Oral/IV:
200 mg/kg per day in 4 divided doses

Pharmacokinetics

Molecular weight (daltons)	129
% Protein binding	<10
% Excreted unchanged in urine	80–90
Volume of distribution (L/kg)	0.6
Half-life – normal/ESRF (hrs)	3–6/75–200

Dose in renal impairment
GFR (mL/min)

20–40	50 mg/kg 12-hourly
10–20	50 mg/kg 24-hourly
<10	50 mg/kg then dose according to levels. Dose 500 mg–1 g daily is usually adequate

Dose in patients undergoing renal replacement therapies

CAPD	Dialysed. Give 50 mg/kg daily in 4 divided doses. Monitor levels
HD	Dialysed. Dose as in GFR = <10 mL/min, given post-dialysis. Monitor trough level pre-dialysis and reduce post-dialysis dose accordingly
CAV/VVHD	Dialysed. Give dose as in GFR = 10–20 mL/min and monitor blood levels pre-dose

Important drug interactions

CYCLOSPORIN

–

POTENTIALLY HAZARDOUS INTERACTIONS WITH OTHER DRUGS

• Cytarabine: monitor flucytosine levels

Administration

RECONSTITUTION

–

ROUTE

• IV peripherally through a blood filter

RATE OF ADMINISTRATION

• 20–40 min

COMMENTS

–

Other information

• Monitor blood levels 24 hrs after therapy commences. Pre-dose level 25–50 micrograms/mL is usually adequate.
  Do not exceed 80 micrograms/mL

• 250 mL intravenous flucytosine infusion contains 34.44 mmol sodium

• Bone marrow suppression is more common in patients with renal impairment

• Tablets available on named-patient basis only

Flumazenil

Clinical use

Reversal of sedative effects of benzodiazepines in anaesthetic, intensive care and diagnostic procedures

Dose in normal renal function

Initially 200 micrograms over 15 sec, then 100 micrograms at 60-sec intervals if required; usual dose range 300–600 micrograms. Maximum dose 1 mg, or 2 mg in intensive care situations. If drowsiness recurs, an IV infusion of 100–400 micrograms/hr may be given

Pharmacokinetics

Molecular weight (daltons)	303
% Protein binding	40–50
% Excreted unchanged in urine	<0.1
Volume of distribution (L/kg)	0.6–1.1
Half-life – normal/ESRF (hrs)	0.7–1.3/–

Dose in renal impairment GFR (mL/min)

20–50	Dose as in normal renal function
10–20	Dose as in normal renal function
<10	Dose as in normal renal function

Dose in patients undergoing renal replacement therapies

CAPD	Unknown dialysability. Dose as in normal renal function
HD	Unknown dialysability. Dose as in normal renal function
CAV/VVHD	Unknown dialysability. Dose as in normal renal function

Important drug interactions

CYCLOSPORIN

–

POTENTIALLY HAZARDOUS INTERACTIONS WITH OTHER DRUGS

–

Administration

RECONSTITUTION

• Infusion: suitable diluents include sodium chloride 0.9% infusion, sodium chloride 0.45% and glucose 2.5% IV infusion, glucose 5% IV infusion

ROUTE

• IV injection, IV infusion

RATE OF ADMINISTRATION

• See 'Dose in normal renal function'

COMMENTS

–

Other information

• The half-life of flumazenil is shorter than those of diazepam and midazolam. Hence patients should be closely monitored to avoid the risk of them becoming re-sedated

Fluorouracil

Clinical use

Antineoplastic agent

Dose in normal renal function

IV infusion:

15 mg/kg/day to a total dose of 12–15 g

IV bolus:

12 mg/kg/day for 3 days, then 6 mg/kg on alternate days or 15 mg/kg once a week

Intra-arterial infusion:

5.0–7.5 mg/kg by continuous 24-hr infusion

Maintenance:

5–15 mg/kg once a week

or consult relevant local chemotherapy protocol

Pharmacokinetics

Molecular weight (daltons)	130
% Protein binding	10
% Excreted unchanged in urine	15
Volume of distribution (L/kg)	0.25–0.5
Half-life – normal/ESRF (hrs)	0.1/unchanged

Dose in renal impairment GFR (mL/min)

20–50	100% of normal dose
10–20	100% of normal dose
<10	100% of normal dose

Dose in patients undergoing renal replacement therapies

CAPD	Some removal likely. Dose as in GFR = <10 mL/min
HD	Some removal likely. Dose as in GFR = <10 mL/min
CAV/VVHD	Some removal likely. Dose as in GFR = 10–20 mL/min

Important drug interactions

CYCLOSPORIN

–

POTENTIALLY HAZARDOUS INTERACTIONS WITH OTHER DRUGS

• Metronidazole and cimetidine inhibit metabolism (increased toxicity)

Administration

RECONSTITUTION

• Consult relevant local protocol

ROUTE

• IV infusion intermittent or continuous, IV injection, intra-arterial, oral

RATE OF ADMINISTRATION

• Consult relevant local protocol

COMMENTS

–

Other information

• Use ideal body weight in patients showing obesity, ascites or oedema

• Roche recommends decreasing the initial dose by $\frac{1}{3}$ to $\frac{1}{2}$ in patients with impaired hepatic or renal function

Fluoxetine

Clinical use

SSRI antidepressant, used for depressive illness, bulimia nervosa, obsessive-compulsive disorder

Dose in normal renal function

20–60 mg daily depending on indication

Pharmacokinetics

Molecular weight (daltons)	346
% Protein binding	94.5
% Excreted unchanged in urine	<10
Volume of distribution (L/kg)	20–42
Half-life – normal/ESRF (hrs)	24–72/unchanged (acute dosing); 4–6 days/– (chronic dosing)

Dose in renal impairment GFR (mL/min)

20–50	Dose as in normal renal function
10–20	Dose as in normal renal function or on alternate days
<10	Dose as in normal renal function on alternate days

Dose in patients undergoing renal replacement therapies

CAPD	Insignificant removal. Dose as in GFR = <10 mL/min
HD	Insignificant removal. Dose as in GFR = <10 mL/min
CAV/VVHD	Insignificant removal. Dose as in GFR = 10–20 mL/min

Important drug interactions

CYCLOSPORIN

–

POTENTIALLY HAZARDOUS INTERACTIONS WITH OTHER DRUGS

- Anticoagulants: effects of warfarin enhanced
- Other antidepressants: enhanced CNS effects of MAOIs (increased risk of toxicity)
- Anti-epileptics: antagonism (lowered convulsive threshold). Plasma concentrations of carbamazepine and phenytoin increased
- Antipsychotics: plasma concentrations of haloperidol and sertindole increased
- Dopaminergics: hypertension and CNS excitation
- Lithium: increased risk of CNS effects (lithium toxicity reported)

Administration

RECONSTITUTION

–

ROUTE

- Oral

RATE OF ADMINISTRATION

–

COMMENTS

–

Other information

- Manufacturer's literature states fluoxetine should not be administered to patients with severe renal failure (GFR <10 mL/min) because accumulation may occur in these patients during chronic treatment (metabolites are excreted renally).
- Levy et al. (1996) [General Hospital Psychiatry 18: 8–13] studied 7 patients undergoing haemodialysis and concluded that the process of HD does not alter the pharmacokinetics of fluoxetine or its major metabolite. All patients received fluoxetine 20 mg per day for 8 weeks

Flurbiprofen

Clinical use

NSAID, used for rheumatic disease and other musculoskeletal disorders; dysmenorrhoea; post-operative analgesia

Dose in normal renal function

Oral/PR:

150–200 mg daily in divided doses, increased in acute conditions to 300 mg daily

Pharmacokinetics

Molecular weight (daltons)	244
% Protein binding	99
% Excreted unchanged in urine	<20
Volume of distribution (L/kg)	0.10
Half-life – normal/ESRF (hrs)	3–5/unchanged

Dose in renal impairment GFR (mL/min)

20–50	Dose as in normal renal function, but avoid if possible
10–20	Dose as in normal renal function but avoid if possible
<10	Dose as in normal renal function, but only if ESRD on dialysis

Dose in patients undergoing renal replacement therapies

CAPD	Removal very unlikely. Dose as in GFR = <10 mL/min
HD	Removal very unlikely. Dose as in GFR = <10 mL/min
CAV/VVHD	Removal very unlikely. Dose as in GFR = 10–20 mL/min

Important drug interactions

CYCLOSPORIN

• Increased risk of renal toxicity

POTENTIALLY HAZARDOUS INTERACTIONS WITH OTHER DRUGS

• Decreased excretion of lithium
• Cytotoxic agents: reduced excretion of methotrexate
• Anticoagulants: effects of warfarin and nicoumalone enhanced
• Antidiabetic agents: effects of sulphonylureas enhanced
• Anti-epileptic agents: effects of phenytoin enhanced
• ACE inhibitors: antagonism of hypotensive effect; increased risk of hyperkalaemia and renal damage
• Uricosurics: probenecid delays excretion of NSAID

Administration

RECONSTITUTION

–

ROUTE

• Oral, PR

RATE OF ADMINISTRATION

–

COMMENTS

–

Other information

• NSAIDs have been reported to cause nephrotoxicity in various forms: interstitial nephritis, nephrotic syndrome and renal failure. In patients with renal, cardiac or hepatic impairment, caution is required since the use of NSAIDs may result in deterioration of renal function
• Inhibition of renal prostaglandin synthesis by NSAIDs may interfere with renal function, especially in the presence of existing renal disease. Avoid if possible; if not, check serum creatinine 48–72 hrs after starting NSAID. If creatinine has increased, discontinue therapy
• Use normal doses in patients with ESRD on dialysis
• Use with caution in renal transplant recipients – can reduce intra-renal autocoid synthesis

Fluvastatin

Clinical use

HMG CoA reductase inhibitor, used for primary hypercholesterolaemia

Dose in normal renal function

Initially 20 mg daily in the evening; usual range 20–40 mg daily, adjusted at intervals of 4 weeks. Maximum 40 mg twice daily

Pharmacokinetics

Molecular weight (daltons)	433.5
% Protein binding	>98
% Excreted unchanged in urine	<1
Volume of distribution (L/kg)	0.42
Half-life – normal/ESRF (hrs)	2.3–2.5/–

Dose in renal impairment GFR (mL/min)

20–50	Dose as in normal renal function
10–20	Dose as in normal renal function
<10	20 mg daily

Dose in patients undergoing renal replacement therapies

CAPD	Removal unlikely. Dose as in GFR = <10 mL/min
HD	Removal unlikely. Dose as in GFR = <10 mL/min
CAV/VVHD	Removal unlikely. Dose as in normal renal function

Important drug interactions

CYCLOSPORIN

• Concomitant treatment with cyclosporin may lead to risk of muscle toxicity

POTENTIALLY HAZARDOUS INTERACTIONS WITH OTHER DRUGS

• Other lipid-lowering drugs and erythromycin: increased risk of serious muscle toxicity

Administration

RECONSTITUTION

–

ROUTE

• Oral

RATE OF ADMINISTRATION

–

COMMENTS

–

Other information

• The Committee on Safety of Medicines has advised that rhabdomyolysis associated with lipid-lowering drugs, such as the fibrates and statins, appears to be rare (approximately 1 case in every 100 000 treatment years), but may be increased in those with renal impairment and possibly in those with hypothyroidism
• Manufacturer's literature indicates fluvastatin is contraindicated in patients with severe renal impairment (creatinine ⩾160 mmol/L)

Folic acid

Clinical use

Folate-deficient megaloblastic anaemia or supplement in HD patients

Dose in normal renal function

5 mg/day for 4 months, then weekly according to response

Pharmacokinetics

Molecular weight (daltons)	441.4
% Protein binding	–
% Excreted unchanged in urine	Varies with daily dose
Volume of distribution (L/kg)	–
Half-life – normal/ESRF (hrs)	2.5/–

Dose in renal impairment GFR (mL/min)

20–50	Dose as in normal renal function
10–20	Dose as in normal renal function
<10	Dose as in normal renal function

Dose in patients undergoing renal replacement therapies

CAPD	Dialysed. Dose as in normal renal function
HD	Dialysed. Dose as in normal renal function. Dose after HD
CAV/VVHD	Dialysed. Dose as in normal renal function

Important drug interactions

CYCLOSPORIN

–

POTENTIALLY HAZARDOUS INTERACTIONS WITH OTHER DRUGS

• Reduces plasma phenytoin levels

Administration

RECONSTITUTION

–

ROUTE

• Oral

RATE OF ADMINISTRATION

–

COMMENTS

–

Other information

• If profusely folate deficient, give 10 mg/day for 1 month, then 5 mg/day
• Most nutritionists recommend 0.5–1 mg folic acid for patients on HD or CAPD; may accumulate in uraemic patients
• Dosage used by dialysis units varies from 5 mg daily to 5 mg once weekly

Folinic acid

Clinical use

Folinic acid rescue; enhancement of 5-fluorouracil cytotoxicity in advanced colorectal cancer; treatment of folate deficiency

Dose in normal renal function

Varies according to indication

Pharmacokinetics

Molecular weight (daltons)	511.5
% Protein binding	54
% Excreted unchanged in urine	–
Volume of distribution (L/kg)	17.5
Half-life – normal/ESRF	32 min/–

Dose in renal impairment GFR (mL/min)

20–50	Dose as in normal renal function
10–20	Dose as in normal renal function
<10	Dose as in normal renal function

Dose in patients undergoing renal replacement therapies

CAPD	Some removal likely. Dose as in normal renal function
HD	Some removal likely. Dose as in normal renal function
CAV/VVHD	Some removal likely. Dose as in normal renal function

Important drug interactions

CYCLOSPORIN

–

POTENTIALLY HAZARDOUS INTERACTIONS WITH OTHER DRUGS

• Folinic acid should not be administered simultaneously with a folic acid antagonist, as this may nullify the effect of the antagonist

Administration

RECONSTITUTION

• For IV infusion compatible with sodium chloride 0.9%, glucose 5%, glucose 10% and sodium chloride 0.9% injection compound, sodium lactate injection

ROUTE

• IM, IV injection, IV infusion, oral

RATE OF ADMINISTRATION

• Because of the calcium content of leucovorin solutions, no more than 160 mg/min should be injected IV

COMMENTS

–

Other information

–

Foscarnet

Clinical use

Antiviral agent, used for treatment of cytomegalovirus retinitis. (Use for other forms of cytomegalovirus and use in patients with serum creatinine >250 micromol/mL is not licensed)

Dose in normal renal function

60 mg/kg every 8 hrs induction dose

Pharmacokinetics

Molecular weight (daltons)	192
% Protein binding	14–17
% Excreted unchanged in urine	85
Volume of distribution (L/kg)	0.22–0.78
Half-life – normal/ESRF (hrs)	36/very long

Dose in renal impairment GFR (mL/min)

Dose according to serum creatinine

20–50	28 mg/kg every 8 hrs
10–20	15 mg/kg every 8 hrs
<10	6 mg/kg every 8 hrs

Dose in patients undergoing renal replacement therapies

CAPD	Dialysed. Dose in accordance with serum creatinine or as in GFR = <10 mL/min
HD	Dialysed. Dose in accordance with serum creatinine or as in GFR = <10 mL/min
CAV/VVHD	Dialysed. Dose in accordance with serum creatinine or as in GFR = 10–20 mL/min

Important drug interactions

CYCLOSPORIN

–

POTENTIALLY HAZARDOUS INTERACTIONS WITH OTHER DRUGS

–

Administration

RECONSTITUTION

• If given peripherally dilute with glucose 5% to a concentration of 12 mg/mL or less

ROUTE

• Centrally (undiluted); peripherally (diluted)

RATE OF ADMINISTRATION

• Continuous infusion over 24 hrs

COMMENTS

• If given peripherally, piggy-back to a glucose 5% infusion running at the same rate as the foscarnet solution

Other information

• Give 20 mg/kg over 30 min followed by daily dose as follows:

S-Creatinine	Dose (mg/kg/24 hrs)
<110	200
111–130	199–129
131–150	129–115
151–170	115–100
171–190	100–86
191–210	86–72
211–230	72–43
231–250	43–21
>250	Not recommended

Treatment is usually continued for 2–3 weeks depending on response

• Some units dose by creatinine clearance/weight as follows:

Clearance (mL/min/kg)	Dose (mg/kg every 8 hrs)
1.6	60
1.5	57
1.4	53
1.3	49
1.2	46
1.1	42
1.0	39
0.9	35
0.8	32
0.7	28
0.6	25
0.5	21
0.4	18

• Maintain adequate hydration to prevent renal toxicity

• Monitor serum calcium and magnesium

• Some units use full-dose ganciclovir plus half-dose foscarnet concomitantly for treatment of resistant CMV disease

Fosinopril

Clinical use

Angiotensin-converting enzyme inhibitor, used for hypertension

Dose in normal renal function

10–40 mg once daily

Pharmacokinetics

Molecular weight (daltons)	586
% Protein binding	95
% Excreted unchanged in urine	<1
Volume of distribution (L/kg)	1.5
Half-life – normal/ESRF (hrs)	11.5–12/12–20

Dose in renal impairment GFR (mL/min)

20–50	Dose as in normal renal function
10–20	Dose as in normal renal function. Start with low dose
<10	Dose as in normal renal function. Start with low dose

Dose in patients undergoing renal replacement therapies

CAPD	Probably not dialysed. Dose as in GFR = <10 mL/min
HD	Probably not dialysed. Dose as in GFR = <10 mL/min
CAV/VVHD	Probably not dialysed. Dose as in GFR = 10–20 mL/min

Important drug interactions

CYCLOSPORIN

• Increased risk of hyperkalaemia

POTENTIALLY HAZARDOUS INTERACTIONS WITH OTHER DRUGS

• Antacids: reduced serum levels and urinary excretion of fosinoprilat

• Diuretics: hyperkalaemia with potassium-sparing diuretics, enhanced hypotensive effects
• Epoetin: increased risk of hyperkalaemia
• Lithium: reduced excretion. Possibility of enhanced lithium toxicity
• Potassium salts: increased risk of hyperkalaemia
• NSAIDs: antagonism of hypotensive effect, increased risk of hyperkalaemia and renal damage
• Anaesthetics: enhanced hypotensive effect

Administration

RECONSTITUTION

–

ROUTE

• Oral

RATE OF ADMINISTRATION

–

COMMENTS

–

Other information

• Any diuretic should preferably be discontinued for several days prior to beginning therapy with fosinopril to reduce the risk of an excessive hypotensive response
• Hepatobiliary elimination compensates for the diminished renal excretion
• Hyperkalaemia and other side-effects are more common in patients with impaired renal function
• Close monitoring of renal function during therapy is necessary in those with renal insufficiency
• Renal failure has been reported in association with ACE inhibitors in patients with renal artery stenosis, post-renal transplant or congestive heart failure
• A high incidence of anaphylactoid reactions has been reported in patients dialysed with high-flux polyacrylonitrile membranes and treated concomitantly with an ACE inhibitor – this combination should therefore be avoided

Frusemide

Clinical use

Loop diuretic

Dose in normal renal function

Oral:

20 mg–2 g daily

IV:

20 mg–1 g daily

Doses titrated to response

Pharmacokinetics

Molecular weight (daltons)	330.8
% Protein binding	95–99
% Excreted unchanged in urine	67
Volume of distribution (L/kg)	0.07–0.2
Half-life – normal/ESRF (hrs)	0.5–1.5/2–10

Dose in renal impairment GFR (mL/min)

20–50	Dose as in normal renal function
10–20	Dose as in normal renal function. Increased doses may be required
<10	Dose as in normal renal function. Increased doses may be required

Dose in patients undergoing renal replacement therapies

CAPD	Removal unlikely. Dose as in GFR = <10 mL/min
HD	Removal unlikely. Dose as in GFR = <10 mL/min
CAV/VVHD	Removal unlikely. Dose as in GFR = 10–20 mL/min

Important drug interactions

CYCLOSPORIN

• Variable reports: increased nephrotoxicity, ototoxicity and hepatotoxicity

POTENTIALLY HAZARDOUS INTERACTIONS WITH OTHER DRUGS

• Lithium: lithium excretion reduced
• ACE inhibitors: enhanced first-dose effect

Administration

RECONSTITUTION

• 250 mg to 50 mL sodium chloride 0.9% or undiluted via CRIP

ROUTE

• IV peripherally or centrally

RATE OF ADMINISTRATION

• 1 hr; not greater than 4 mg/min

COMMENTS

• Increased danger of ototoxicity and nephrotoxicity if infused at faster rate than approximately 4 mg/min
• Maximum dose by infusion: 1 g/24 hrs
• Protect from light

Other information

• 500 mg orally ≡ 250 mg IV
• Excreted by tubular secretion, therefore in severe renal impairment (GFR 5–10 mL/min) higher doses may be required due to a reduction in the number of functioning nephrons
• Oliguria: start 250 mg daily, increasing 4–6 hourly to a maximum single dose of 2 g (rarely used)
• Frusemide acts within 1 hr of oral administration (after IV peak effect within 30 min). Diuresis is complete within 6 hrs

Fusidic acid

Clinical use

Antibacterial agent

Dose in normal renal function

Oral:

480 mg every 8 hrs (equivalent to 500 mg sodium fusidate every 8 hrs)

IV:

480 mg every 8 hrs (equivalent to 500 mg sodium fusidate every 8 hrs)

Pharmacokinetics

Molecular weight (daltons)	526
% Protein binding	95
% Excreted unchanged in urine	<10
Volume of distribution (L/kg)	6.79–14.73
Half-life – normal/ESRF (hrs)	10–15/unchanged

Dose in renal impairment GFR (mL/min)

20–50	Dose as in normal renal function
10–20	Dose as in normal renal function
<10	Dose as in normal renal function

Dose in patients undergoing renal replacement therapies

CAPD	Not dialysed. Dose as in normal renal function
HD	Not dialysed. Dose as in normal renal function
CAV/VVHD	Not dialysed. Dose as in normal renal function

Important drug interactions

CYCLOSPORIN

–

POTENTIALLY HAZARDOUS INTERACTIONS WITH OTHER DRUGS

–

Administration

RECONSTITUTION

• Use buffered solution provided, then dilute in 500 mL sodium chloride 0.9%

ROUTE

• IV peripherally over 6 hrs

RATE OF ADMINISTRATION

–

COMMENTS

• Unlicensed administration: 500 mg/10 mL buffered solution diluted to 100 mL and given via a central line over 2–6 hrs

Other information

• 500 mg reconstituted with buffer contains 3.1 mmol sodium
• Can be administered neat via central line (unlicensed)

Gabapentin

Clinical use

Anti-epileptic, used for adjunctive treatment of partial seizures with or without secondary generalisation

Dose in normal renal function

300 mg on day 1, 300 mg twice daily on day 2, 300 mg 3 times daily on day 3, then increased according to response to 1.2 g daily (in 3 equally divided doses). If necessary may be further increased in steps of 300 mg daily to a maximum of 2.4 g daily. Usual range 0.9–1.2 g daily; maximum period between doses should not exceed 12 hrs.

Pharmacokinetics

Molecular weight (daltons)	171.2
% Protein binding	<3
% Excreted unchanged in urine	≈100
Volume of distribution (L/kg)	1.0
Half-life – normal/ESRF (hrs)	5–7/–

Dose in renal impairment GFR (mL/min)

60–90	400 mg 3 times daily
30–60	300 mg twice daily
15–30	300 mg once daily
<15	300 mg on alternate days

Dose in patients undergoing renal replacement therapies

CAPD	Probably dialysed. Dose as in GFR <15 mL/min
HD	Probably dialysed. Loading dose of 300–400 mg in patients who have never received gabapentin. Maintenance dose of 200–300 mg after each HD session
CAV/VVHD	Probably dialysed. Dose as in GFR <15 mL/min

Important drug interactions

CYCLOSPORIN

–

POTENTIALLY HAZARDOUS INTERACTIONS WITH OTHER DRUGS

• Antacids reduce absorption

Administration

RECONSTITUTION

–

ROUTE

• Oral

RATE OF ADMINISTRATION

–

COMMENTS

–

Other information

• Can cause false-positive readings with some urinary protein tests

Ganciclovir

Clinical use

Antiviral agent. Used IV for treatment of life- or sight-threatening cytomegalovirus (CMV) in immunocompromised people and for CMV prophylaxis in immunosuppressed patients secondary to organ transplantation. Used orally for maintenance treatment of CMV retinitis in AIDS patients (licensed), prophylaxis and maintenance against other CMV infection (unlicensed use)

Dose in normal renal function

IV treatment:

induction: 5 mg/kg 12-hourly for 14–21 days

maintenance: 6 mg/kg per day for 5 days per week or 5 mg/kg per day for 7 days per week

prevention: as per treatment except induction length 7–14 days

Oral:

1000 mg 3 times per day

Pharmacokinetics

Molecular weight (daltons)	277
% Protein binding	<2
% Excreted unchanged in urine	90–100
Volume of distribution (L/kg)	0.47
Half-life – normal/ESRF (hrs)	2.9/30

Dose in normal renal impairment GFR (mL/min)

20–50	See 'Other information'
10–20	See 'Other information'
<10	See 'Other information'

Dose in patients undergoing renal replacement therapies

CAPD	Oral and IV: dose as in GFR = <10 mL/min
HD	Dialysable. IV: 1.25 mg/kg per day, given post-dialysis on dialysis days. PO: 500 mg 3 times a week, given post-dialysis on dialysis days
CAV/VVHD	IV: give 2.5 mg/kg per day. PO: give 500 mg once daily

Important drug interactions

CYCLOSPORIN

–

POTENTIALLY HAZARDOUS INTERACTIONS WITH OTHER DRUGS

- Increased risk of myelosuppression with other myelosuppressive drugs
- Profound myelosuppression with zidovudine
- Generalised seizures reported with imipenen-cilastatin

Administration

RECONSTITUTION

- Reconstitute 1 vial (500 mg) with 10 mL water for injection (50 mg/mL). Then transfer dose to 100 mL sodium chloride 0.9%

ROUTE

- IV peripherally in fast-flowing vein or centrally – see below

RATE OF ADMINISTRATION

- Over 1 hr

COMMENTS

- May give 50% dose over 15 min after HD in washback (unlicensed)

Other information

- IV dosage:

Serum creatinine (micromol/L)	Creatinine clearance (mL/min)	Dose (mg/kg/hr)
<124	>50	5 mg/kg 12-hourly
125–225	25–50	2.5 mg/kg 12-hourly
226–398	10–25	2.5 mg/kg 24-hourly
>398	<10	1.25 mg/kg 24-hourly

- Oral dose:

Creatinine clearance (mL/min)	Dose
⩾70	1000 mg 3 times a day
50–69	1500 mg daily
25–49	1000 mg daily
10–24	500 mg daily
<10	500 mg 3 times a week

- Monitor patient for myelosuppression, particularly in patients receiving prophylactic co-trimoxazole therapy
- Predialysis therapeutic blood levels in range 5–12 mg/L
- Not to be infused in concentrations over 10 mg/mL peripherally

Gemfibrozil

Clinical use

Hyperlipidaemias of types IIa, IIb, III, IV and V

Dose in normal renal function

1.2 g daily, usually in 2 divided doses;
range 0.9–1.5 g daily

Pharmacokinetics

Molecular weight (daltons)	250
% Protein binding	95
% Excreted unchanged in urine	<5
Volume of distribution (L/kg)	–
Half-life – normal/ESRF (hrs)	1.5/1.5–2.4

Dose in renal impairment
GFR (mL/min)

20–50	Initially 900 mg daily
10–20	Initially 900 mg daily. Monitor carefully
<10	Initially 900 mg daily. Monitor carefully

Dose in patients undergoing renal replacement therapies

CAPD	Not dialysable. Dose as in GFR = <10 mL/min
HD	Not dialysable. Dose as in GFR = <10 mL/min
CAV/VVHD	Not dialysable. Dose as in GFR = 10–20 mL/min

Important drug interactions

CYCLOSPORIN

• Parke-Davis has one report on file of an interaction with cyclosporin where serum cyclosporin levels were decreased. No effects on muscle were noted

POTENTIALLY HAZARDOUS INTERACTIONS WITH OTHER DRUGS

• Enhanced anticoagulant effect seen with nicoumalone, phenindione and warfarin

Administration

RECONSTITUTION

–

ROUTE

• Oral

RATE OF ADMINISTRATION

–

COMMENTS

–

Other information

• Adverse effects have not been reported in patients with renal disease, but such patients should start treatment at 900 mg daily, which may be increased after careful assessment of response and renal function

• Rare cases of rhabdomyolysis may be increased in those with renal impairment

• Approximately 60–70% is excreted in the urine as both conjugated and unconjugated drug

• Gemfibrozil alone has caused myalgia and myositis, but the effects appear to occur much more frequently and are more severe when an HMG CoA reductase inhibitor is also used. The combination is therefore not recommended

Gentamicin

Clinical use

Antibacterial agent

Dose in normal renal function

3–7 mg/kg (ideal body weight) daily (divided into 1–4 doses). CAPD peritonitis – see local policy and below

Pharmacokinetics

Molecular weight (daltons)	1418
% Protein binding	0–20
% Excreted unchanged in urine	95
Volume of distribution (L/kg)	0.23–0.26
Half-life – normal/ESRF (hrs)	2/20–60

Dose in renal impairment GFR (mL/min)

See 'Other information' for dosage for dialysis and for single daily dosing regimen

30–70	80 mg 12-hourly (60 mg if <60 kg)
10–30	80 mg 24-hourly (60 mg if <60 kg)
5–10	80 mg 48-hourly (60 mg if <60 kg) or post-dialysis if on HD

Dose in patients undergoing renal replacement therapies

CAPD	Dialysable. CAPD clearance is about 3 mL/min. Dose as in GFR = 5–10 mL/min. Monitor levels
HD	Dialysable. Dose as in GFR = 5–10 mL/min. Give after dialysis
CAV/VVHD	Dialysable. Dose as in GFR = 10–30 mL/min and measure levels

Important drug interactions

CYCLOSPORIN

• Increased risk of nephrotoxicity

POTENTIALLY HAZARDOUS INTERACTIONS WITH OTHER DRUGS

• Muscle relaxants: effect of tubocurarine enhanced
• Cytotoxics: increased risk of nephrotoxicity with cisplatin
• Cholinergics: antagonism of effect of neostigmine and pyridostigmine

Administration

RECONSTITUTION

–

ROUTE

• Bolus IV injection or short infusion – maximum 100 mL

RATE OF ADMINISTRATION

• Bolus IV: over not less than 3 min. Short infusion: over not less than 20 min

COMMENTS

–

Other information

• Adjustment for renal impairment: dialysis – 80 mg (or up to 2 mg/kg) post-dialysis
• Single daily dosing regimen:

GFR >80:   5.1 mg/kg every 24 hrs
GFR 60–80: 4.0 mg/kg every 24 hrs
GFR 40–60: 3.5 mg/kg every 24 hrs
GFR 30–40: 2.5 mg/kg every 24 hrs
GFR 20–30: 4.0 mg/kg every 48 hrs
GFR 10–20: 3.0 mg/kg every 48 hrs
GFR <10:   2.0 mg/kg every 48 hrs

• Concurrent penicillins may result in subtherapeutic blood levels
• Monitor blood levels. 1-hr post-dose peak levels must not exceed 10 mg/L. Pre-dose trough levels should be less than 2 mg/L
• Empirical IP therapy for CAPD peritonitis in conjunction with vancomycin. A common regimen used is gentamicin 4–5 mg/L + vancomycin IP at a dose of 1–2 g stat on days 1 and 7 of course. Monitoring of blood levels is advisable, as absorption is increased by inflamed peritoneum
• Potential nephrotoxicity of the drug may worsen residual renal function

Glibenclamide

Clinical use

Non-insulin dependent diabetes mellitus

Dose in normal renal function

Initially 5 mg daily (elderly patients 2.5 mg) adjusted according to response; maximum 15 mg daily

Pharmacokinetics

Molecular weight (daltons)	494
% Protein binding	98–99
% Excreted unchanged in urine	<5
Volume of distribution (L/kg)	0.15–0.2
Half-life – normal/ESRF (hrs)	5–10/–

Dose in renal impairment GFR (mL/min)

20–50	Initial dose of 1.25–2.5 mg once a day. Monitor closely
10–20	Initial dose of 1.25–2.5 mg once a day. Monitor closely
<10	Initial dose of 1.25–2.5 mg once a day. Use with caution with continuous monitoring

Dose in patients undergoing renal replacement therapies

CAPD	Not dialysable. Dose as in GFR = <10 mL/min
HD	Low dialysability. Dose as in GFR = <10 mL/min
CAV/VVHD	Unknown dialysability. Dose as in GFR = 10–20 mL/min

Important drug interactions

CYCLOSPORIN

–

POTENTIALLY HAZARDOUS INTERACTIONS WITH OTHER DRUGS

- Analgesics: azapropazone, phenylbutazone and possibly other NSAIDs enhance effect
- Antibacterials: chloramphenicol, co-trimoxazole, 4-quinolones, sulphonamides and trimethoprim enhance effect
- Antifungals: fluconazole and miconazole increase glibenclamide plasma concentration
- Uricosurics: sulphinpyrazone enhances effect of glibenclamide

Administration

RECONSTITUTION

–

ROUTE

- Oral

RATE OF ADMINISTRATION

–

COMMENTS

- Take with breakfast

Other information

- The metabolites of glibenclamide are only weakly hypoglycaemic; this is not clinically relevant where renal and hepatic functions are normal. If creatinine clearance is <10 mL/min, accumulation of metabolite and unchanged drug in plasma may cause prolonged hyperglycaemia
- Company information states that use is contraindicated in serious renal impairment
- Compensatory excretion via bile in faeces occurs in renal impairment

Gliclazide

Clinical use

Non-insulin dependent diabetes mellitus

Dose in normal renal function

Initially 40–80 mg daily, adjusted according to response up to 160 mg as a single dose, with breakfast; higher doses divided.
Maximum 320 mg daily

Pharmacokinetics

Molecular weight (daltons)	323
% Protein binding	85–95
% Excreted unchanged in urine	<5
Volume of distribution (L/kg)	0.24
Half-life – normal/ESRF (hrs)	8–11/prolonged

Dose in renal impairment GFR (mL/min)

20–50	Initially 20–40 mg daily. Use with caution and monitor
10–20	Initially 20–40 mg daily. Use with caution and monitor
<10	Initially 20–40 mg daily. Use with great caution and monitor closely

Dose in patients undergoing renal replacement therapies

CAPD	Dialysability unlikely. Dose as in GFR = <10 mL/min
HD	Dialysability unlikely. Dose as in GFR = <10 mL/min
CAV/VVHD	Unknown dialysability. Dose as in GFR = 10–20 mL/min

Important drug interactions

CYCLOSPORIN

–

POTENTIALLY HAZARDOUS INTERACTIONS WITH OTHER DRUGS

• Analgesics: azapropazone, phenylbutazone and possibly other NSAIDs enhance effect
• Antibacterials: chloramphenicol, co-trimoxazole, 4-quinolones, sulphonamides and trimethoprim enhance effect
• Antifungals: fluconazole and miconazole increase gliclazide plasma concentration
• Uricosurics: sulphinpyrazone enhances effect

Administration

RECONSTITUTION

–

ROUTE

• Oral

RATE OF ADMINISTRATION

–

COMMENTS

–

Other information

• Care should be exercised in patients with hepatic and/or renal impairment and a small starting dose should be used with careful patient monitoring
• Manufacturer contraindicates prescribing of Diamicron in severe renal impairment, which they define as creatinine clearance below 40 mL/min

Glipizide

Clinical use

Non-insulin-dependent diabetes mellitus

Dose in normal renal function

Initially 2.5–5 mg daily, adjusted according to response; maximum 40 mg daily; up to 15 mg may be given as a single dose before breakfast; higher doses divided

Pharmacokinetics

Molecular weight (daltons)	445
% Protein binding	97
% Excreted unchanged in urine	4.5–7
Volume of distribution (L/kg)	0.13–0.16
Half-life – normal/ESRF (hrs)	3–7/–

Dose in renal impairment GFR (mL/min)

20–50	Initially 2.5 mg daily. Use with caution
10–20	Initially 2.5 mg daily. Use with caution
<10	Contraindicated

Dose in patients undergoing renal replacement therapies

CAPD	Dialysability insignificant. However, contraindicated if GFR <10 mL/min
HD	Dialysability insignificant. However, contraindicated if GFR <10 mL/min
CAV/VVHD	Dialysability insignificant. Dose as in GFR = 10–20 mL/min

Important drug interactions

CYCLOSPORIN

–

POTENTIALLY HAZARDOUS INTERACTIONS WITH OTHER DRUGS

- Azapropazone, phenylbutazone and possibly other NSAIDs enhance effect of sulphonylureas
- Antibacterials: chloramphenicol, co-trimoxazole, 4-quinolones, sulphonamides and trimethoprim enhance effect
- Antifungals (fluconazole and miconazole) increase glipizide plasma concentration
- Sulphinpyrazone enhances effect

Administration

RECONSTITUTION

–

ROUTE

- Oral

RATE OF ADMINISTRATION

–

COMMENTS

–

Other information

- Manufacturer does not recommend the use of Glibenese in patients with renal insufficiency
- Renal or hepatic insufficiency may cause elevated blood levels of glipizide with increased risk of serious hypoglycaemic reactions

Griseofulvin

Clinical use

Antifungal agent, used for dermatophyte infections
of the skin, scalp, hair and nails

Dose in normal renal function

500 mg daily, in divided doses or as a single dose;
in severe infection dose may be doubled

Pharmacokinetics

Molecular weight (daltons)	353
% Protein binding	84
% Excreted unchanged in urine	1
Volume of distribution (L/kg)	1.6
Half-life – normal/ESRF (hrs)	9.5–21/20

Dose in renal impairment GFR (mL/min)

20–50	Dose as in normal renal function
10–20	Dose as in normal renal function
<10	Dose as in normal renal function

Dose in patients undergoing renal replacement therapies

CAPD	Not dialysable. Dose as in normal renal function
HD	Not dialysable. Dose as in normal renal function
CAV/VVHD	Not dialysable. Dose as in normal renal function

Important drug interactions

CYCLOSPORIN

• Griseofulvin possibly reduces plasma cyclosporin
concentration (there are two reports of such an
interaction in the literature)

POTENTIALLY HAZARDOUS INTERACTIONS WITH
OTHER DRUGS

• Anticoagulants: metabolism of nicoumalone and
warfarin accelerated (reduced anticoagulant
effect)

• Metabolism of oral contraceptives accelerated
(reduced contraceptive effect)

Administration

RECONSTITUTION

–

ROUTE

• Oral

RATE OF ADMINISTRATION

–

COMMENTS

–

Other information

• Use with extreme caution in patients with
systemic lupus erythematosus

Haloperidol

Clinical use

Sedative in severe anxiety, intractable hiccup, nausea and vomiting, schizophrenia and other psychoses

Dose in normal renal function

Anxiety / hiccup:
1.5–3.0 mg 2–3 times daily
Nausea and vomiting:
0.5–2.0 mg daily
Schizophrenia:
1.5–5.0 mg 2–3 times daily, up to 120 mg daily in resistant cases

Pharmacokinetics

Molecular weight (daltons)	375.9
% Protein binding	90–92
% Excreted unchanged in urine	1
Volume of distribution (L/kg)	14–30
Half-life – normal/ESRF (hrs)	10–40/–

Dose in renal impairment GFR (mL/min)

20–50	Dose as in normal renal function
10–20	Dose as in normal renal function
<10	Start with lower doses. For single doses use 100% of normal dose. Avoid repeated dosage because of accumulation

Dose in patients undergoing renal replacement therapies

CAPD	Not dialysed. Dose as in GFR = <10 mL/min
HD	Not dialysed. Dose as in GFR = <10 mL/min
CAV/VVHD	Not dialysed. Dose as in normal renal function

Important drug interactions

CYCLOSPORIN

–

POTENTIALLY HAZARDOUS INTERACTIONS WITH OTHER DRUGS

• Anaesthetics: enhanced hypotensive effects
• Antidepressants: increased effect and side-effects
• Anti-epileptics: increased metabolism of haloperidol with carbamazepine; lowered seizure threshold
• Astemizole/terfenadine: increased risk of arrhythmias

Administration

RECONSTITUTION

–

ROUTE

• Oral, IM or IV (by slow bolus)

RATE OF ADMINISTRATION

–

COMMENTS

–

Other information

• May cause hypotension and excessive sedation
• Increased CNS sensitivity in renally impaired patients. Start with small doses – metabolites may accumulate
• Equivalent IV/IM dose = 40% of oral dose

Hydralazine

Clinical use

Vasodilator antihypertensive agent

Dose in normal renal function

Oral:

25–50 mg twice daily. Maximum daily dose 100 mg in slow acetylators and women, 200 mg in fast acetylators

IV:

slow IV injection: 5–10 mg over 20 min. Repeat after 20–30 min if necessary

infusion: 200–300 micrograms/min initially reducing to 50–150 micrograms/min

Pharmacokinetics

Molecular weight (daltons)	197
% Protein binding	87
% Excreted unchanged in urine	25
Volume of distribution (L/kg)	0.5–0.9
Half-life – normal/ESRF (hrs)	2–4.5/7–16

Dose in renal impairment GFR (mL/min)

20–50	Start with small dose and adjust in accordance with response
10–20	Start with small dose and adjust in accordance with response
<10	Start with small dose and adjust in accordance with response

Dose in patients undergoing renal replacement therapies

CAPD	Not dialysable. Dose as in GFR = <10 mL/min
HD	Not dialysable. Dose as in GFR = <10 mL/min
CAV/VVHD	Not dialysable. Dose as in GFR = 10–20 mL/min

Important drug interactions

CYCLOSPORIN

–

POTENTIALLY HAZARDOUS INTERACTIONS WITH OTHER DRUGS

• Anaesthetics: increased hypotensive effects

Administration

RECONSTITUTION

• 20 mg with 1 mL water for injection, then dilute with 10 mL sodium chloride 0.9% for IV injection or 500 mL sodium chloride 0.9% for IV infusion

ROUTE

• Oral, IV peripherally

RATE OF ADMINISTRATION

• As above

COMMENTS

–

Other information

• Avoid long-term use due to accumulation of metabolites in severe renal insufficiency and dialysis patients

Hydrocortisone acetate

Clinical use

Corticosteroid, used for local inflammation of joints and soft tissue

Dose in normal renal function

5–50 mg according to joint size

Pharmacokinetics

Molecular weight (daltons)	404.5
% Protein binding	>90
% Excreted unchanged in urine	0
Volume of distribution (L/kg)	0.4–0.7
Half-life – normal/ESRF (hrs)	1.5–2.0/–

Dose in renal impairment GFR (mL/min)

20–50	Dose as in normal renal function
10–20	Dose as in normal renal function
<10	Dose as in normal renal function

Dose in patients undergoing renal replacement therapies

CAPD	Low dialysability. Dose as in normal renal function
HD	Low dialysability. Dose as in normal renal function
CAV/VVHD	Low dialysability. Dose as in normal renal function

Important drug interactions

CYCLOSPORIN

–

POTENTIALLY HAZARDOUS INTERACTIONS WITH OTHER DRUGS

- Rifampicin: increased metabolism of hydrocortisone
- Anti-epileptics: increased metabolism of hydrocortisone

Administration

RECONSTITUTION

–

ROUTE

- Intra-articular, peri-articular

RATE OF ADMINISTRATION

–

COMMENTS

–

Other information

- Used for its local effects. Systemic absorption occurs slowly

Hydrocortisone sodium succinate

Clinical use

Corticosteroid, used as anti-inflammatory agent in respiratory, gastrointestinal and endocrine disorders and allergic states

Dose in normal renal function

100–500 mg 3–4 times in 24 hrs or as required

Pharmacokinetics

Molecular weight (daltons)	484.5
% Protein binding	90–95
% Excreted unchanged in urine	0
Volume of distribution (L/kg)	0.4–0.7
Half-life – normal/ESRF (hrs)	1.5–2/–

Dose in renal impairment GFR (mL/min)

20–50	Dose as in normal renal function
10–20	Dose as in normal renal function
<10	Dose as in normal renal function

Dose in patients undergoing renal replacement therapies

CAPD	Low dialysability. Dose as in normal renal function
HD	Low dialysability. Dose as in normal renal function
CAV/VVHD	Low dialysability. Dose as in normal renal function

Important drug interactions

CYCLOSPORIN

• Convulsions reported with concurrent use

POTENTIALLY HAZARDOUS INTERACTIONS WITH OTHER DRUGS

• Rifampicin accelerates metabolism of hydrocortisone
• Anti-epileptics: carbamazepine, phenobarbitone, phenytoin and primidone accelerate metabolism
• Amphotericin: increased risk of hypokalaemia

Administration

RECONSTITUTION

• IV injection, IM injection: add 2 mL of sterile water for injection
• IV infusion: add not more than 2 mL water for injection, then add to 100–1000 mL (not less than 100 mL) glucose 5% or sodium chloride 0.9%

ROUTE

• IV injection, IV infusion, IM

RATE OF ADMINISTRATION

• IV bolus: 2–3 min

COMMENTS

–

Other information

• Non-plasma-protein bound hydrocortisone is removed by HD
• One study has shown that plasma clearance rates of hydrocortisone during haemodialysis were 30–63% higher than after dialysis.
No recommendations exist to indicate that dosing should be altered to take account of this

Hydroxyurea

Clinical use

Antineoplastic agent

Dose in normal renal function

20–30 mg/kg daily, or 80 mg/kg every third day.
Consult local protocol

Pharmacokinetics

Molecular weight (daltons)	76
% Protein binding	Minimal
% Excreted unchanged in urine	35–50
Volume of distribution (L/kg)	0.5
Half-life – normal/ESRF (hrs)	2–6/–

Dose in renal impairment
GFR (mL/min)

20–50	100% of normal dose and titrate to response
10–20	50% of normal dose and titrate to response
<10	20% of normal dose and titrate to response

Dose in patients undergoing renal replacement therapies

CAPD	Probably dialysed. Dose as in GFR = <10 mL/min
HD	Probably dialysed. Dose as in GFR = <10 mL/min
CAV/VVHD	Probably dialysed. Dose as in GFR = 10–20 mL/min

Important drug interactions

CYCLOSPORIN

–

POTENTIALLY HAZARDOUS INTERACTIONS WITH OTHER DRUGS

–

Administration

RECONSTITUTION

–

ROUTE

• Oral

RATE OF ADMINISTRATION

–

COMMENTS

–

Other information

• Full blood count, renal and hepatic function should be determined repeatedly during treatment

• Dosage should be based on the patient's actual or ideal weight, whichever is less

• Hydroxyurea has been associated with impairment of renal tubular function and accompanied by elevation in serum uric acid, BUN and creatinine levels

• The following formula can be used to determine the fraction of normal dose used for renally impaired patients:

Fraction of normal dose = (normal dose) x $\{[f (k_r-1)] + 1\}$

where f = fraction of the original dose excreted as active or toxic moiety (f = 0.35 for hydroxyurea); k_r = patient's creatinine clearance (mL/min) divided by 120 mL/min

• Administer with caution to patients with marked renal dysfunction; such patients may rapidly develop visual and auditory hallucinations and pronounced haematologic toxicity

Hydroxyzine

Clinical use

Antihistamine, used for pruritus

Dose in normal renal function

25 mg at night increasing as necessary to 3–4 times a day

Pharmacokinetics

Molecular weight (daltons)	448 (hydrochloride)
% Protein binding	–
% Excreted unchanged in urine	0
Volume of distribution (L/kg)	19.5
Half-life – normal/ESRF (hrs)	14–20/–

Dose in renal impairment GFR (mL/min)

20–50	Dose as in normal renal function
10–20	Start with small dose, e.g. 25 mg at night and increase to 2–3 times a day if necessary
<10	Start with small dose, e.g. 25 mg at night and increase to 2–3 times a day if necessary

Dose in patients undergoing renal replacement therapies

CAPD	Removal unlikely. Dose as in GFR = <10 mL/min
HD	Not dialysable. Dose as in GFR = <10 mL/min
CAV/VVHD	Not dialysable. Dose as in GFR = 10–20 mL/min

Important drug interactions

CYCLOSPORIN

–

POTENTIALLY HAZARDOUS INTERACTIONS WITH OTHER DRUGS

–

Administration

RECONSTITUTION

–

ROUTE

• Oral

RATE OF ADMINISTRATION

–

COMMENTS

–

Other information

• Increased possibility of side-effects, particularly drowsiness

Ibuprofen

Clinical use

NSAID, used for pain and inflammation in rheumatic disease and other musculoskeletal disorders

Dose in normal renal function

Adult: initially 1.2–1.8 g daily in 3–4 divided doses, after food. Maximum 2.4 g daily

Pharmacokinetics

Molecular weight (daltons)	206
% Protein binding	90–99
% Excreted unchanged in urine	<10
Volume of distribution (L/kg)	0.15–0.17
Half-life – normal/ESRF (hrs)	2–3.2/unchanged

Dose in renal impairment GFR (mL/min)

20–50	Dose as in normal renal function, but avoid long-term use in severe renal insufficiency and dialysis patients
10–20	Dose as in normal renal function, but avoid long-term use in severe renal insufficiency and dialysis patients
<10	Dose as in normal renal function, but only use if ESRD on dialysis

Dose in patients undergoing renal replacement therapies

CAPD	Not dialysable. Dose as in normal renal function
HD	Not dialysable. Dose as in normal renal function
CAV/VVHD	Not dialysable. Dose as in normal renal function

Important drug interactions

CYCLOSPORIN

• Increased risk of nephrotoxicity

POTENTIALLY HAZARDOUS INTERACTIONS WITH OTHER DRUGS

• Lithium: excretion reduced
• Cytotoxic agents: reduced excretion of methotrexate
• Anticoagulants: effects of warfarin and nicoumalone enhanced
• Antidiabetic agents: effects of sulphonylureas enhanced
• ACE inhibitors: antagonism of hypotensive effect; increased risk of renal damage and hyperkalaemia
• Anti-epileptic agents: effects of phenytoin enhanced

Administration

RECONSTITUTION

–

ROUTE

• Oral

RATE OF ADMINISTRATION

–

COMMENTS

–

Other information

• Inhibition of renal prostaglandin synthesis by NSAIDs may interfere with renal function, especially in the presence of existing renal disease. Avoid if possible; if not, check serum creatinine 48–72 hrs after starting NSAID. If raised, discontinue NSAID therapy
• Use normal doses in patients with ESRD on dialysis
• Use with caution in renal transplant recipients – can reduce intra-renal autocoid synthesis

Ifosfamide

Clinical use

Antineoplastic agent, used for tumours of lung, ovary, cervix, breast, testis and in soft tissue sarcoma

Dose in normal renal function

Usual total dose for each course is either 8–12 g/m², equally divided as single daily doses over 3–5 days, or 5–6 g/m² (maximum 10 g) given as a 24-hr infusion

Pharmacokinetics

Molecular weight (daltons)	261
% Protein binding	0
% Excreted unchanged in urine	15
Volume of distribution (L/kg)	0.4–0.64
Half-life – normal/ESRF (hrs)	4–10/–

Dose in renal impairment GFR (mL/min)

20–50	75% of normal dose
10–20	75% of normal dose
<10	50% of normal dose

Dose in patients undergoing renal replacement therapies

CAPD	Dialysed. Dose as in GFR = <10 mL/min. Following dose do not perform CAPD exchange for 12 hrs
HD	Dialysed. Dose as in GFR = <10 mL/min. Dose at minimum of 12 hrs before HD session
CAV/VVHD	Dialysed. Dose as in GFR = 10–20 mL/min

Important drug interactions

CYCLOSPORIN

–

POTENTIALLY HAZARDOUS INTERACTIONS WITH OTHER DRUGS

• Ifosfamide possibly enhances effect of warfarin

Administration

RECONSTITUTION

• Reconstitute 1-g vial with 12.5 mL water for injection. Reconstitute 2-g vial with 25 mL water for injection. The resultant solution of 8% ifosfamide should NOT be injected directly into the vein

ROUTE

• IV injection: dilute to less than a 4% solution
• IV infusion: dilute as detailed below

RATE OF ADMINISTRATION

• IV infusion: infuse in glucose 5% or sodium chloride 0.9% over 30–120 min; or inject directly into a fast-running infusion; or make up in 3 L of glucose 5% or sodium chloride 0.9%, each litre should be given over 8 hrs

COMMENTS

–

Other information

• Nephrotoxicity may occur with oliguria, raised uric acid, increased BUN and serum creatinine, and decreased creatinine clearance
• Ifosfamide is known to be more nephrotoxic than cyclophosphamide, hence greater caution is advised
• Data sheet contraindicates the use of ifosfamide if serum creatinine is >120 micromol/L
• If patient is anuric and on dialysis, neither the ifosfamide nor its metabolites nor mesna should appear in the urinary tract. The use of mesna may therefore be unnecessary, although this would be a clinical decision
• If the patient is passing urine, mesna should be given to prevent urothelial toxicity

Iloprost

Clinical use

Prostacyclin analogue for relief of pain, promotion of ulcer healing and limb salvage in patients with severe peripheral arterial ischaemia

Dose in normal renal function

Dose is adjusted according to individual tolerability within the range of 0.5–2.0 nanograms/kg/min over 6 hrs daily, or continuous infusions at a rate of 0.5–1.0 nanogram/kg/min

Pharmacokinetics

Molecular weight (daltons)	360.5
% Protein binding	≈60
% Excreted unchanged in urine	<5
Volume of distribution (L/kg)	0.7
Half-life – normal/ESRF (hrs)	0.3–0.5/–

Dose in renal impairment GFR (mL/min)

20–50	Dose as in normal renal function
10–20	Dose as in normal renal function
<10	Dose as in normal renal function

Dose in patients undergoing renal replacement therapies

CAPD	Unknown dialysability. Dose as in normal renal function
HD	Unknown dialysability. Dose as in normal renal function
CAV/VVHD	Unknown dialysability. Dose as in normal renal function

Important drug interactions

CYCLOSPORIN

–

POTENTIALLY HAZARDOUS INTERACTIONS WITH OTHER DRUGS

- Beta-blockers, ACE inhibitors, vasodilators: additive antihypertensive effect
- Heparin, warfarin: increased risk of bleeding as iloprost inhibits platelet aggregation
- NSAIDs, phosphodiesterase inhibitors: additive inhibition of platelet aggregation

Administration

RECONSTITUTION

- Dilute 0.1 mg with 500 mL sodium chloride 0.9% or glucose 5%. Final concentration = 0.2 micrograms iloprost/mL

ROUTE

- IV infusion via peripheral vein or central venous catheter

RATE OF ADMINISTRATION

- Infuse 0.1 mg over 6 hrs daily (see below)

COMMENTS

- Treatment should be started at an infusion rate of 10 mL/hr for 30 min, which corresponds to a dose of 0.5 nanograms/kg/min for a patient of 65 kg. Then increase the dose in steps of 10 mL/hr every 30 min up to a rate of 40 mL/hr (50 mL/hr if patient's body weight is more than 75 kg). Depending on the occurrence of side-effects, such as headache and nausea, or an undesired drop in BP, the infusion rate should be reduced until the tolerable dose is found. If side-effects are severe, the infusion should be interrupted. For the rest of the treatment period, therapy should be continued with the dose found to be tolerated in the first 2–3 days

Other information

- BP and heart rate must be measured at the start of the infusion and after every increase in dose
- Duration of treatment is up to 4 weeks. Shorter treatment periods (3–5 days) are often sufficient in Raynaud's phenomenon
- Iloprost infusions can also be used to control blood pressure during a scleroderma hypertensive crisis
- For fluid-restricted patients, dilute 0.1 mg iloprost with 50 mL sodium chloride 0.9% and run at a rate of 1–4 mL/hr
- Toxic by inhalation, contact with skin and if swallowed

Imipenem/cilastatin (Primaxin)

Clinical use

Antibacterial agent

Dose in normal renal function

Mild infection:

250 mg every 6 hrs

Moderate infection: 500 mg every 8 hrs

Severe, fully susceptible infection:

500 mg every 6 hrs

Severe pseudomonal infection or other less susceptible infection:

1 g every 6–8 hrs

Pharmacokinetics

Molecular weight (daltons)	imipenem: 317; cilastatin: 380
% Protein binding	imipenem: 13–21; cilastatin: 35
% Excreted unchanged in urine	imipenem: 20–70; cilastatin: 60–70
Volume of distribution (L/kg)	imipenem: 0.17–0.30; cilastatin: 0.22
Half-life – normal/ESRF (hrs)	imipenem: 1/4; cilastatin: 1/15–24

Dose in renal impairment GFR (mL/min)

20–50	500 mg–1 g every 8 hrs
10–20	500 mg–1 g every 12 hrs
<10	250 mg (or 3.5 mg/kg, whichever is lower) every 12 hrs

Dose in patients undergoing renal replacement therapies

CAPD	Dialysed. Dose as in GFR = <10 mL/min
HD	Dialysed. Dose as in GFR = <10 mL/min
CAV/VVHD	Dialysed. Dose as in GFR = 10–20 mL/min

Important drug interactions

CYCLOSPORIN

• Variable reports of increase/no change in cyclosporin levels and of neurotoxicity

POTENTIALLY HAZARDOUS INTERACTIONS WITH OTHER DRUGS

• Convulsions reported with concomitant administration of ganciclovir

Administration

RECONSTITUTION

• 250 mg with 50 mL, 500 mg with 100 mL sodium chloride 0.9% (in some units 500 mg with 50 mL)

ROUTE

• IV peripherally or centrally (500 mg/50 mL given centrally)

RATE OF ADMINISTRATION

• 250 or 500 mg dose over 20 min. 1 g over 40 min

COMMENTS

–

Other information

• Risk of adverse neurological effects, e.g. convulsions. Extreme caution required in patients with history of CNS disease
• Cilastatin can accumulate in patients with impaired renal function
• Sodium content 2.8 mmol/g
• Imipenem is administered with cilastatin to prevent metabolism of imipenem within the kidney
• Non-renal clearance in acute renal failure is less than in chronic renal failure
• Patients with GFR <5 mL/min should not receive drug unless HD is started within 48 hrs

Imipramine hydrochloride

Clinical use

Tricyclic antidepressant

Dose in normal renal function

25 mg up to 3 times daily increasing stepwise to 150–200 mg

Pharmacokinetics

Molecular weight (daltons)	317
% Protein binding	86–96
% Excreted unchanged in urine	<2
Volume of distribution (L/kg)	21
Half-life – normal/ESRF (hrs)	12–24/–

Dose in renal impairment GFR (mL/min)

20–50	Dose as in normal renal function
10–20	Dose as in normal renal function
<10	Dose as in normal renal function

Dose in patients undergoing renal replacement therapies

CAPD	Not dialysed. Dose as in normal renal function
HD	Not dialysed. Dose as in normal renal function
CAV/VVHD	Not dialysed. Dose as in normal renal function

Important drug interactions

CYCLOSPORIN

–

Potentially hazardous interactions with other drugs

- Alcohol: enhanced sedative effect
- Anti-arrhythmics: increased risk of ventricular arrhythmias
- Other antidepressants: CNS excitation and hypertension with MAOIs
- Anti-epileptics: convulsive threshold lowered
- Beta-blockers: increased risk of ventricular arrhythmias
- Antihistamines: increased antimuscarinic and sedative effects. Increased risk of ventricular arrhythmias
- Antihypertensives: enhanced hypotensive effect
- Antimalarials: increased risk of ventricular arrhythmias
- Sympathomimetics: hypertension and arrhythmias

Administration

RECONSTITUTION

–

ROUTE

- Oral

RATE OF ADMINISTRATION

–

COMMENTS

–

Other information

- Imipramine is metabolised to active metabolite desipramine, which has <1% urinary excretion

Indapamide

Clinical use

Essential hypertension

Dose in normal renal function

2.5–5 mg daily in the morning

Pharmacokinetics

Molecular weight (daltons)	375
% Protein binding	76–79
% Excreted unchanged in urine	<5
Volume of distribution (L/kg)	0.3–1.3
Half-life – normal/ESRF (hrs)	14–18/unchanged

Dose in renal impairment GFR (mL/min)

20–50	Dose as in normal renal function
10–20	Dose as in normal renal function
<10	Dose as in normal renal function

Dose in patients undergoing renal replacement therapies

CAPD	Not dialysable. Dose as in normal renal function
HD	Not dialysable. Dose as in normal renal function
CAV/VVHD	Not dialysable. Dose as in normal renal function

Important drug interactions

CYCLOSPORIN

–

POTENTIALLY HAZARDOUS INTERACTIONS WITH OTHER DRUGS

- Anti-arrhythmics: hypokalaemia leads to increased cardiac toxicity
- Antihistamines: increased risk of cardiac arrhythmias
- Antihypertensives: increased risk of hypokalaemia
- Antimalarials: increased risk of cardiac arrhythmias
- Cardiac glycosides: risk of hypokalaemia
- Lithium: increased lithium levels

Administration

RECONSTITUTION

–

ROUTE

- Oral

RATE OF ADMINISTRATION

–

COMMENTS

–

Other information

- If pre-existing renal insufficiency is aggravated, stop indapamide
- Doses greater than 2.5 mg daily are not recommended
- Caution is needed if hypokalaemia develops
- Ineffective in ESRF
- Studies in functionally anephric patients for 1 month undergoing chronic haemodialysis have not shown evidence of drug accumulation, despite the fact that indapamide is not dialysable

Insulin, soluble (Actrapid or Humulin S)

Clinical use

Emergency management of hyperkalaemia; hyperglycaemia; control of diabetes mellitus

Dose in normal renal function

Variable

Pharmacokinetics

Molecular weight (daltons)	5808
% Protein binding	5
% Excreted unchanged in urine	0
Volume of distribution (L/kg)	0.15
Half-life – normal/ESRF (hrs)	2–4/13

Dose in renal impairment GFR (mL/min)

20–50	Variable
10–20	Variable
<10	Variable

Dose in patients undergoing renal replacement therapies

CAPD	Not dialysed. Dose according to clinical response
HD	Not dialysed. Dose according to clinical response
CAV/VVHD	Not dialysed. Dose according to clinical response

Important drug interactions

CYCLOSPORIN

–

POTENTIALLY HAZARDOUS INTERACTIONS WITH OTHER DRUGS

–

Administration

RECONSTITUTION

• Add 25 iu insulin to 50 mL 50% glucose

ROUTE

• IV via CRIP

RATE OF ADMINISTRATION

• Over 30 min

COMMENTS

• Continue infusing insulin/glucose solution at rate of 10 mL/hr according to serum potassium
• Add 50 iu insulin to 500 mL 10% glucose and adjust rate according to blood glucose levels

Other information

• Monitor blood glucose
• Prior to insulin/glucose infusion, give IV 20 mL 10% calcium gluconate to protect myocardium and 50–100 mL 8.4% sodium bicarbonate to correct acidosis
• Commence calcium resonium 15 g 4 times a day orally
• Insulin is metabolised renally, therefore requirements are reduced in ESRF

Ipratropium bromide

Clinical use

Anticholinergic bronchodilator, used for reversible airways obstruction, particularly in chronic bronchitics

Dose in normal renal function

Depends on presentation used: nebuliser solution – 100–500 micrograms up to 4 times daily

Pharmacokinetics

Molecular weight (daltons)	430
% Protein binding	–
% Excreted unchanged in urine	2.8
Volume of distribution (L/kg)	4.6
Half-life – normal/ESRF (hrs)	1.6–3.8/–

Dose in renal impairment GFR (mL/min)

20–50	Dose as in normal renal function
10–20	Dose as in normal renal function
<10	Dose as in normal renal function

Dose in patients undergoing renal replacement therapies

CAPD	Unknown dialysability. Dose as in normal renal function
HD	Unknown dialysability. Dose as in normal renal function
CAV/VVHD	Unknown dialysability. Dose as in normal renal function

Important drug interactions

CYCLOSPORIN

–

POTENTIALLY HAZARDOUS INTERACTIONS WITH OTHER DRUGS

–

Administration

RECONSTITUTION

• Nebuliser: the dose of nebuliser solution may need to be diluted in order to obtain a final volume suitable for the nebuliser. Sterile sodium chloride 0.9% should be used if dilution is required

ROUTE

• Inhaled

RATE OF ADMINISTRATION

• Nebuliser: according to nebuliser

COMMENTS

–

Other information

• Following inhalation, only a small amount of ipratropium reaches the systemic circulation. Any swallowed drug is poorly absorbed from the gastrointestinal tract

Iron dextran 5% solution (unlicensed product)

Clinical use

Prophylaxis (when oral treatment is not effective or contraindicated) or treatment of iron deficiency during epoetin therapy especially if serum ferritin is very low (<50 nanograms/mL)

Dose in normal renal function

Dose of iron dextran as mL 5% solution (women) = [0.0476 x w x (T–H)] + 6

Dose of iron dextran as mL 5% solution (men) = [0.0476 x w x (T–H)] + 14

where w = patient weight in kg (or ideal body weight if obese) and H is the haemoglobin level in g/dL and T = target haemoglobin level (11 g/dL for renal patients as a guide)

A test dose is essential. Give 0.5 mL diluted with 4–5 mL of patient's blood slowly and observe for 30 min for anaphylaxis. Have resuscitative equipment and drugs at hand (adrenaline, chlorpheniramine and hydrocortisone)

Pharmacokinetics

Molecular weight (daltons)	73 000
% Protein binding	0
% Excreted unchanged in urine	<1
Volume of distribution (L/kg)	0.031–0.055
Half-life – normal/ESRF (hrs)	36–72/–

Dose in renal impairment GFR (mL/min)

20–50	Dose as in normal renal function
10–20	Dose as in normal renal function
<10	Dose as in normal renal function

Dose in patients undergoing renal replacement therapies

CAPD	Not dialysed. Dose as in normal renal function
HD	Not dialysed. Dose as in normal renal function
CAV/VVHD	Not dialysed. Dose as in normal renal function

Important drug interactions

CYCLOSPORIN

–

POTENTIALLY HAZARDOUS INTERACTIONS WITH OTHER DRUGS

–

Administration

RECONSTITUTION

–

ROUTE

• IV peripherally

RATE OF ADMINISTRATION

• 1 mL/min

COMMENTS

• Keep under strict supervision during and for 1 hr after infusion

Other information

• Do not give to patients with history of asthma

• If patients with a history of allergy must be given iron dextran, give adequate antihistamine cover prior to administration

• Providing the patient can tolerate iron dextran (test dose), give the total dose required at a rate of 1 mL/min. Keep under strict supervision during infusion and for 1 hr after

• There is less thrombophlebitis if it is diluted in sodium chloride 0.9%

• The dose of iron dextran varies widely from 100 mg per dialysis session for 6–10 sessions, to single doses of 500 mg to 1 g

• The majority of renal units in the UK use iron saccharate, as it is associated with a lower incidence of side-effects compared with iron dextran

Isoniazid

Clinical use

Antibacterial agent, used for treatment and prophylaxis of tuberculosis in 'at risk' immunocompromised patients

Dose in normal renal function

300 mg daily

Pharmacokinetics

Molecular weight (daltons)	137
% Protein binding	4–30
% Excreted unchanged in urine	5–30
Volume of distribution (L/kg)	0.75
Half-life – normal/ESRF (hrs)	0.7–4/8–17 (depends on acetylator status)

Dose in renal impairment GFR (mL/min)

20–50	300 mg daily
10–20	300 mg daily
<10	200–300 mg daily

Dose in patients undergoing renal replacement therapies

CAPD	Dialysed. Dose as in GFR = <10 mL/min
HD	Dialysed. Dose as in GFR = <10 mL/min. Give dose post-dialysis
CAV/VVHD	Probably dialysed. Dose as in normal renal function

Important drug interactions

CYCLOSPORIN

–

POTENTIALLY HAZARDOUS INTERACTIONS WITH OTHER DRUGS

• Anti-epileptics: metabolism of carbamazepine, ethosuximide and phenytoin inhibited (enhanced effect); also with carbamazepine, isoniazid hepatotoxicity possibly increased

Administration

RECONSTITUTION

• Dilute with water for injection

ROUTE

• Oral, IM, IV, intrapleural or intrathecal

RATE OF ADMINISTRATION

• Not critical. Give by IV infusion or by slow bolus over 1–2 hrs

COMMENTS

–

Other information

• Adjust dose accordingly if hepatic illness, slow/fast acetylator status identified
• Pyridoxine HCl 10 mg daily has been recommended for prophylaxis of peripheral neuritis

Isosorbide mononitrate

Clinical use

Vasodilator, used for treatment and prophylaxis of angina. Adjunct in congestive heart failure

Dose in normal renal function

20–120 mg daily in divided doses

Pharmacokinetics

Molecular weight (daltons)	191
% Protein binding	72
% Excreted unchanged in urine	10–20
Volume of distribution (L/kg)	1.5–4
Half-life – normal/ESRF (hrs)	0.15–0.5/4

Dose in renal impairment GFR (mL/min)

20–50	Dose as in normal renal function
10–20	Dose as in normal renal function
<10	Dose as in normal renal function

Dose in patients undergoing renal replacement therapies

CAPD	Not dialysed. Dose as in normal renal function
HD	Dialysed. Dose as in normal renal function. Dose after haemodialysis
CAV/VVHD	Probably dialysed. Dose as in normal renal function

Important drug interactions

CYCLOSPORIN

–

POTENTIALLY HAZARDOUS INTERACTIONS WITH OTHER DRUGS

–

Administration

RECONSTITUTION

–

ROUTE

• Oral

RATE OF ADMINISTRATION

–

COMMENTS

–

Other information

• Tolerance may develop. This may be minimised by having nitrate-'free' periods

Isosorbide dinitrate

Clinical use

Vasodilator, used for prophylaxis and treatment of angina and left ventricular failure

Dose in normal renal function

Sublingual:
5–10 mg
Oral:
angina, 30–120 mg daily in divided doses
IV: 2–10 mg/hr

Pharmacokinetics

Molecular weight (daltons)	236
% Protein binding	16–40
% Excreted unchanged in urine	<2
Volume of distribution (L/kg)	1.4–8.6
Half-life – normal/ESRF (hrs)	0.5–1/–

Dose in renal impairment GFR (mL/min)

20–50	Dose as in normal renal function
10–20	Dose as in normal renal function
<10	Dose as in normal renal function

Dose in patients undergoing renal replacement therapies

CAPD	Not dialysed. Dose as in normal renal function
HD	Not dialysed. Dose as in normal renal function
CAV/VVHD	Unknown dialysability. Dose as in normal renal function

Important drug interactions

CYCLOSPORIN

–

POTENTIALLY HAZARDOUS INTERACTIONS WITH OTHER DRUGS

–

Administration

RECONSTITUTION

• Dilute using sodium chloride 0.9% or glucose 5% to 1 mg/10 mL or 2 mg/10 mL. Final volume 500 mL

ROUTE

• Oral, S/L, IV infusion

RATE OF ADMINISTRATION

• 1 mg/10 mL; 60 mL/hr ≡ 6 mg/hr
• 2 mg/10 mL; 30 mL/hr ≡ 6 mg/hr

COMMENTS

• The use of PVC giving sets and containers should be avoided since significant losses of the active ingredient by absorption can occur

Other information

• Isosorbide dinitrate undergoes extensive first-pass metabolism, mainly in the liver. The major metabolites are isosorbide-2-mononitrate and isosorbide-5-mononitrate; both possess vasodilatory activity and may contribute to the activity of the parent compound. Both metabolites have longer half-lives than the parent compound

Isotretinoin

Clinical use

Treatment of nodulo-cystic and conglobate acne and severe acne which has failed to respond to an adequate course of systemic antibiotic

Dose in normal renal function

0.5 mg/kg daily in 1–2 divided doses initially. Range 0.1–1 mg/kg/day

Pharmacokinetics

Molecular weight (daltons)	300
% Protein binding	99.5
% Excreted unchanged in urine	50
Volume of distribution (L/kg)	1.5
Half-life – normal/ESRF (hrs)	10–20/–

Dose in renal impairment GFR (mL/min)

<50   Contraindicated. See 'Other information'

Dose in patients undergoing renal replacement therapies

CAPD	Not dialysed. Dose as in GFR = <50 mL/min
HD	Not dialysed. Dose as in GFR = <50 mL/min
CAV/VVHD	Not dialysed. Dose as in GFR = <50 mL/min

Important drug interactions

CYCLOSPORIN

–

POTENTIALLY HAZARDOUS INTERACTIONS WITH OTHER DRUGS

• Rare cases of benign intracranial hypertension have been reported after isotretinoin and after tetracyclines. Supplementary treatment with tetracyclines is therefore contraindicated

Administration

RECONSTITUTION

–

ROUTE

• Oral, topical (0.5% gel)

RATE OF ADMINISTRATION

–

COMMENTS

–

Other information

• Patients on haemodialysis have been treated successfully on 10–20 mg daily or 20 mg on alternate days
• Since the drug is highly protein bound, it is not expected to be significantly removed by dialysis

Ispaghula husk (Fybogel and Fybogel Orange)

Clinical use

Treatment of constipation and of patients requiring a high-fibre regimen

Dose in normal renal function

One sachet (3.5 g) in water twice daily

Pharmacokinetics

Molecular weight (daltons)	–
% Protein binding	0
% Excreted unchanged in urine	0
Volume of distribution (L/kg)	Not absorbed
Half-life – normal/ESRF (hrs)	Not absorbed

Dose in renal impairment GFR (mL/min)

20–50	Dose as in normal renal function
10–20	Dose as in normal renal function
<10	Dose as in normal renal function

Dose in patients undergoing renal replacement therapies

CAPD	Not dialysed. Dose as in normal renal function
HD	Not dialysed. Dose as in normal renal function
CAV/VVHD	Not dialysed. Dose as in normal renal function

Important drug interactions

CYCLOSPORIN

–

POTENTIALLY HAZARDOUS INTERACTIONS WITH OTHER DRUGS

–

Administration

RECONSTITUTION

–

ROUTE

• Oral

RATE OF ADMINISTRATION

–

COMMENTS

• Fybogel should be stirred into 150 mL water and taken as quickly as possible, preferably after meals
• Additional fluid intake should be maintained

Other information

• Fybogel is low in sodium and potassium, containing approximately 0.4 mmol sodium and 0.7 mmol potassium per sachet
• Fybogel is sugar- and gluten-free
• Fybogel contains aspartame (contributes to the phenylalanine intake and may affect control of phenylketonuria)
• Fluid restrictions for dialysis patients can render this treatment inappropriate

Ispaghula husk (Regulan)

Clinical use

Treatment of constipation and of patients requiring a high-fibre regimen

Dose in normal renal function

One sachet in water 1–3 times daily

Pharmacokinetics

Molecular weight (daltons)	–
% Protein binding	0
% Excreted unchanged in urine	0
Volume of distribution (L/kg)	Not absorbed
Half-life – normal/ESRF (hrs)	Not absorbed

Dose in renal impairment GFR (mL/min)

20–50	Dose as in normal renal function
10–20	Dose as in normal renal function
<10	Dose as in normal renal function

Dose in patients undergoing renal replacement therapies

CAPD	Not dialysed. Dose as in normal renal function
HD	Not dialysed. Dose as in normal renal function
CAV/VVHD	Not dialysed. Dose as in normal renal function

Important drug interactions

CYCLOSPORIN

–

POTENTIALLY HAZARDOUS INTERACTIONS WITH OTHER DRUGS

–

Administration

RECONSTITUTION

–

ROUTE

• Oral

RATE OF ADMINISTRATION

–

COMMENTS

• The measured dose of Regulan should be stirred into 150 mL cool water and taken immediately
• Additional fluid intake should be maintained

Other information

• Original flavour contains 3.6 g ispaghula husk BP, 0.23 mmol sodium, 6.4 mmol potassium, 3.5 kCal sucrose per sachet and is gluten-free
• Orange and lemon/lime flavours contain 3.4 g ispaghula husk BP, 0.3 mmol sodium, <1 mmol potassium per sachet and are gluten- and sugar-free. They also contain aspartame (contributes to the phenylalanine intake and may affect control of phenylketonuria)
• Fluid restrictions in dialysis patients can render this treatment inappropriate

Isradipine

Clinical use

Calcium-channel blocker, used for essential hypertension

Dose in normal renal function

Initially 2.5 mg twice daily, increased if necessary after 3–4 weeks to 5 mg twice daily

Pharmacokinetics

Molecular weight (daltons)	371
% Protein binding	95
% Excreted unchanged in urine	<5
Volume of distribution (L/kg)	3–4
Half-life – normal/ESRF (hrs)	1.9–4.8/10–11

Dose in renal impairment GFR (mL/min)

20–50	Dose as in normal renal function
10–20	Dose as in normal renal function
<10	Dose as in normal renal function

Dose in patients undergoing renal replacement therapies

CAPD	Not dialysed. Dose as in normal renal function
HD	Not dialysed. Dose as in normal renal function
CAV/VVHD	Not dialysed. Dose as in normal renal function

Important drug interactions

CYCLOSPORIN

–

POTENTIALLY HAZARDOUS INTERACTIONS WITH OTHER DRUGS

- Anaesthetics: isoflurane enhances hypotensive effect of isradipine
- Antibacterials: rifampicin possibly increases the metabolism of isradipine
- Anti-epileptics: effect of isradipine is reduced by carbamazepine, phenobarbitone, phenytoin and primidone
- Antihypertensives: enhanced hypotensive effect
- Ritonavir: possibly increased levels of isradipine
- Theophylline: possible increase in theophylline levels

Administration

RECONSTITUTION

–

ROUTE

- Oral

RATE OF ADMINISTRATION

–

COMMENTS

–

Other information

- In elderly patients, or where hepatic or renal function is impaired, initial dose should be 1.25 mg twice daily. Dose should be increased according to the requirements of the individual patient

Itraconazole

Clinical use

Antifungal agent

Dose in normal renal function

100–200 mg every 12–24 hrs according to indication

Pharmacokinetics

Molecular weight (daltons)	706
% Protein binding	99.8
% Excreted unchanged in urine	<0.03
Volume of distribution (L/kg)	10.7
Half-life – normal/ESRF (hrs)	20–25/25

Dose in renal impairment GFR (mL/min)

20–50	Dose as in normal renal function
10–20	Dose as in normal renal function
<10	Dose as in normal renal function

Dose in patients undergoing renal replacement therapies

CAPD	Not dialysed. Dose as in normal renal function
HD	Not dialysed. Dose as in normal renal function
CAV/VVHD	Not dialysed. Dose as in normal renal function

Important drug interactions

CYCLOSPORIN

• Metabolism of cyclosporin inhibited (increased plasma cyclosporin levels)

POTENTIALLY HAZARDOUS INTERACTIONS WITH OTHER DRUGS

• Antibacterials: rifampicin accelerates metabolism of itraconazole
• Anticoagulants: effect of warfarin and nicoumalone enhanced
• Anti-epileptics: plasma concentrations of itraconazole reduced by phenytoin
• Antihistamines: itraconazole inhibits astemizole and terfenadine metabolism (avoid concomitant use – cardiac toxicity reported)
• Anxiolytics and hypnotics: plasma concentration of midazolam increased by itraconazole
• Cardiac glycosides: plasma concentrations of digoxin increased
• Cisapride: risk of ventricular arrhythmias – avoid
• Lipid-lowering drugs: itraconazole increases risk of myopathy with simvastatin – avoid

Administration

RECONSTITUTION

–

ROUTE

• Oral

RATE OF ADMINISTRATION

–

COMMENTS

–

Other information

• The oral bioavailability of itraconazole may be lower in some patients with renal insufficiency, e.g. those receiving CAPD. Monitoring of itraconazole plasma levels and dose adaptation are advisable. Manufacturer offers no guidelines for dose alteration
• Manufacturer advises no dose alterations required in renal impairment as the drug is extensively metabolised in the liver and pharmacokinetics are unchanged in patients with ESRF compared to normal

Ketoprofen

Clinical use

NSAID, used for pain and mild inflammation in rheumatic disease and other musculoskeletal disorders; acute gout, dysmenorrhoea

Dose in normal renal function

100–200 mg daily in 2–4 divided doses

Pharmacokinetics

Molecular weight (daltons)	254
% Protein binding	94–99
% Excreted unchanged in urine	<1
Volume of distribution (L/kg)	0.11
Half-life– normal/ESRF (hrs)	1.5–4/unchanged

Dose in renal impairment GFR (mL/min)

20–50	Dose as in normal renal function, but avoid if possible
10–20	Dose as in normal renal function, but avoid if possible
<10	Dose as in normal renal function, but only use if ESRD on dialysis

Dose in patients undergoing renal replacement therapies

CAPD	Unlikely to be dialysed. Dose as in GFR = <10 mL/min
HD	Unlikely to be dialysed. Dose as in GFR = <10 mL/min
CAV/VVHD	Unlikely to be dialysed. Dose as in GFR = 10–20 mL/min

Important drug interactions

CYCLOSPORIN

• Increased risk of nephrotoxicity

POTENTIALLY HAZARDOUS INTERACTIONS WITH OTHER DRUGS

• ACE inhibitors: antagonism of hypotensive effect. Increased risk of renal damage and hyperkalaemia
• Anticoagulants: effects of warfarin and nicoumalone enhanced
• Antidiabetics: effects of sulphonylureas enhanced
• Methotrexate: excretion reduced
• Lithium: excretion reduced

Administration

RECONSTITUTION

–

ROUTE

• Oral, IM, rectal. The injection must not be given by the IV route

RATE OF ADMINISTRATION

–

COMMENTS

• IM: maximum 200 mg in 24 hrs. Injection should not be used for longer than 3 days. Dose 50–100 mg every 4 hrs (see maximum). Administer by deep IM injection into the upper, outer quadrant of the buttock

Other information

• Combined oral and rectal treatment, maximum total daily dose 200 mg
• Inhibition of renal prostaglandin synthesis by NSAIDs may interfere with renal function, especially in the presence of existing renal disease. Avoid if possible; if not, check serum creatinine 48–72 hrs after starting NSAID. If raised, discontinue NSAID therapy
• Use normal doses in patients with ESRD on dialysis
• Use with caution in renal transplant recipients – can reduce intra-renal autocoid synthesis
• NSAIDs decrease platelet aggregation
• Associated with nephrotic syndrome, interstitial nephritis, hyperkalaemia and sodium retention

Ketorolac

Clinical use

Short-term management of moderate-to-severe acute post-operative pain

Dose in normal renal function

Post-operative:

Oral:

10 mg every 4–6 hrs (elderly patients every 6–8 hrs). Maximum 40 mg daily; maximum duration 7 days

IM/IV:

initially 10 mg, then 10–30 mg every 4–6 hrs prn (every 2 hrs in initial post-operative period). Maximum 90 mg daily (elderly patients and patients less than 50 kg: maximum 60 mg daily). Maximum duration 2 days

Pharmacokinetics

Molecular weight (daltons)	376
% Protein binding	>99
% Excreted unchanged in urine	5–10
Volume of distribution (L/kg)	0.13–0.25
Half-life – normal/ESRF (hrs)	IM dose: 3.5–9.2/5.9–19.2

Dose in renal impairment GFR (mL/min)

20–50	Maximum 60 mg daily
10–20	Avoid if possible. Use small doses and monitor closely
<10	Avoid if possible. Use small doses and monitor closely

Dose in patients undergoing renal replacement therapies

CAPD	Unlikely to be dialysed. Dose as in GFR = <10 mL/min
HD	Unlikely to be dialysed. Dose as in GFR = <10 mL/min
CAV/VVHD	Unknown dialysability. Dose as in GFR = 10–20 mL/min

Important drug interactions

CYCLOSPORIN

• Increased risk of nephrotoxicity

POTENTIALLY HAZARDOUS INTERACTIONS WITH OTHER DRUGS

• ACE inhibitors: increased risk of renal damage and increased risk of hyperkalaemia, antagonism of hypotensive effect
• Other NSAIDs: avoid concomitant administration of two or more NSAIDs
• Anticoagulants: effect of warfarin and nicoumalone possibly enhanced, increased risk of haemorrhage with parenteral ketorolac
• Antidiabetics: effects of sulphonylureas possibly enhanced
• Methotrexate: excretion of methotraxate reduced
• Lithium: excretion of lithium reduced (avoid concomitant use)
• Probenecid: delays excretion of ketorolac
• Oxpentifylline: risk of ketorolac-associated bleeding increased
• Anti-epileptics: effect of phenytoin possibly enhanced

Administration

RECONSTITUTION

• Compatible with sodium chloride 0.9%, glucose 5%, Ringer's, lactated Ringer's or Plasma-Lyte solutions

ROUTE

• Oral, IM, IV – IV/IM preparation is not for epidural or spinal administration

RATE OF ADMINISTRATION

• IV: administer IV bolus over no less than 15 sec

COMMENTS

–

Other information

- Drugs that inhibit prostaglandin biosynthesis (including NSAIDs) have been reported to cause nephrotoxicity, including, but not limited to, glomerular nephritis, interstitial nephritis, renal papillary necrosis, nephrotic syndrome and acute renal failure. In patients with renal, cardiac or hepatic impairment, caution is required since the use of NSAIDs may result in deterioration of renal function

- Ketorolac and its metabolites are excreted primarily by the kidney

- Reported renal side-effects include increased urinary frequency, oliguria, acute renal failure, hyponatraemia, hyperkalaemia, haemolytic uraemic syndrome, flank pain (with or without haematuria), raised serum urea and creatinine, and interstitial nephritis

Labetalol

Clinical use

Beta-adrenoreceptor blocker, used for hypertensive crisis and hypertension

Dose in normal renal function

Oral:

100–800 mg 2–3 times daily. Usual dose 200 mg twice a day

IV:

15–120 mg/hr

Pharmacokinetics

Molecular weight (daltons)	365 (hydrochloride)
% Protein binding	50
% Excreted unchanged in urine	5
Volume of distribution (L/kg)	5.6
Half-life – normal/ESRF (hrs)	3–9/unchanged

Dose in renal impairment GFR (mL/min)

20–50	Dose as in normal renal function
10–20	Dose as in normal renal function
<10	Dose as in normal renal function

Dose in patients undergoing renal replacement therapies

CAPD	Not dialysed. Dose as in normal renal function
HD	Not dialysed. Dose as in normal renal function
CAV/VVHD	Probably not dialysed. Dose as in normal renal function

Important drug interactions

CYCLOSPORIN

–

POTENTIALLY HAZARDOUS INTERACTIONS WITH OTHER DRUGS

–

Administration

RECONSTITUTION

• 200 mg labetalol (40 mL) to 200 mL glucose 5%

ROUTE

• IV peripherally

RATE OF ADMINISTRATION

• 2 mg/min initially, then titrate according to response

COMMENTS

• *Bolus dosing in crisis*: 50 mg IV over 1 min. Repeat at 5-min intervals to maximum 200 mg

Other information

• No adverse effects on renal function
• No accumulation in renal impairment
• Hypoglycaemia can occur in dialysis patients

Lacidipine

Clinical use

Calcium-channel blocker, used for hypertension

Dose in normal renal function

Initially 2 mg as a single daily dose, increased after 3–4 weeks to 4 mg daily, then if necessary to 6 mg daily

Pharmacokinetics

Molecular weight (daltons)	456
% Protein binding	>95
% Excreted unchanged in urine	0
Volume of distribution (L/kg)	0.9–2.3
Half-life – normal/ESRF (hrs)	13–19/–

Dose in renal impairment GFR (mL/min)

20–50	Dose as in normal renal function
10–20	Dose as in normal renal function
<10	Dose as in normal renal function

Dose in patients undergoing renal replacement therapies

CAPD	Unknown dialysability. Dose as in normal renal function
HD	Unknown dialysability. Dose as in normal renal function
CAV/VVHD	Unknown dialysability. Dose as in normal renal function

Important drug interactions

CYCLOSPORIN

• 10 kidney transplant patients on cyclosporin, prednisolone and azathioprine were given 4 mg lacidipine daily. A very small increase in the trough serum levels (+6%) and AUC (+14%) of the cyclosporin occurred

POTENTIALLY HAZARDOUS INTERACTIONS WITH OTHER DRUGS

• Anaesthetics: isoflurane enhances hypotensive effect of lacidipine interactions
• Antihypertensives: enhanced hypotensive effect
• Anti-epileptics: effects decreased by carbamazepine, phenobarbitone, phenytoin and primidone
• Theophylline: effect of theophylline possibly enhanced

Administration

RECONSTITUTION

–

ROUTE

• Oral

RATE OF ADMINISTRATION

–

COMMENTS

–

Other information

–

Lactulose

Clinical use

Constipation, hepatic encephalopathy

Dose in normal renal function

Constipation:

15–30 mL twice daily

Hepatic encephalopathy:

30–50 mL 3 times daily adjusted to produce
2–3 soft stools daily

Pharmacokinetics

Molecular weight (daltons)	342
% Protein binding	–
% Excreted unchanged in urine	<3
Volume of distribution (L/kg)	N/A – not absorbed
Half-life – normal/ESRF (hrs)	–

Dose in renal impairment GFR (mL/min)

20–50	Dose as in normal renal function
10–20	Dose as in normal renal function
<10	Dose as in normal renal function

Dose in patients undergoing renal replacement therapies

CAPD	Not dialysed. Dose as in normal renal function
HD	Not dialysed. Dose as in normal renal function
CAV/VVHD	Not dialysed. Dose as in normal renal function

Important drug interactions

CYCLOSPORIN

–

POTENTIALLY HAZARDOUS INTERACTIONS WITH
OTHER DRUGS

–

Administration

RECONSTITUTION

–

ROUTE

• Oral

RATE OF ADMINISTRATION

–

COMMENTS

–

Other information

• May take up to 72 hrs to work
• Not significantly absorbed from gastrointestinal tract
• Safe for diabetics
• Osmotic and bulking effect

Lamotrigine

Clinical use

Monotherapy and adjunctive treatment of partial seizures and primary and secondary generalised tonic-clonic seizures

Dose in normal renal function

25–200 mg daily in divided doses, according to clinical indication. Maximum 500 mg daily

Pharmacokinetics

Molecular weight (daltons)	256
% Protein binding	55
% Excreted unchanged in urine	<10
Volume of distribution (L/kg)	0.92–1.22
Half-life – normal/ESRF (hrs)	24–35/50

Dose in renal impairment GFR (mL/min)

20–50	Caution. Start with low doses and monitor closely
10–20	Caution. Start with low doses and monitor closely
<10	Caution. Start with low doses and monitor closely

Dose in patients undergoing renal replacement therapies

CAPD	Unknown dialysability. Dose as in GFR = <10 mL/min
HD	Not efficiently removed. Dose as in GFR = <10 mL/min
CAV/VVHD	Unknown dialysability. Dose as in GFR = 10–20 mL/min

Important drug interactions

CYCLOSPORIN

–

POTENTIALLY HAZARDOUS INTERACTIONS WITH OTHER DRUGS

• Other anti-epileptics: concomitant administration of two or more anti-epileptics may enhance toxicity without a corresponding increase in anti-epileptic effect; moreover, interactions between individual anti-epileptics can complicate monitoring of treatment

Administration

RECONSTITUTION

–

ROUTE

• Oral

RATE OF ADMINISTRATION

–

COMMENTS

–

Other information

• There is no experience of treatment with lamotrigine of patients with renal failure. Pharmacokinetic studies using single doses in subjects with renal failure indicate that lamotrigine pharmacokinetics are little affected, but plasma concentrations of the major glucuronide metabolite increase almost 8-fold due to reduced renal clearance

• The 2-N-glucuronide is inactive and accounts for 75–90% of the drug metabolised present in the urine. Although the metabolite is inactive the consequences of accumulation are unknown; hence the manufacturer advises caution with the use of lamotrigine in renal impairment

• The half-life of lamotrigine is affected by other drugs, it is reduced to 14 hrs when given with enzyme-inducing drugs, e.g. carbamazepine and phenytoin, and is increased to approximately 70 hrs when co-administered with sodium valproate alone

Lansoprazole

Clinical use

Benign gastric ulcer, duodenal ulcer, duodenal ulcer or gastritis associated with *H. pylori*, reflux oesophagitis

Dose in normal renal function

15–30 mg daily in the morning; duration dependent on indication

Pharmacokinetics

Molecular weight (daltons)	369
% Protein binding	99.8
% Excreted unchanged in urine	0
Volume of distribution (L/kg)	16–32
Half-life – normal/ESRF (hrs)	1–2/unchanged

Dose in renal impairment GFR (mL/min)

20–50	Dose as in normal renal function
10–20	Dose as in normal renal function
<10	Dose as in normal renal function

Dose in patients undergoing renal replacement therapies

CAPD	Unknown dialysability. Dose as in normal renal function
HD	Not dialysed. Dose as in normal renal function
CAV/VVHD	Unknown dialysability, probably not removed. Dose as in normal renal function

Important drug interactions

CYCLOSPORIN

• Theoretically interaction unlikely – little information available

POTENTIALLY HAZARDOUS INTERACTIONS WITH OTHER DRUGS

–

Administration

RECONSTITUTION

–

ROUTE

• Oral

RATE OF ADMINISTRATION

–

COMMENTS

–

Other information

• Lansoprazole is metabolised substantially by the liver; no dose adjustment is necessary in renal impairment. The recommended dose should not be exceeded

Liothyronine (tri-iodothyronine)

Clinical use

Hypothyroidism

Dose in normal renal function

Oral:

20 micrograms daily increased to 60 micrograms in 2–3 divided doses

IV:

5–20 micrograms every 4–12 hrs, or 50 micrograms initially then 25 micrograms every 8 hrs reducing to 25 micrograms twice a day

Pharmacokinetics

Molecular weight (daltons)	651
% Protein binding	<99
% Excreted unchanged in urine	2.5
Volume of distribution (L/kg)	0.1–0.2
Half-life – normal/ESRF (hrs)	16–48/–

Dose in renal impairment GFR (mL/min)

<50   Dose as in normal renal function

Dose in patients undergoing renal replacement therapies

CAPD	Not dialysed. Dose as in normal renal function
HD	Not dialysed. Dose as in normal renal function
CAV/VVHD	Not dialysed. Dose as in normal renal function

Important drug interactions

CYCLOSPORIN

–

POTENTIALLY HAZARDOUS INTERACTIONS WITH OTHER DRUGS

• Anticoagulants: it is likely that the effect of nicoumalone, phenindione and warfarin is enhanced

Administration

RECONSTITUTION

• Dissolve with 1–2 mL water for injection

ROUTE

• IV

RATE OF ADMINISTRATION

• Slow bolus

COMMENTS

• Alkaline solution – may cause irritation if given IM

Other information

• Protein-losing states, such as nephrotic syndrome, will result in a decrease in total T3 and T4

• Thyroxine (T4) is the drug of choice in hypothyroidism, but T3 can be used due to its rapid onset of action

• Elderly patients should receive smaller initial doses

Lisinopril

Clinical use

Angiotensin-converting enzyme inhibitor, used for hypertension, congestive heart failure and following myocardial infarction in haemodynamically stable patients

Dose in normal renal function

Hypertension and congestive heart failure:

initially 2.5 mg daily; maintenance dose depends on indication, maximum 40 mg daily

Pharmacokinetics

Molecular weight (daltons)	441
% Protein binding	0–10
% Excreted unchanged in urine	80–90
Volume of distribution (L/kg)	1.3–1.5
Half-life – normal/ESRF (hrs)	11–12/40–50

Dose in renal impairment GFR (mL/min)

20–50	50–75% of the normal dose
10–20	50–75% of the normal dose and titrate according to response
<10	25–50% of the normal dose and titrate according to response

Dose in patients undergoing renal replacement therapies

CAPD	Unknown dialysability. Dose as in GFR = <10 mL/min. Adjust according to response
HD	Removed by dialysis. Dose as in GFR = <10 mL/min. Adjust according to response
CAV/VVHD	Unknown dialysability. Dose as in GFR = 10–20 mL/min. Adjust according to response

Important drug interactions

CYCLOSPORIN

• Increased risk of hyperkalaemia

POTENTIALLY HAZARDOUS INTERACTIONS WITH OTHER DRUGS

• Anaesthetics: enhanced hypotensive effect
• NSAIDs: antagonism of hypotensive effect; hyperkalaemia; increased risk of renal damage
• Diuretics: enhanced hypotensive effect; hyperkalaemia with potassium-sparing diuretics
• Epoetin: increased risk of hyperkalaemia
• Lithium: ACE inhibitors reduce excretion of lithium
• Potassium salts: increased risk of hyperkalaemia

Administration

RECONSTITUTION

–

ROUTE

• Oral

RATE OF ADMINISTRATION

–

COMMENTS

–

Other information

• Close monitoring of renal function during therapy is necessary in those with renal insufficiency
• Renal failure has been reported in association with ACE inhibitors, mainly in patients with severe congestive heart failure, renal artery stenosis or post renal transplant
• A high incidence of anaphylactoid reactions has been reported in patients dialysed with high-flux polyacrylonitrile membranes and treated concomitantly with an ACE inhibitor. This combination should therefore be avoided
• Hyperkalaemia and other side-effects are more common in patients with impaired renal function

Lithium carbonate

Clinical use

Treatment and prophylaxis of mania, manic-depressive illness and recurrent depression; aggressive or self-mutilating behaviour

Dose in normal renal function

See individual preparations. Adjust according to lithium plasma concentrations

Pharmacokinetics

Molecular weight (daltons)	74
% Protein binding	0
% Excreted unchanged in urine	95
Volume of distribution (L/kg)	0.5–0.9
Half-life – normal/ESRF (hrs)	14–28/40

Dose in renal impairment GFR (mL/min)

	Contraindicated in renal impairment
20–50	Avoid if possible or reduce dose and monitor plasma concentration carefully
10–20	Avoid if possible or reduce dose and monitor plasma concentration carefully
<10	Avoid if possible or reduce dose and monitor plasma concentration carefully

Dose in patients undergoing renal replacement therapies

CAPD	Dialysable in lithium intoxication. Dose as in GFR = <10 mL/min
HD	Dialysable in lithium intoxication. Dose as in GFR = <10 mL/min
CAV/VVHD	Unknown dialysability. Dose as in GFR = 10–20 mL/min

Important drug interactions

CYCLOSPORIN

–

POTENTIALLY HAZARDOUS INTERACTIONS WITH OTHER DRUGS

• ACE inhibitors: lithium excretion reduced
• NSAIDs: excretion of lithium reduced
• Antidepressants (SSRIs): increased risk of CNS effects
• Methyldopa: neurotoxicity may occur without increased plasma lithium levels
• Diuretics: lithium excretion reduced by loop diuretics, potassium-sparing diuretics and thiazides. Lithium excretion increased by acetazolamide
• Sumatriptan: increases risk of CNS toxicity

Administration

RECONSTITUTION

–

ROUTE

• Oral

RATE OF ADMINISTRATION

–

COMMENTS

• Different preparations vary widely in bioavailability; a change in the preparation used requires the same precautions as initiation of treatment

Other information

• Doses are adjusted to achieve plasma concentrations of 0.4–1.0 mmol Li^+ /L (lower end of range for maintenance therapy and elderly patients) on samples taken 12 hrs after the preceding dose
• Long-term treatment may result in permanent changes in kidney histology and impairment of renal function. High serum concentration of lithium, including episodes of acute lithium toxicity, may aggravate these changes. The minimum clinically effective dose of lithium should always be used
• Bennett suggests 25–50% of normal dose if GFR <10 mL/min and 50–75% of normal dose if GFR between 10–50 mL/min. Closely monitor lithium plasma concentrations
• Lithium generally should not be used in patients with severe renal disease because of increased risk of toxicity
• Dialysability: serum lithium concentrations rebound within 5–8 hrs post haemodialysis because of redistribution of the drug, often necessitating repeated courses of haemodialysis. Peritoneal dialysis is less effective at removing lithium and is only used if haemodialysis is not possible
• Up to ⅓ of patients on lithium may develop polyuria, usually due to lithium blocking the effect of ADH. This reaction is reversible on withdrawal of lithium therapy

Loperamide

Clinical use

Antidiarrhoeal agent

Dose in normal renal function

4 mg stat, then 2 mg after each loose stool, maximum 16 mg daily

Pharmacokinetics

Molecular weight (daltons)	514 (hydrochloride)
% Protein binding	80
% Excreted unchanged in urine	<10
Volume of distribution (L/kg)	–
Half-life – normal/ESRF (hrs)	7–15/–

Dose in renal impairment GFR (mL/min)

20–50	Dose as in normal renal function
10–20	Dose as in normal renal function
<10	Dose as in normal renal function

Dose in patients undergoing renal replacement therapies

CAPD	Probably not dialysable. Dose as in normal renal function
HD	Probably not dialysable. Dose as in normal renal function
CAV/VVHD	Probably not dialysable. Dose as in normal renal function

Important drug interactions

CYCLOSPORIN

–

POTENTIALLY HAZARDOUS INTERACTIONS WITH OTHER DRUGS

–

Administration

RECONSTITUTION

–

ROUTE

• Oral

RATE OF ADMINISTRATION

–

COMMENTS

–

Other information

–

Lorazepam

Clinical use

Benzodiazepine: short-term use in anxiety or insomnia; status epilepticus; peri-operative

Dose in normal renal function

Anxiety:

1–4 mg daily in divided doses

Insomnia associated with anxiety:

1–2 mg at bedtime

Pharmacokinetics

Molecular weight (daltons)	321
% Protein binding	85
% Excreted unchanged in urine	<5
Volume of distribution (L/kg)	0.9–1.3
Half-life – normal/ESRF (hrs)	5–10/32–70

Dose in renal impairment GFR (mL/min)

20–50	Dose as in normal renal function
10–20	Dose as in normal renal function
<10	Dose as in normal renal function

Dose in patients undergoing renal replacement therapies

CAPD	Unknown dialysability. Dose as in normal renal function
HD	Not dialysed. Dose as in normal renal function
CAV/VVHD	Unknown dialysability. Dose as in normal renal function

Important drug interactions

CYCLOSPORIN

–

POTENTIALLY HAZARDOUS INTERACTIONS WITH OTHER DRUGS

–

Administration

RECONSTITUTION

• Dilute 1:1 with sodium chloride 0.9% or water for injection

ROUTE

• Oral, IV, IM

RATE OF ADMINISTRATION

• Slow IV bolus

COMMENTS

• Onset of effect after IM injection is similar to oral administration
• IV route preferred to IM route

Other information

• Patients with impaired renal or hepatic function should be monitored frequently and have their dosage adjusted carefully according to response. Lower doses may be sufficient in these patients
• Lorazepam as intact drug is not removed by dialysis. The glucuronide metabolite is highly dialysable, but is pharmacologically inactive
• Increased CNS sensitivity in patients with renal impairment

Mefenamic acid

Clinical use

NSAID, used for mild to moderate rheumatic pain, dysmenorrhoea and menorrhagia

Dose in normal renal function

500 mg 3 times daily

Pharmacokinetics

Molecular weight (daltons)	241
% Protein binding	99
% Excreted unchanged in urine	<6
Volume of distribution (L/kg)	1.3
Half-life – normal/ESRF (hrs)	2–4/unchanged

Dose in renal impairment GFR (mL/min)

20–50	250–500 mg 3 times a day, but avoid if possible
10–20	250–500 mg 3 times a day, but avoid if possible
<10	250 mg 3 times a day, but only use if ESRD on dialysis

Dose in patients undergoing renal replacement therapies

CAPD	Unlikely to be dialysed. Dose as in GFR = <10 mL/min
HD	Not dialysed. Dose as in normal renal function
CAV/VVHD	Unlikely to be dialysed. Dose as in GFR = 10–20 mL/min

Important drug interactions

CYCLOSPORIN

• Increased risk of nephrotoxicity

POTENTIALLY HAZARDOUS INTERACTIONS WITH OTHER DRUGS

• ACE inhibitors: antagonism of hypotensive effect; increased risk of renal damage and hyperkalaemia
• Antidiabetic agents: effects of sulphonylureas enhanced
• Cytotoxic agents: reduced excretion of methotrexate
• Lithium: excretion reduced
• Anticoagulants: effects of warfarin and nicoumalone enhanced
• Anti-epileptic agents: effects of phenytoin enhanced

Administration

RECONSTITUTION

–

ROUTE

• Oral

RATE OF ADMINISTRATION

–

COMMENTS

–

Other information

• As with other prostaglandin inhibitors, allergic glomerulonephritis has occurred occasionally. There have also been reports of acute interstitial nephritis with haematuria and proteinuria and occasionally nephrotic syndrome
• Inhibition of renal prostaglandin synthesis by NSAIDs may interfere with renal function, especially in the presence of existing renal disease. Avoid use if possible; if not, check serum creatinine 48–72 hrs after starting NSAID. If raised, discontinue NSAID therapy
• Use normal doses in patients with ESRD on dialysis
• Use with caution in renal transplant recipients – can reduce intra-renal autocoid synthesis

Melphalan

Clinical use

Antineoplastic agent, used for myelomatosis, solid tumours and lymphoma

Dose in normal renal function

Orally:
150–300 micrograms/kg daily for 4–6 days, repeated after 4–8 weeks

IV administration:
16–200 mg/m^2 according to indication and local protocol

Pharmacokinetics

Molecular weight (daltons)	305
% Protein binding	90
% Excreted unchanged in urine	12
Volume of distribution (L/kg)	0.6–0.75
Half-life – normal/ESRF (hrs)	1.1–1.4/4–6

Dose in renal impairment GFR (mL/min)

20–50	See 'Other information'
10–20	See 'Other information'
<10	See 'Other information'

Dose in patients undergoing renal replacement therapies

CAPD	Unknown dialysability. Dose as in GFR = <10 mL/min
HD	Unknown dialysability. Dose as in GFR = <10 mL/min
CAV/VVHD	Unknown dialysability. Dose as in GFR = 10–20 mL/min

Important drug interactions

CYCLOSPORIN

• Increased risk of nephrotoxicity

POTENTIALLY HAZARDOUS INTERACTIONS WITH OTHER DRUGS

–

Administration

RECONSTITUTION

• Reconstitute with 10 mL of diluent provided
• Further dilution with 0.9% sodium chloride

ROUTE

• Oral, IV

RATE OF ADMINISTRATION

• Inject slowly into a fast-running infusion solution or via an infusion bag

COMMENTS

–

Other information

• Melphalan clearance, although variable, is decreased in renal impairment

• Currently available pharmacokinetic data do not justify an absolute recommendation on dosage reduction when administering melphalan tablets to patients with renal impairment, but it may be prudent to use a reduced dosage initially until tolerance is established

• When melphalan injection is used at conventional IV dosage (8–40 mg/m^2 BSA), it is recommended that the initial dose should be reduced by 50% in patients with moderate to severe renal impairment and subsequent dosage determined by the degree of haematological suppression

• For high IV doses of melphalan (100–240 mg/m^2 BSA), the need for dose reduction depends on the degree of renal impairment, whether autologous bone marrow stem cells are reinfused and therapeutic need. High-dose melphalan is not recommended in patients with more severe renal impairment (EDTA clearance < 30 mL/min)

• It should be borne in mind that dose reduction of melphalan in renal impairment is somewhat arbitrary. At moderate doses, where melphalan is used as part of a combined regimen, dosage reductions of up to 50% may be appropriate. However, at high doses, e.g. conditioning for bone marrow transplant, there is a risk of underdosing the patient and not achieving the desired therapeutic effect, so the dose should be reduced with caution in these instances

• Adequate hydration and forced diuresis may be necessary in patients with poor renal function

• In myeloma patients with renal damage, temporary but significant increases in blood urea levels have been observed during melphalan therapy

Mercaptopurine

Clinical use

Antineoplastic agent, used for acute leukaemias

Dose in normal renal function

Usual dose is 2.5 mg/kg/day, but the dose and duration of administration depend on the nature and dosage of other cytotoxic agents given in conjunction with mercaptopurine

Pharmacokinetics

Molecular weight (daltons)	170
% Protein binding	20
% Excreted unchanged in urine	8–21
Volume of distribution (L/kg)	0.1–1.7
Half-life – normal/ESRF (hrs)	0.9–1.5/–

Dose in renal impairment GFR (mL/min)

20–50	Caution – reduce dose. See 'Other information'
10–20	Caution – reduce dose. See 'Other information'
<10	Caution – reduce dose. See 'Other information'

Dose in patients undergoing renal replacement therapies

CAPD	Unknown dialysability. Dose as in GFR = <10 mL/min
HD	Not dialysable. Dose as in GFR = <10 mL/min
CAV/VVHD	Unknown dialysability. Dose as in GFR = 10–20 mL/min

Important drug interactions

CYCLOSPORIN

–

POTENTIALLY HAZARDOUS INTERACTIONS WITH OTHER DRUGS

• Allopurinol: decreases rate of catabolism of mercaptopurine – reduce dose of mercaptopurine to ¼ of normal dose

Administration

RECONSTITUTION

–

ROUTE

• Oral

RATE OF ADMINISTRATION

–

COMMENTS

–

Other information

• Mercaptopurine is extensively metabolised and excreted via the kidneys, and the active metabolites have a longer half-life than the parent drug. Manufacturer recommends consideration be given to reducing the dose in patients with impaired hepatic or renal function, although no specific dosing guidelines are available

• A recent study on anti-cancer drug renal toxicity and elimination concluded that the dose of 6-mercaptopurine does not require modification in patients with decreased renal function (except in conjunction with allopurinol). This study also gives % excreted unchanged in urine as 21% (*Cancer Treatment Reviews* (1995) **21**: 33–64)

Mesalazine

Clinical use

Induction and maintenance of remission in ulcerative colitis

Dose in normal renal function

Acute attack:

1.5–4.0 g daily in divided doses

Maintenance:

750 mg–1.5 g daily in divided doses

Pharmacokinetics

Molecular weight (daltons)	153
% Protein binding	40–50
% Excreted unchanged in urine	–
Volume of distribution (L/kg)	–
Half-life – normal/ESRF (hrs)	1.0/–

Dose in renal impairment GFR (mL/min)

20–50   Caution – use only if necessary. Start with low dose and increase according to response

10–20   Caution – use only if necessary. Start with low dose and monitor closely

<10   Caution – use only if necessary. Start with low dose and monitor closely

Dose in patients undergoing renal replacement therapies

CAPD	Unknown dialysability. Dose as in GFR = <10 mL/min
HD	Unknown dialysability. Dose as in GFR = <10 mL/min
CAV/VVHD	Unknown dialysability. Dose as in GFR = 10–20 mL/min

Important drug interactions

CYCLOSPORIN

–

POTENTIALLY HAZARDOUS INTERACTIONS WITH OTHER DRUGS

–

Administration

RECONSTITUTION

–

ROUTE

• Oral, PR

RATE OF ADMINISTRATION

–

COMMENTS

–

Other information

• Mesalazine is excreted rapidly by the kidney, mainly as its metabolite N-acetyl-5-aminosalicylic acid. Nephrotoxicity has been reported

• Mesalazine is best avoided in patients with established renal impairment, but if necessary should be used with caution and the patient carefully monitored

Mesna

Clinical use

Prophylaxis of urothelial toxicity in patients treated with ifosfamide or cyclophosphamide

Dose in normal renal function

Dose and timing depend on cytotoxic agent and on route of administration of mesna

Pharmacokinetics

Molecular weight (daltons)	164
% Protein binding	<10
% Excreted unchanged in urine	16–32
Volume of distribution (L/kg)	0.65
Half-life – normal/ESRF (hrs)	0.25–0.5/–

Dose in renal impairment GFR (mL/min)

20–50	See 'Other information'
10–20	–
<10	–

Dose in patients undergoing renal replacement therapies

CAPD	Unknown dialysability. Dose as in GFR = <10 mL/min
HD	Probably dialysed. Dose as in GFR = <10 mL/min
CAV/VVHD	Unknown dialysability. Dose as in GFR = 10–20 mL/min

Important drug interactions

CYCLOSPORIN

–

POTENTIALLY HAZARDOUS INTERACTIONS WITH OTHER DRUGS

–

Administration

RECONSTITUTION

• Compatible with sodium chloride 0.9%

ROUTE

• Oral, IV bolus, IV infusion

RATE OF ADMINISTRATION

• IV bolus: over 15–30 min
• IV infusion: over 12–24 hrs

COMMENTS

• Mesna injection can be administered orally in orange juice or cola to improve palatability

Other information

• Urinary output should be maintained at 100 mL/hr (as required for oxazaphosphorine treatment)
• The dose of mesna is dependent on the dose of oxazaphosphorine, e.g. reduce dose of cyclophosphamide to 50% normal dose if GFR <10 mL/min, hence dose of mesna will consequently be reduced
• From what is known about the pharmacokinetics and mechanism of action of mesna, its availability in the urinary tract depends on renal function
• In the case of completely anuric patients (extremely rare), neither cyclophosphamide nor its metabolites should appear in the urinary tract; the use of mesna concomitantly may therefore be unnecessary in anuric patients. If there is any risk of cyclophosphamide or its metabolites entering the urinary tract, mesna should probably be given to prevent urothelial toxicity
• Limited kinetic information would suggest that mesna would be eliminated by haemodialysis

Methadone hydrochloride

Clinical use

Treatment of opioid drug addiction; analgesic for moderate to severe pain

Dose in normal renal function

Opioid addiction:

10–20 mg daily increasing by 10–20 mg per day until there are no signs of withdrawal or intoxication. Reduce gradually

Analgesia:

5–10 mg every 6–8 hrs

Pharmacokinetics

Molecular weight (daltons)	346
% Protein binding	60–90
% Excreted unchanged in urine	33
Volume of distribution (L/kg)	3–6
Half-life – normal/ESRF (hrs)	13–58/–

Dose in renal impairment GFR (mL/min)

20–50	Dose as in normal renal function
10–20	Dose as in normal renal function
<10	50% of normal dose. Titrate according to response

Dose in patients undergoing renal replacement therapies

CAPD	Insignificant amount removed. Dose as in GFR = <10 mL/min
HD	Insignificant amount removed. Dose as in GFR = <10 mL/min
CAV/VVHD	Unknown dialysability. Dose as in normal renal function

Important drug interactions

CYCLOSPORIN

–

POTENTIALLY HAZARDOUS INTERACTIONS WITH OTHER DRUGS

- MAOIs: possible CNS excitation or depression
- Antivirals: methadone possibly increases plasma concentration of zidovudine
- Dopaminergics: hyperpyrexia and CNS toxicity reported with selegiline and opioids

Administration

RECONSTITUTION

–

ROUTE

- Oral, IM, SC

RATE OF ADMINISTRATION

–

COMMENTS

- Methadone is probably not suitable for use as an analgesic for patients with severe renal impairment

Other information

- Overdosage with methadone can be reversed using naloxone

Methotrexate

Clinical use

Antineoplastic agent, used for neoplastic disease, severe uncontrolled psoriasis and severe rheumatoid arthritis

Dose in normal renal function

Rheumatoid arthritis:

5–10 mg per week

Psoriasis: 10–25 mg orally once weekly, adjusted to response

Neoplastic disease:

dose by weight or surface area according to specific indication

Pharmacokinetics

Molecular weight (daltons)	454
% Protein binding	45–60
% Excreted unchanged in urine	80–90
Volume of distribution (L/kg)	0.76–1.0
Half-life – normal/ESRF (hrs)	8–12/increased

Dose in renal impairment GFR (mL/min)

20–50	50–100% of normal dose
10–20	50% of normal dose
<10	Contraindicated

Dose in patients undergoing renal replacement therapies

CAPD	Not dialysed. Contraindicated
HD	Not dialysed. Haemodialysis clearance is 38–40 mL/min. Contraindicated
CAV/VVHD	Unknown dialysability. Dose as in GFR = 10–20 mL/min

Important drug interactions

CYCLOSPORIN

• Methotrexate may inhibit the clearance of cyclosporin or its metabolites

• Cyclosporin may inhibit methotrexate elimination

POTENTIALLY HAZARDOUS INTERACTIONS WITH OTHER DRUGS

• NSAIDs: increased risk of toxicity

• Antibacterials: antifolate effect increased with co-trimoxazole and trimethoprim. Penicillin reduces excretion of methotrexate – increased risk of toxicity

• Acitretin: plasma concentration of methotrexate increased

• Probenecid: excretion of methotrexate reduced

Administration

RECONSTITUTION

• Methotrexate compatible with glucose 5%, sodium chloride 0.9%, compound sodium lactate, or Ringer's solution

ROUTE

• Oral, IM, IV (bolus injection or infusion), intrathecal, intra-arterial, intraventricular

RATE OF ADMINISTRATION

• Slow IV injection

COMMENTS

• High-dose methotrexate may cause precipitation of methotrexate or its metabolites in renal tubules. A high fluid throughput and alkalinisation of urine, using sodium bicarbonate if necessary, is recommended

Other information

• Calcium folinate (calcium leucovorin) is a potent agent for neutralising the immediate toxic effects of methotrexate on the haematopoietic system. Calcium folinate rescue may begin 24, 32 or 36 hrs post start of methotrexate therapy, according to local protocol. Doses of up to 120 mg may be given over 12–24 hrs by IM or IV injection or infusion, followed by 12–15 mg IM, or 15 mg orally every 6 hrs for the next 48 hrs

• Renal function should be closely monitored throughout treatment

• An approximate correction for renal function may be made by reducing the dose in proportion to the reduction in creatinine clearance based on a normal Clcreat of 60 mL/min/m^2

Methyldopa

Clinical use

Hypertension

Dose in normal renal function

250–500 mg 3 times a day. Maximum daily dose 3g

Pharmacokinetics

Molecular weight (daltons)	238 (hydrate)
% Protein binding	10–20
% Excreted unchanged in urine	25–40
Volume of distribution (L/kg)	0.5
Half-life – normal/ESRF (hrs)	1.5–6/6–16

Dose in renal impairment GFR (mL/min)

20–50	250–500mg 3 times a day
10–20	250–500mg 2–3 times a day
<10	250–500mg once or twice a day

Dose in patients undergoing renal replacement therapies

CAPD	Dialysed. Dose as in GFR = <10 mL/min
HD	Dialysed. Dose as in GFR = <10 mL/min
CAV/VVHD	Probably dialysed. Dose as in GFR = 10–20 mL/min

Important drug interactions

CYCLOSPORIN

–

POTENTIALLY HAZARDOUS INTERACTIONS WITH OTHER DRUGS

- Anaesthetics: enhanced hypotensive effect
- Lithium: neurotoxicity (without increased plasma lithium concentrations)

Administration

RECONSTITUTION

- Add dose to 100 mL glucose 5%

ROUTE

- Oral/IV peripherally

RATE OF ADMINISTRATION

- 30 min

COMMENTS

–

Other information

- Active metabolites with long half-life
- Interferes with serum creatinine measurement
- Orthostatic hypotension more common in renally impaired patients

Methylprednisolone

Clinical use

Corticosteroid, used for suppression of inflammatory and allergic disorders. Immunosuppressant

Dose in normal renal function

Oral:

2–40 mg daily

IM/IV:

10–500 mg

Graft rejection:

up to 1 g daily for up to 3 days

Pharmacokinetics

Molecular weight (daltons)	375
% Protein binding	50–77
% Excreted unchanged in urine	2.6–7.2
Volume of distribution (L/kg)	1.0–1.5
Half-life – normal/ESRF (hrs)	1.9–6.0/unchanged

Dose in renal impairment GFR (mL/min)

20–50	Dose as in normal renal function
10–20	Dose as in normal renal function
<10	Dose as in normal renal function

Dose in patients undergoing renal replacement therapies

CAPD	Dialysed. Dose as in normal renal function
HD	Dialysed. Dose as in normal renal function, after haemodialysis
CAV/VVHD	Probably significant dialysability. Dose as in normal renal function

Important drug interactions

CYCLOSPORIN

• Levels of cyclosporin increased

POTENTIALLY HAZARDOUS INTERACTIONS WITH OTHER DRUGS

• Rifampicin accelerates metabolism
• Anti-epileptics: carbamazepine, phenobarbitone, phenytoin and primidone accelerate metabolism
• Antifungals: increased risk of hypokalaemia with amphotericin

Administration

RECONSTITUTION

• Use solvent supplied (Solu-medrone) or see manufacturer's recommendations

ROUTE

• IV peripherally or centrally

RATE OF ADMINISTRATION

• 30 min

COMMENTS

• Rapid bolus injection may be associated with arrhythmias or cardiovascular collapse

Other information

• A single dose of 1 g is often given at transplantation
• Three 1-g doses at 24-hr intervals are often used as first line for reversal of acute rejection episodes. (Some units use 300–500 mg daily for 3 days)
• Anecdotally possesses less mineralocorticoid activity than equipotent doses of prednisolone

Metoclopramide

Clinical use

Nausea and vomiting

Dose in normal renal function

10–20 mg 3–4 times daily. The use of
metoclopramide in patients under 20 years
should be restricted

Pharmacokinetics

Molecular weight (daltons)	354 (hydrochloride)
% Protein binding	40
% Excreted unchanged in urine	10–22
Volume of distribution (L/kg)	2–3.4
Half-life – normal/ESRF (hrs)	2.5–5.4/14–15

Dose in renal impairment GFR (mL/min)

20–50	Dose as in normal renal function
10–20	75% of normal dose 3–4 times daily
<10	50% of normal dose 3–4 times daily

Dose in patients undergoing renal replacement therapies

CAPD	Not dialysed. Dose as in GFR = <10 mL/min
HD	Dialysed. Dose as in GFR = <10 mL/min
CAV/VVHD	Probably not dialysed. Dose as in GFR = 10–20 mL/min

Important drug interactions

CYCLOSPORIN

• Increased cyclosporin blood levels

POTENTIALLY HAZARDOUS INTERACTIONS WITH
OTHER DRUGS

–

Administration

RECONSTITUTION

–

ROUTE

• Oral, IV, IM

RATE OF ADMINISTRATION

• 1–2 min

COMMENTS

–

Other information

• Increased risk of extrapyramidal reactions in
severe renal impairment

Metolazone

Clinical use

Hypertension, oedema. Acts synergistically with loop diuretics

Dose in normal renal function

Oedema:

5–10 mg increased to 20 mg daily. Maximum 80 mg daily

Hypertension:

5 mg initially. Maintenance 5 mg on alternate days

Pharmacokinetics

Molecular weight (daltons)	366
% Protein binding	95
% Excreted unchanged in urine	70
Volume of distribution (L/kg)	1.6
Half-life – normal/ESRF (hrs)	4–20/–

Dose in renal impairment GFR (mL/min)

20–50	Dose as in normal renal function
10–20	Dose as in normal renal function
<10	Dose as in normal renal function

Dose in patients undergoing renal replacement therapies

CAPD	Unknown dialysability. Dose as in normal renal function
HD	Not dialysed. Dose as in normal renal function
CAV/VVHD	Probably not dialysed. Dose as in normal renal function

Important drug interactions

CYCLOSPORIN

- Impaired renal function

POTENTIALLY HAZARDOUS INTERACTIONS WITH OTHER DRUGS

- Lithium excretion reduced
- Antihypertensives: enhanced hypotensive effect
- Antihistamines: hypokalaemia increases risk of ventricular arrhythmias with astemizole and terfenadine
- Cardiac glycosides: increased toxicity if hypokalaemia occurs

Administration

RECONSTITUTION

–

ROUTE

- Oral

RATE OF ADMINISTRATION

–

COMMENTS

–

Other information

- May result in profound diuresis. Monitor patient's fluid balance carefully
- Monitor for hypokalaemia
- In patients with creatinine clearance less than 50 mL/min there is no clinical evidence of accumulation

Metoprolol

Clinical use

Beta-adrenoreceptor blocker, used for
hypertension, angina and cardiac arrhythmias

Dose in normal renal function

Oral:
50–100 mg 2–3 times daily
IV:
5–15 mg

Pharmacokinetics

Molecular weight (daltons)	685 (tartrate)
% Protein binding	8–12
% Excreted unchanged in urine	5
Volume of distribution (L/kg)	5.5
Half-life – normal/ESRF (hrs)	3.5/2.5–4.5

Dose in renal impairment GFR (mL/min)

20–50	Dose as in normal renal function
10–20	Start with small doses/normal interval
<10	Start with small doses/normal interval

Dose in patients undergoing renal replacement therapies

CAPD	Not dialysed. Start with small doses
HD	Dialysed. Start with small doses
CAV/VVHD	Probably dialysed. Start with small doses and titrate in accordance with response

Important drug interactions

CYCLOSPORIN

–

POTENTIALLY HAZARDOUS INTERACTIONS WITH OTHER DRUGS

- Anaesthetics: enhance hypotensive effect
- Anti-arrhythmics: increased risk of myocardial depression and bradycardia. Amiodarone increased risk of bradycardia and AV block
- Antihypertensives: enhanced effect
- Calcium-channel blockers: increased risk of bradycardia and AV block with diltiazem. Care if used with nifedipine. Asystole, severe hypotension and heart failure with verapamil
- Sympathomimetics: severe hypertension, e.g. with adrenaline and noradrenaline. Severe hypertension also possible with sympathomimetics in anorectics and cough and cold remedies

Administration

RECONSTITUTION

–

ROUTE

- Oral, IV

RATE OF ADMINISTRATION

- For bolus injection 1–2 mg/min or by continuous infusion via CRIP

COMMENTS

- A total dose of 10–15 mg is usually sufficient

Other information

- Can cause hypoglycaemia in dialysis patients
- Almost all of the drug is excreted as inactive metabolites. Accumulation of the metabolites will occur in renal failure, but does not seem to cause any side-effects

Metronidazole

Clinical use

Antibiotic, used for anaerobic and protozoal infections

Dose in normal renal function

Oral:

200–400 mg every 8–12 hrs

IV:

500 mg every 8 hrs

PR:

1 g every 8–12 hrs

Pharmacokinetics

Molecular weight (daltons)	171
% Protein binding	20
% Excreted unchanged in urine	20
Volume of distribution (L/kg)	0.76–1.02
Half-life – normal/ESRF (hrs)	6–14/7–21

Dose in renal impairment GFR (mL/min)

20–50	Dose as in normal renal function
10–20	Dose as in normal renal function
<10	Normal dose every 12 hrs

Dose in patients undergoing renal replacement therapies

CAPD	Not dialysed. Dose as in GFR = <10 mL/min
HD	Dialysed. Dose as in normal renal function
CAV/VVHD	Unknown dialysability. Dose as in normal renal function

Important drug interactions

CYCLOSPORIN

• Raised blood level of cyclosporin

POTENTIALLY HAZARDOUS INTERACTIONS WITH OTHER DRUGS

• Effects of warfarin and nicoumalone enhanced
• Anti-epileptics: metabolism of phenytoin inhibited. Phenobarbitone accelerates metabolism of metronidazole
• Alcohol: disulfiram-like reaction

Administration

RECONSTITUTION

–

ROUTE

• Oral, PR, IV

RATE OF ADMINISTRATION

• IV: 5 mL/min, i.e. 500 mg over 20 min

COMMENTS

–

Other information

• Active metabolites have long half-life in renal impairment
• Increased incidence of gastrointestinal tract reactions and vestibular toxicity in renal failure
• Drug-induced lupus is a rare adverse drug reaction
• Rectally: dose frequency reduced to 12 hrs after 3 days
• 500 mg/100 mL infusion provides 14 mmol sodium

Mexiletine hydrochloride

Clinical use

Ventricular arrhythmias, especially after myocardial infarction

Dose in normal renal function

Oral:
400 mg loading dose followed by 200–250 mg 3–4 times daily commencing 2 hrs after the loading dose
IV injection:
100–250 mg followed by infusion of 250 mg as a 0.1% solution over 2 hrs, then 500 micrograms/min thereafter

Pharmacokinetics

Molecular weight (daltons)	216
% Protein binding	50–70
% Excreted unchanged in urine	10
Volume of distribution (L/kg)	5.5–6.6
Half-life – normal/ESRF (hrs)	8–13/16

Dose in renal impairment GFR (mL/min)

20–50	Dose as in normal renal function
10–20	Dose as in normal renal function
<10	50% of normal dose and titrate according to response

Dose in patients undergoing renal replacement therapies

CAPD	Removal insignificant. Dose as in GFR = <10 mL/min
HD	Removal insignificant. Dose as in GFR = <10 mL/min
CAV/VVHD	Removal insignificant. Dose as in normal renal function

Important drug interactions

CYCLOSPORIN

–

POTENTIALLY HAZARDOUS INTERACTIONS WITH OTHER DRUGS

• Anti-arrhythmics: increased myocardial depression with any combination of anti-arrhythmics

Administration

RECONSTITUTION

• Add 250 mg (10 mL) mexiletine to 500 mL of infusion solution, e.g. sodium chloride 0.9%, glucose 5%, sodium bicarbonate 1.4%, sodium lactate (M/6), sodium chloride 0.9% with potassium chloride 0.3% or 0.6%

ROUTE

• Oral, IV infusion

RATE OF ADMINISTRATION

–

COMMENTS

• Mexiletine should never be injected in bolus form

Other information

• Mexiletine has a narrow therapeutic index. Its therapeutic effect has been correlated with plasma concentrations of 0.5–2 micrograms/mL
• Mexiletine is metabolised in the liver and is excreted in the urine, mainly in the form of metabolites
• Rate of elimination is increased with acidic urine
• Injection can be given orally. However, due to local anaesthetic effect, care is needed with hot foods

Miconazole

Clinical use

Antifungal agent

Dose in normal renal function

Oral tablets:

250 mg every 6 hrs for 10 days or up to 2 days after symptoms clear

Oral gel:

5–10 mL in mouth, after food, 4 times daily

Pharmacokinetics

Molecular weight (daltons)	416
% Protein binding	90
% Excreted unchanged in urine	1
Volume of distribution (L/kg)	20
Half-life – normal/ESRF (hrs)	20–24/unchanged

Dose in renal impairment
GFR (mL/min)

20–50	Dose as in normal renal function
10–20	Dose as in normal renal function
<10	Dose as in normal renal function

Dose in patients undergoing renal replacement therapies

CAPD	Unlikely to be significantly removed. Dose as in normal renal function
HD	Not dialysed. Dose as in normal renal function
CAV/VVHD	Unlikely to be significantly removed. Dose as in normal renal function

Important drug interactions

CYCLOSPORIN

• Possibly increased plasma cyclosporin concentrations

POTENTIALLY HAZARDOUS INTERACTIONS WITH OTHER DRUGS

• Anticoagulants: effect of nicoumalone and warfarin enhanced
• Cisapride: ventricular arrhythmias reported, avoid concomitant use
• Anti-epileptics: effect of phenytoin enhanced
• Astemizole and terfenadine: avoid concomitant use
• Antidiabetics: plasma concentrations of sulphonylureas increased
• Tacrolimus: possibly increased tacrolimus concentration

Administration

RECONSTITUTION

–

ROUTE

• Oral tablets and oral gel

RATE OF ADMINISTRATION

–

COMMENTS

• Oral gel absorbed

Other information

• Miconazole is metabolised in the liver to inactive metabolites; 10–20% of an oral dose is excreted in the urine as metabolites. About 50% of an oral dose may be excreted mainly unchanged in the faeces
• There is little absorption through skin or mucous membranes when miconazole nitrate is applied topically

Midazolam

Clinical use

Benzodiazepine, used for sedation with amnesia, and in conjunction with local anaesthesia; premedication, induction

Dose in normal renal function

Sedation:

IV injection over 30 sec, 2 mg followed after 2 min by increments of 0.5–1 mg if sedation not adequate; usual range 2.5–7.5 mg

See data sheet for dosing guidelines in other indications

Pharmacokinetics

Molecular weight (daltons)	362
% Protein binding	93–96
% Excreted unchanged in urine	<1
Volume of distribution (L/kg)	1.0–6.6
Half-life – normal/ESRF (hrs)	1.2–12.3/ unchanged

Dose in renal impairment GFR (mL/min)

20–50	Dose as in normal renal function
10–20	Dose as in normal renal function
<10	50% of normal dose

Dose in patients undergoing renal replacement therapies

CAPD	Unknown dialysability. Dose as in GFR = <10 mL/min
HD	Unknown dialysability. Dose as in GFR = <10 mL/min
CAV/VVHD	Unknown dialysability. Dose as in normal renal function

Important drug interactions

CYCLOSPORIN

• In-vitro studies suggested that cyclosporin could inhibit the metabolism of midazolam. However, blood cyclosporin concentrations in patients given cyclosporin to prevent graft rejection were considered too low to result in an interaction

POTENTIALLY HAZARDOUS INTERACTIONS WITH OTHER DRUGS

• Erythromycin: increased plasma midazolam concentration with profound sedation
• Antifungals: itraconazole, ketoconazole and possibly fluconazole increase plasma concentration of midazolam (prolonged sedative effect)

Administration

RECONSTITUTION

• Compatible with glucose 5%, sodium chloride 0.9%, glucose 4% with sodium chloride 0.18%

ROUTE

• IV, IM

RATE OF ADMINISTRATION

• 1–10 mL/hr according to response

COMMENTS

–

Other information

• Protein binding of midazolam is decreased in ESRD, hence more unbound drug is available to produce CNS effects; therefore a decrease in dose is recommended
• CSM has received reports of respiratory depression, sometimes associated with severe hypotension, following intravenous administration
• Caution with use for sedation in severe renal impairment, especially when used with opiates and/or neuromuscular blocking agents – monitor sedation and titrate to response
• Increased CNS sensitivity in patients with renal impairment
• One study reports midazolam as having a sieving coefficient of 0.06 and unlikely to be removed by haemofiltration

Minoxidil

Clinical use

Severe hypertension, in addition to a diuretic and a beta-blocker

Dose in normal renal function

Initially 5 mg (elderly patients 2.5 mg) daily in 1–2 doses increased by 5–10 mg every 3 or more days; maximum 50 mg daily

Pharmacokinetics

Molecular weight (daltons)	209
% Protein binding	0
% Excreted unchanged in urine	15–20
Volume of distribution (L/kg)	2–3
Half-life – normal/ESRF (hrs)	2.8–4.2/8.9

Dose in renal impairment GFR (mL/min)

<50	Start with small doses and titrate according to response. See 'Other information'

Dose in patients undergoing renal replacement therapies

CAPD	Unknown dialysability. Dose as in GFR = <50 mL/min
HD	Dialysed. Dose as in GFR = <50 mL/min
CAV/VVHD	Unknown dialysability. Dose as in GFR = <50 mL/min

Important drug interactions

CYCLOSPORIN

–

POTENTIALLY HAZARDOUS INTERACTIONS WITH OTHER DRUGS

• Anaesthetics: enhanced hypotensive effect

Administration

RECONSTITUTION

–

ROUTE

• Oral

RATE OF ADMINISTRATION

–

COMMENTS

–

Other information

• A study of the pharmacokinetics of minoxidil in patients with varying degrees of renal impairment found that the non-renal clearance was also impaired as renal function worsened. Substantial accumulation of minoxidil might occur in these patients during multiple-dose therapy. It is advised that minoxidil therapy be initiated with smaller doses or a longer dose interval in patients with significant renal impairment

• Minoxidil is a peripheral vasodilator and should be given in conjunction with a diuretic to control salt and water retention and a beta-blocker to control reflex tachycardia. Patients on dialysis do not need to be given minoxidil in conjunction with a diuretic

• Following topical application between 0.3% and 4.5% of the total applied dose of minoxidil is absorbed from intact scalp

Misoprostol

Clinical use

Benign gastric and duodenal ulceration and
NSAID-associated ulceration; prophylaxis of
NSAID-induced ulceration

Dose in normal renal function

Treatment:
800 micrograms daily in 2 or 4 divided doses
Prophylaxis:
200–800 micrograms daily in divided doses

Pharmacokinetcs

Molecular weight (daltons)	382.5
% Protein binding	85 (as misoprostol acid)
% Excreted unchanged in urine	<1
Volume of distribution (L/kg)	–
Half-life – normal/ESRF (hrs)	0.5/– (as misoprostol acid)

Dose in renal impairment
GFR (mL/min)

20–50	Dose as in normal renal function
10–20	Dose as in normal renal function
<10	Dose as in normal renal function

Dose in patients undergoing renal replacement therapies

CAPD	Unknown dialysability. Dose as in normal renal function
HD	Unknown dialysability. Dose as in normal renal function
CAV/VVHD	Unknown dialysability. Dose as in normal renal function

Important drug interactions

CYCLOSPORIN

–

POTENTIALLY HAZARDOUS INTERACTIONS WITH
OTHER DRUGS

–

Administration

RECONSTITUTION

–

ROUTE

• Oral

RATE OF ADMINISTRATION

–

COMMENTS

–

Other information

• Plasma concentrations of misoprostol are
generally undetectable due to its rapid metabolic
conversion to misoprostol acid

• Although there is an approximate doubling of
half-life, maximum plasma concentration and area
under the curve in patients with varying degrees
of renal impairment, dosing adjustment is not
usually necessary. If renal patients are unable to
tolerate it, then the dose can be reduced

Mitomycin C

Clinical use

Antitumour antibiotic used in a range of neoplastic conditions

Dose in normal renal function

IV:

10–20 mg/m^2 or 0.06–0.15 mg/kg given at 1–6-weekly intervals depending on concurrent therapy and bone marrow recovery

For instillation into bladder:

20–40 mg potency

Pharmacokinetics

Molecular weight (daltons)	334
% Protein binding	–
% Excreted unchanged in urine	10
Volume of distribution (L/kg)	0.5
Half-life – normal/ESRF (hrs)	0.5–1/–

Dose in renal impairment GFR (mL/min)

20–50	Dose as in normal renal function
10–20	Dose as in normal renal function
<10	75% of normal dose

Dose in patients undergoing renal replacement therapies

CAPD	Unknown dialysability. Dose as in GFR = <10 mL/min
HD	Unknown dialysability. Dose as in GFR = <10 mL/min
CAV/VVHD	Unknown dialysability. Dose as in normal renal function

Important drug interactions

CYCLOSPORIN

–

POTENTIALLY HAZARDOUS INTERACTIONS WITH OTHER DRUGS

–

Administration

RECONSTITUTION

• Reconstitute with water for injection or 20% glucose solution; 5 mL for the 2-mg vial, at least 10 mL for the 10-mg vial and at least 20 mL for the 20-mg vial

ROUTE

• IV injection, intra-arterial, bladder instillation

RATE OF ADMINISTRATION

• Bolus injection over 3–5 min

COMMENTS

–

Other information

• A syndrome of thrombotic microangiopathy resembling the haemolytic-uraemic syndrome has been seen in patients receiving mitomycin, either alone or, more frequently, combined with other agents. Symptoms of haemolysis and renal failure may be complemented by ATN and cardiovascular problems, pulmonary oedema and neurological symptoms

• The percentage dose excreted in the urine increases with increasing dose

• The principal toxicity of Mitomycin C is bone marrow suppression. The nadir is usually around 4 weeks after treatment and toxicity is cumulative, with increasing risk after each course of treatment

Mivacurium

Clinical use

Non-depolarising muscle relaxant of short duration

Dose in normal renal function

IV injection:

70–250 micrograms/kg; maintenance 100 micrograms/kg every 15 min

IV infusion:

maintenance of block 8–10 micrograms/kg/min adjusted to maintenance dose of 6–7 micrograms/kg/min according to response

Pharmacokinetics

Molecular weight (daltons)	940
% Protein binding	–
% Excreted unchanged in urine	<7
Volume of distribution (L/kg)	0.1–0.3
Half-life – normal/ESRF (hrs)	0.03–0.08/–

Dose in renal impairment GFR (mL/min)

20–50	Adjust to response. Slower infusion rate may be required
10–20	Adjust to response. Slower infusion rate may be required
<10	Reduce dose. See 'Other information'

Dose in patients undergoing renal replacement therapies

CAPD	Unknown dialysability. Adjust infusion to response
HD	Unknown dialysability. Adjust infusion to response
CAV/VVHD	Unknown dialysability. Adjust infusion to response

Important drug interactions

CYCLOSPORIN

–

POTENTIALLY HAZARDOUS INTERACTIONS WITH OTHER DRUGS

• Anti-arrhythmics: procainamide and quinidine enhance muscle relaxant effect

• Antibacterials: effect enhanced by aminoglycosides, azlocillin, clindamycin, colistin and piperacillin

• Botulinum toxin: neuromuscular blockade enhanced, risk of toxicity

Administration

RECONSTITUTION

• Compatible with sodium chloride 0.9%; glucose 5%, sodium chloride 0.18% and glucose 4%; lactated Ringer's

• Dilute to 500 micrograms/mL

ROUTE

• IV bolus, IV infusion

RATE OF ADMINISTRATION

• IV bolus: doses of up to 0.15 mg/kg may be administered over 5–15 sec. Higher doses should be administered over 30 sec

COMMENTS

• Compatible with fentanyl, alfentanil, droperidol and midazolam

Other information

• Spontaneous recovery is complete in approximately 15 min and is independent of dose administered

• In patients with ESRD the clinically effective duration of block produced by 0.15 mg/kg is approximately 1.5 times longer than in patients with normal renal function. Subsequently, dosage should be adjusted according to individual clinical response

• The results from a study which compared 20 anephric patients with 20 healthy patients also highlight the need for reduced dosages of Mivacron in patients with renal failure; patients with renal failure had a slightly shorter time to maximum depression of T1/T0, a slower recovery of T1/T0 to 5% (15.3 vs. 9.8 min), required a slower infusion rate (6.3 vs. 10.4 micrograms/kg/min) and experienced slower spontaneous recovery (12.2 vs. 7.7 min). The manufacturer has no specific guidelines as to the extent of dose reduction required

Morphine

Clinical use

Opiate analgesic

Dose in normal renal function

5–20 mg every 4 hrs (higher in very severe pain or terminal illness)

Pharmacokinetics

Molecular weight (daltons)	759 (sulphate)
% Protein binding	20–30
% Excreted unchanged in urine	10
Volume of distribution (L/kg)	3.5
Half-life – normal/ESRF (hrs)	1–4/unchanged

Dose in renal impairment GFR (mL/min)

20–50	75% of normal dose
10–20	Use small doses, e.g. 2.5–5 mg
<10	Use small doses, e.g. 1.25–2.5 mg

Dose in patients undergoing renal replacement therapies

CAPD	Probably not dialysed. Dose as in GFR = <10 mL/min
HD	Dialysed, active metabolite removed significantly. Dose as in GFR = <10 mL/min
CAV/VVHD	Dialysed. Dose as in GFR = 10–20 mL/min

Important drug interactions

CYCLOSPORIN

–

POTENTIALLY HAZARDOUS INTERACTIONS WITH OTHER DRUGS

• MAOIs: avoid concomitant use. CNS excitation or depression (hypertension or hypotension)
• Selegiline: hyperpyrexia and CNS toxicity reported

Administration

RECONSTITUTION

• Water for injection. Small volume if SC

ROUTE

• Oral, SC, IM, IV

RATE OF ADMINISTRATION

• IV: 2 mg/min (titrate according to response)

COMMENTS

• Very soluble

Other information

• Extreme caution with all opiates in patients with impaired renal function
• Potential accumulation of morphine 6-glucuronide (an active, renally excreted metabolite more potent than morphine). The half-life of morphine 6-glucuronide is increased from 3–5 hrs in normal renal function to about 50 hrs in ESRD
• Ensure naloxone is readily available
• Some units avoid slow-release oral preparations as any side-effects may be prolonged

Muromonab CD3 (OKT3) (unlicensed drug)

Clinical use

Steroid-resistant acute transplant rejection, prophylaxis of rejection in sensitised patients

Dose in normal renal function

5 mg daily for 5–14 days (10 days most common)

Pharmacokinetics

Molecular weight (daltons)	50 000 (heavy chain) + 25 000 (light chain)
% Protein binding	–
% Excreted unchanged in urine	–
Volume of distribution (L/kg)	0.093
Half-life – normal/ESRF (hrs)	18–36/–

Dose in normal renal impairment GFR (mL/min)

20–50	Dose as in normal renal function
10–20	Dose as in normal renal function
<10	Dose as in normal renal function

Dose in patients undergoing renal replacement therapies

CAPD	Unlikely to be dialysed. Dose as in normal renal function
HD	Not dialysed. Dose as in normal renal function
CAV/VVHD	Unknown dialysability. Dose as in normal renal function

Important drug interactions

CYCLOSPORIN

• Increases cyclosporin plasma levels

POTENTIALLY HAZARDOUS INTERACTIONS WITH OTHER DRUGS

• Indomethacin: may increase risk of encephalopathy
• Volatile anaesthetics/drugs that decrease cardiac contractility: increase risk of developing cardiovascular problems

Administration

RECONSTITUTION

–

ROUTE

• IV peripherally

RATE OF ADMINISTRATION

• Fast – over less than 1 min

COMMENTS

• Doctor administration recommended

Other information

• Ensure patient is not fluid overloaded prior to administration
• Possible future scope for dose titration according to CD3 or absolute T-cell count
• Reduce or stop other immunosuppressant therapy during treatment and resume 3 days prior to cessation of OKT3
• IV methylprednisolone sodium succinate 8 mg/kg given 1–4 hrs prior to the first dose of OKT3 is strongly recommended to decrease the incidence and severity of reactions to the first dose. Paracetamol and antihistamine given concomitantly with OKT3 may also help to reduce some early reactions
• Side-effects pronounced. **Warn patient**

Mycophenolate mofetil (MMF)

Clinical use

Prophylaxis against acute transplant rejection

Dose in normal renal function

1.0–1.5 g twice a day

Pharmacokinetics

Molecular weight (daltons)	320
% Protein binding	97
% Excreted unchanged in urine	<1
Volume of distribution (L/kg)	3.6–4.0
Half-life – normal/ESRF (hrs)	11–18/–

Dose in renal impairment GFR (mL/min)

20–50	Dose as in normal renal function
10–20	1.0 g twice a day
<10	1.0 g twice a day

Dose in patients undergoing renal replacement therapies

CAPD	Not dialysed. Dose as in GFR = <10 mL/min
HD	Not dialysed. Dose as in GFR = <10 mL/min
CAV/VVHD	Not dialysed. Dose as in normal renal function

Important drug interactions

CYCLOSPORIN

–

POTENTIALLY HAZARDOUS INTERACTIONS WITH OTHER DRUGS

- Antivirals: higher plasma concentrations of both mycophenolate mofetil and aciclovir when the two are prescribed concomitantly
- Antacids: absorption of MMF decreased in the presence of magnesium and aluminium salts
- Cholestyramine: 40% reduction in oral bioavailability of MMF
- Oral contraception: may have decreased efficacy with long-term use of MMF

Administration

RECONSTITUTION

–

ROUTE

- Oral

RATE OF ADMINISTRATION

–

COMMENTS

–

Other information

- MMF rapidly undergoes complete presystemic absorption to mycophenolic acid (MPA) which in turn is metabolised to MPA glucuronide. This undergoes extensive enterohepatic recirculation, hence a secondary increase in MPA plasma levels is seen 6–12 hrs post-dose
- If neutrophil count drops below 1.3×10^3/microL, consider suspending MMF therapy
- No dosage reduction is required in the event of a transplant rejection episode

Nabumetone

Clinical use

NSAID, used for osteoarthritis and rheumatoid arthritis

Dose in normal renal function

1 g at night, in severe conditions 0.5–1g in the morning as well; elderly patients 0.5–1g daily

Pharmacokinetics

Molecular weight (daltons)	228
% Protein binding	>99
% Excreted unchanged in urine	<1
Volume of distribution (L/kg)	0.11
Half-life – normal/ESRF (hrs)	24/unchanged

Dose in renal impairment
GFR (mL/min)

20–50	Dose as in normal renal function, but avoid if possible
10–20	0.5–1g daily, but avoid if possible
<10	0.5–1g daily, but avoid if possible

Dose in patients undergoing renal replacement therapies

CAPD	Dose as in GFR = <10 mL/min
HD	Dose as in GFR = <10 mL/min
CAV/VVHD	Dose as in GFR = 10–20 mL/min

Important drug interactions

CYCLOSPORIN

• Increased risk of nephrotoxicity

POTENTIALLY HAZARDOUS INTERACTIONS WITH OTHER DRUGS

• ACE inhibitors: antagonism of hypotensive effect. Possible increased risk of renal damage and hyperkalaemia
• Anticoagulants: anticoagulant effect of warfarin and nicoumalone possibly increased

• Lithium: excretion of lithium reduced
• Methotrexate: excretion of methotrexate possibly reduced, increased risk of toxicity
• Sulphonylureas: effect of sulphonylurea possibly enhanced
• Phenytoin: effect of phenytoin possibly enhanced

Administration

RECONSTITUTION

–

ROUTE

• Oral

RATE OF ADMINISTRATION

–

COMMENTS

–

Other information

• Nabumetone is absorbed from the gastrointestinal tract and rapidly metabolised in the liver to the principal active metabolite 6-methoxy-2-naphythylacetic acid (6-MNA). The metabolite is a potent inhibitor of prostaglandin synthesis. Excretion of the metabolite is predominantly in the urine. The data sheet recommends a dose reduction for Clcr <30 mL/min. However, an article published recently concluded that dosage adjustments may not be necessary with decreased renal function. The authors found an increase in the elimination half-life of 6-MNA. However, they stated that the increased half-life in patients with renal failure is offset by changes in the apparent volume of distribution that prevent the accumulation of 6-MNA (Brier ME et al. (1995) Clinical Pharmacology and Therapeutics 57(6): 622–7)
• Inhibition of renal prostaglandin synthesis by NSAIDs may interfere with renal function, especially in the presence of existing renal disease. Avoid if possible; if not, check serum creatinine 48–72 hrs after starting NSAID. If increased, discontinue NSAID therapy
• Use normal doses in patients with ESRD on dialysis
• Use with caution in renal transplant recipients – can reduce intra-renal autocoid synthesis

Nadolol

Clinical use

Beta-adrenoreceptor blocker, used for management of angina pectoris, hypertension, arrhythmias, migraine, thyrotoxicosis

Dose in normal renal function

40–240 mg daily

Pharmacokinetics

Molecular weight (daltons)	309
% Protein binding	30
% Excreted unchanged in urine	90
Volume of distribution (L/kg)	1.9
Half-life – normal/ESRF (hrs)	19/45

Dose in renal impairment GFR (mL/min)

>50	Dose as in normal renal function
31–50	Normal dose every 24–36 hrs
10–30	50% of dose every 24–48 hrs
<10	25% of dose every 40–60 hrs

Dose in patients undergoing renal replacement therapies

CAPD	Dialysed. Dose as in GFR = <10 mL/min
HD	Dialysed. Dose as in GFR = <10 mL/min
CAV/VVHD	Dialysed. Dose as in GFR = 10–30 mL/min

Important drug interactions

CYCLOSPORIN

–

POTENTIALLY HAZARDOUS INTERACTIONS WITH OTHER DRUGS

• Anaesthetics: enhanced hypotensive effect
• Anti-arrhythmics: increased risk of myocardial depression and bradycardia
• Antihypertensives: enhanced hypotensive effect
• Calcium-channel blockers: increased risk of bradycardia and AV block with diltiazem; severe hypotension and heart failure occasionally with nifedipine; asystole, severe hypotension and heart failure with verapamil
• Sympathomimetics: severe hypertension

Administration

RECONSTITUTION

–

ROUTE

• Oral

RATE OF ADMINISTRATION

–

COMMENTS

–

Other information

• Data-sheet guidelines for increasing dosing interval for patients with renal impairment may be impractical with respect to patient compliance
• Unlike most other beta-blockers, nadolol is not metabolised and is excreted unchanged mainly by the kidneys

Naloxone

Clinical use

Reversal of opioid-induced respiratory depression

Dose in normal renal function

See 'Other information'

Pharmacokinetics

Molecular weight (daltons)	364 (hydrochloride)
% Protein binding	54
% Excreted unchanged in urine	<5
Volume of distribution (L/kg)	2–3
Half-life – normal/ESRF (hrs)	1–1.5/unchanged

Dose in renal impairment GFR (mL/min)

20–50	Dose as in normal renal function
10–20	Dose as in normal renal function
<10	Dose as in normal renal function

Dose in patients undergoing renal replacement therapies

CAPD	Unknown dialysability. Dose as in normal renal function
HD	Unknown dialysability. Dose as in normal renal function
CAV/VVHD	Unknown dialysability. Dose as in normal renal function

Important drug interactions

CYCLOSPORIN

–

POTENTIALLY HAZARDOUS INTERACTIONS WITH OTHER DRUGS

–

Administration

RECONSTITUTION

–

ROUTE

• IV, IM or SC. IV more rapid response

RATE OF ADMINISTRATION

• Rapid if bolus injection

COMMENTS

–

Other information

• IV post-operative use: give 1.5–3 micrograms/kg. If response inadequate, increments of 100 micrograms every 2 min. Further dose by IM injection if needed OR dilute 400 micrograms in 100 mL sodium chloride 0.9% or glucose 5% (4 micrograms/mL) and give by continuous infusion. Titrate dose according to response

• Opioid overdosage: an initial dose of 400–2000 micrograms IV. If the desired degree of counter action and improvement in respiratory function is not obtained, it may be repeated at 2–3-min intervals (if no response after 10 mg then question the diagnosis of opioid-induced toxicity) or give as an infusion

Naproxen

Clinical use

NSAID, used for rheumatic disease (including juvenile arthritis) and other musculoskeletal disorders; dysmenorrhoea; acute gout

Dose in normal renal function

500–1250 mg daily in 2–3 divided doses

Pharmacokinetics

Molecular weight (daltons)	230
% Protein binding	99
% Excreted unchanged in urine	<1
Volume of distribution (L/kg)	0.14–0.18
Half-life – normal/ESRF (hrs)	12–15/unchanged

Dose in renal impairment GFR (mL/min)

20–50	Dose as in normal renal function, but avoid if possible
10–20	Dose as in normal renal function, but avoid if possible
<10	Dose as in normal renal function, but only use if ESRD on dialysis

Dose in patients undergoing renal replacement therapies

CAPD	Slightly dialysed. Dose as in GFR = <10 mL/min
HD	Slightly dialysed. Dose as in GFR = <10 mL/min
CAV/VVHD	Slightly dialysed. Dose as in GFR = 10–20 mL/min

Important drug interactions

CYCLOSPORIN

• Increased risk of nephrotoxicity

POTENTIALLY HAZARDOUS INTERACTIONS WITH OTHER DRUGS

• Lithium: excretion reduced
• Cytotoxic agents: reduced excretion of methotrexate
• Anticoagulants: effects of warfarin and nicoumalone enhanced
• Antidiabetic agents: effects of sulphonylureas enhanced
• Anti-epileptic agents: effects of phenytoin enhanced
• ACE inhibitors: antagonism of hypotensive effect; increased risk of renal damage and hyperkalaemia

Administration

RECONSTITUTION

–

ROUTE

• Oral, PR

RATE OF ADMINISTRATION

–

COMMENTS

• Enteric coated preps: swallow whole, do not chew. Do not take indigestion remedies or phosphate-binders at the same time of day

Other information

• Naproxen is associated with an intermediate risk of side-effects
• Naproxen is eliminated to a large extent (95%) as metabolites by urinary excretion via glomerular filtration. The remainder is excreted via the faeces
• Inhibition of renal prostaglandin synthesis by NSAIDs may interfere with renal function, especially in the presence of existing renal disease. Avoid if possible; if not, check serum creatinine 48–72 hrs after starting NSAID. If raised, discontinue NSAID therapy
• Use normal doses in patients with ESRD on dialysis
• Use with caution in renal transplant recipients – can reduce intra-renal autocoid synthesis

Neostigmine

Clinical use

Myasthenia gravis, antagonist to non-depolarising neuromuscular blockade; paralytic ileus; post-operative urinary retention

Dose in normal renal function

In myasthenia gravis:

neostigmine bromide 15–30 mg at suitable intervals throughout day, total daily dose 75–300 mg; neostigmine methylsulphate, IM, SC, 1–2.5 mg, usual total daily dose 5–20 mg

Pharmacokinetics

Molecular weight (daltons)	223
% Protein binding	0–25
% Excreted unchanged in urine	67
Volume of distribution (L/kg)	0.5–1.0
Half-life – normal/ESRF (hrs)	1.3/3.0

Dose in renal impairment GFR (mL/min)

20–50	50–100% of normal dose
10–20	50% of normal dose
<10	25% of normal dose

Dose in patients undergoing renal replacement therapies

CAPD	Unknown dialysability. Dose as in GFR = <10 mL/min
HD	Unknown dialysability. Dose as in GFR = <10 mL/min
CAV/VVHD	Unknown dialysability. Dose as in GFR = 10–20 mL/min

Important drug interactions

CYCLOSPORIN

–

POTENTIALLY HAZARDOUS INTERACTIONS WITH OTHER DRUGS

• Aminoglycosides, clindamycin and colistin antagonise effects of neostigmine

Administration

RECONSTITUTION

–

ROUTE

• Neostigmine bromide: oral
• Neostigmine methylsulphate: SC, IM, IV

RATE OF ADMINISTRATION

• IV: very slowly

COMMENTS

–

Other information

• Neostigmine 0.5 mg IV = 1–1.15 mg IM or SC = 15 mg orally
• When used for reversal of non-depolarising neuromuscular blockade, atropine (1–2 mg IV) or glycopyrronium should be given before or with neostigmine in order to prevent bradycardia, excessive salivation and other muscarinic actions of neostigmine
• The physicochemical nature of neostigmine may tend to encourage its removal by various renal replacement therapies

Netilmicin

Clinical use

Antibacterial agent

Dose in normal renal function

IM, IV:
4–7.5 mg/kg daily, as a single daily dose or in divided doses every 8 or 12 hrs

Pharmacokinetics

Molecular weight (daltons)	1442
% Protein binding	<5
% Excreted unchanged in urine	95
Volume of distribution (L/kg)	0.16–0.3
Half-life – normal/ESRF (hrs)	1–3/35–72

Dose in renal impairment
GFR (mL/min)

20–50	25–55% of normal dose daily. Monitor levels
10–20	15–20% of normal dose daily. Monitor levels
<10	10% of normal dose daily. Monitor levels

Dose in patients undergoing renal replacement therapies

CAPD	Dialysed. IV: 2 mg/kg on alternate days. IP: 7.5–10 mg/L per exchange. Monitor levels
HD	Dialysed. Administer 2 mg/kg at the end of each dialysis session. Monitor levels
CAV/VVHD	Dialysed. Dose as in GFR = 10–20 mL/min. Monitor netilmicin levels

Important drug interactions

CYCLOSPORIN

• Increased risk of nephrotoxicity

POTENTIALLY HAZARDOUS INTERACTIONS WITH OTHER DRUGS

• Botulinum toxin: neuromuscular block enhanced
• Cisplatin: increased risk of nephrotoxicity and ototoxicity
• Loop diuretics: increased risk of ototoxicity
• Muscle relaxants: effects of non-depolarising muscle relaxants enhanced
• Parasympathomimetics: antagonised by aminoglycosides

Administration

RECONSTITUTION

• 50–200 mL of sterile water for injection, sodium chloride 0.9%, glucose 5% or 10%

ROUTE

• IM, IP, IV bolus or infusion

RATE OF ADMINISTRATION

• IV bolus: administer over 3–5 min
• IV infusion: administer over 0.5–2 hrs

COMMENTS

• IM and IV dose are identical. Calculate on mg/kg lean body weight, or actual weight, whichever is lower

Other information

• Netilmicin serum concentrations should be monitored and used for basis of dosage adjustment, otherwise follow guidelines in data sheet according to serum creatinine/creatinine clearance
• Once-daily administration of netilmicin may lead to transient peak concentrations of 20–30 micrograms/mL. Other dosage regimens will result in peak levels not exceeding 12 micrograms/mL. Prolonged levels above 16 micrograms/mL should be avoided. If trough levels are monitored they will usually be 3 micrograms/mL or less with the recommended dosage. Increasing trough concentrations above 4 micrograms/mL should be avoided
• Removed by PD if given IV/IM

Nicardipine

Clinical use

Calcium-channel blocker, used for prophylaxis and treatment of angina; mild to moderate hypertension

Dose in normal renal function

60–120 mg daily given in 3 divided doses

Pharmacokinetics

Molecular weight (daltons)	516
% Protein binding	98–99
% Excreted unchanged in urine	<1
Volume of distribution (L/kg)	0.7–1.7
Half-life – normal/ESRF (hrs)	5.0–8.6/unchanged

Dose in renal impairment GFR (mL/min)

20–50	Dose as in normal renal function
10–20	Dose as in normal renal function. Start with small doses
<10	Dose as in normal renal function. Start with small doses

Dose in patients undergoing renal replacement therapies

CAPD	Unlikely to be dialysed. Dose as in GFR = <10 mL/min
HD	Unlikely to be dialysed. Dose as in GFR = <10 mL/min
CAV/VVHD	Unknown dialysability. Dose as in GFR = 10–20 mL/min

Important drug interactions

CYCLOSPORIN

• May increase blood cyclosporin concentration

POTENTIALLY HAZARDOUS INTERACTIONS WITH OTHER DRUGS

• Carbamazepine, phenobarbitone, phenytoin and primidone may reduce effect of nicardipine
• Alpha-blockers: increased risk of first-dose hypotensive effect
• Digoxin: plasma level may be increased
• Theophylline: levels may increase

Administration

RECONSTITUTION

–

ROUTE

• Oral

RATE OF ADMINISTRATION

–

COMMENTS

• Administration of nicardipine with food appears to reduce the bioavailability and delay the achievement of peak plasma concentrations

Other information

• Nicardipine is extensively metabolised in the liver and is excreted in the urine and faeces, mainly as inactive metabolites
• Nicardipine blood levels may also be elevated in some renally impaired patients. Therefore, start with a low dose and titrate to BP and response. The dose interval may also need to be extended to 12-hourly

Nicoumalone

Clinical use

Anticoagulant

Dose in normal renal function

8–12 mg on day 1; 4–8 mg on day 2; maintenance dose usually 1–8 mg daily according to INR

Pharmacokinetics

Molecular weight (daltons)	353
% Protein binding	>98
% Excreted unchanged in urine	<0.2
Volume of distribution (L/kg)	0.16–0.18 R(+) enantiomer; 0.22–0.34 S(−) enantiomer
Half-life – normal/ESRF (hrs)	8–11/–

Dose in renal impairment GFR (mL/min)

20–50	Dose as in normal renal function
10–20	Dose as in normal renal function
<10	Dose as in normal renal function

Dose in patients undergoing renal replacement therapies

CAPD	Unknown dialysability. Dose as in normal renal function
HD	Unknown dialysability. Dose as in normal renal function
CAV/VVHD	Unknown dialysability. Dose as in normal renal function

Important drug interactions

CYCLOSPORIN

–

POTENTIALLY HAZARDOUS INTERACTIONS WITH OTHER DRUGS

• Increased INR: alcohol, analgesics, anti-arrhythmics, cholestyramine, antibacterials, antidepressants (SSRI), anti-epileptics (phenytoin, valproate), antifungals (imidazoles), proguanil, antiplatelet agents, cytotoxics (ifosfamide), disulfiram, hormone antagonists, lipid-lowering drugs, thyroxine, ulcer-healing drugs, uricosuric agents

• Decreased INR: cholestyramine, rifampicin, anti-epileptics (carbamazipine, phenobarbitone, primidone, phenytoin), griseofulvin, aminoglutethimide, oestrogens and progestogens, retinoids, sucralfate, vitamin K

Administration

RECONSTITUTION

–

ROUTE

• Oral

RATE OF ADMINISTRATION

–

COMMENTS

–

Other information

• Nicoumalone prolongs the thromboplastin time within approximately 36–72 hrs

• Decreased protein binding in uraemia

• Titrate dose to end-point INR

Nifedipine

Clinical use

Calcium-channel blocker, used for prophylaxis and treatment of angina, hypertension

Dose in normal renal function

Oral:
5–20 mg 2–4 times daily
Long Acting 30–90 mg daily

Pharmacokinetics

Molecular weight (daltons)	346.3
% Protein binding	98
% Excreted unchanged in urine	<1
Volume of distribution (L/kg)	0.3–1.2
Half-life – normal/ESRF (hrs)	4–6/5–7

Dose in renal impairment GFR (mL/min)

20–50	Dose as in normal renal function
10–20	Dose as in normal renal function. Start with small doses
<10	Dose as in normal renal function. Start with small doses

Dose in patients undergoing renal replacement therapies

CAPD	Not dialysed. Dose as in GFR = <10 mL/min
HD	Dialysed. Dose as in GFR = <10 mL/min
CAV/VVHD	Unknown dialysability. Dose as in GFR = 10–20 mL/min

Important drug interactions

CYCLOSPORIN

• May increase cyclosporin level, but not a problem in practice. Nifedipine concentration may increase

POTENTIALLY HAZARDOUS INTERACTIONS WITH OTHER DRUGS

• Phenytoin: plasma concentration increased
• Beta-blockers: occasionally severe hypertension and heart failure
• Digoxin: plasma level may be increased
• Nifedipine may impair glucose tolerance
• Alpha-blockers: increased risk of first-dose hypotensive effect
• Rifampicin: reduces plasma concentration
• Theophylline levels may increase

Administration

RECONSTITUTION

–

ROUTE

• Oral

RATE OF ADMINISTRATION

–

COMMENTS

–

Other information

• Protein binding decreased in severe renal impairment
• Acute renal dysfunction reported
• Increased incidence of side-effects (headache, flushing, dizziness and peripheral oedema) in patients with ESRD
• For acute use: bite capsule then swallow contents with 10–50 mL water

Nimodipine

Clinical use

Calcium-channel blocker, used for prevention and treatment of ischaemic neurological deficits following subarachnoid haemorrhage

Dose in normal renal function

Prevention orally:

60 mg every 4 hrs (total daily dose 360 mg)

Treatment via central catheter:

1 mg/hr initially. Increased after 2 hrs to 2 mg/hr. If BP unstable, weight <70 kg: start with 0.5 mg/hr or less if necessary

Pharmacokinetics

Molecular weight (daltons)	418
% Protein binding	98
% Excreted unchanged in urine	<10
Volume of distribution (L/kg)	0.9–2.3
Half-life – normal/ESRF (hrs)	1–2.8/22

Dose in renal impairment GFR (mL/min)

20–50	Dose as in normal renal function
10–20	Dose as in normal renal function
<10	Dose as in normal renal function

Dose in patients undergoing renal replacement therapies

CAPD	Unknown dialysability. Dose as in normal renal function
HD	Unknown dialysability. Dose as in normal renal function
CAV/VVHD	Unknown dialysability. Dose as in normal renal function

Important drug interactions

CYCLOSPORIN

–

POTENTIALLY HAZARDOUS INTERACTIONS WITH OTHER DRUGS

- Anti-epileptics: effect reduced by carbamazepine, phenobarbitone, phenytoin and primidone
- Alpha-blockers: increased risk of first-dose hypotensive effect
- Theophylline levels may increase

Administration

RECONSTITUTION

- Nimodipine solution must not be added to an infusion bag or bottle and must not be mixed with other drugs

ROUTE

- Oral, IV

RATE OF ADMINISTRATION

- IV: first 2 hrs – 1 mg (5 mL) nimodipine 1 mg/hr; after 2 hrs – infuse 2 mg (10 mL) nimodipine/hr

COMMENTS

- Nimodipine solution should be administered only via a bypass into a running drip (40 mL/hr) of either sodium chloride 0.9% or glucose 5%
- In the event of nimodipine tablets and solution being administered sequentially, the total duration of treatment should not exceed 21 days

Other information

- Nimodipine solution reacts with PVC. Polyethylene tubes are supplied
- Patients with known renal disease and/or who are receiving nephrotoxic drugs should have renal function monitored closely during IV treatment

Nitrazepam

Clinical use

Benzodiazepine, used as hypnotic

Dose in normal renal function

5–10 mg at bedtime; elderly (or debilitated) patients 2.5–5 mg

Pharmacokinetics

Molecular weight (daltons)	281
% Protein binding	85
% Excreted unchanged in urine	<5
Volume of distribution (L/kg)	1.9–2.4
Half-life – normal/ESRF (hrs)	18–50/unchanged

Dose in renal impairment GFR (mL/min)

20–50	Dose as in normal renal function
10–20	Dose as in normal renal function
<10	Dose as in normal renal function. Start with small doses

Dose in patients undergoing renal replacement therapies

CAPD	Unlikely to be dialysed. Dose as in GFR = <10 mL/min
HD	Unlikely to be dialysed. Dose as in GFR = <10 mL/min
CAV/VVHD	Unlikely to be dialysed. Dose as in normal renal function

Important drug interactions

CYCLOSPORIN

–

POTENTIALLY HAZARDOUS INTERACTIONS WITH OTHER DRUGS

–

Administration

RECONSTITUTION

–

ROUTE

• Oral

RATE OF ADMINISTRATION

–

COMMENTS

–

Other information

• Mild to moderate renal insufficiency does not alter the kinetics of nitrazepam
• ESRD patients will be more susceptible to adverse effects (drowsiness, sedation, unsteadiness)

Nitrofurantoin

Clinical use

Antibacterial agent

Dose in normal renal function

Treatment:
50–100 mg every 6 hrs
Prophylaxis:
50–100 mg at night

Pharmacokinetics

Molecular weight (daltons)	238
% Protein binding	20–70
% Excreted unchanged in urine	30–40
Volume of distribution (L/kg)	0.3–0.7
Half-life – normal/ESRF (hrs)	0.5/1.0

Dose in renal impairment GFR (mL/min)

20–50	Contraindicated
10–20	Contraindicated
<10	Contraindicated

Dose in patients undergoing renal replacement therapies

CAPD	Dialysed. Avoid – contraindicated
HD	Dialysed. Avoid – contraindicated
CAV/VVHD	Dialysed. Avoid – contraindicated

Important drug interactions

CYCLOSPORIN

–

POTENTIALLY HAZARDOUS INTERACTIONS WITH OTHER DRUGS

–

Administration

RECONSTITUTION

–

ROUTE

• Oral

RATE OF ADMINISTRATION

–

COMMENTS

• Urine may be coloured dark yellow or brown
• Macrocrystalline form has slower dissolution and absorption rates, produces lower serum concentration and takes longer to achieve peak concentration in the urine

Other information

• Avoid nitrofurantoin in patients with impaired renal function (GFR <60mL/min), as the drug is ineffective due to inadequate urine concentration and toxic plasma concentrations can occur causing adverse effects, e.g. neuropathy, blood dyscrasias
• Nitrofurantoin gives false-positive urinary glucose (if testing for reducing substances)

Nizatidine

Clinical use

H$_2$-receptor antagonist

Dose in normal renal function

Oral:
150–600 mg daily
IV:
300–480 mg daily

Pharmacokinetics

Molecular weight (daltons)	332
% Protein binding	28–35
% Excreted unchanged in urine	54–65
Volume of distribution (L/kg)	0.8–1.3
Half-life – normal/ESRF (hrs)	1.3–1.6/5.3–11.0

Dose in renal impairment GFR (mL/min)

20–50	150 mg daily (50% of normal dose)
<20	150 mg on alternate days (25% of normal dose)

Dose in patients undergoing renal replacement therapies

CAPD	Unknown dialysability. Dose as in GFR = <20 mL/min
HD	Unknown dialysability. Dose as in GFR = <20 mL/min
CAV/VVHD	Unknown dialysability. Dose as in GFR = <20 mL/min

Important drug interactions

CYCLOSPORIN

–

POTENTIALLY HAZARDOUS INTERACTIONS WITH OTHER DRUGS

–

Administration

RECONSTITUTION

• Sodium chloride 0.9%, glucose 5%

ROUTE

• Oral or IV

RATE OF ADMINISTRATION

• Continuous IV infusion: dilute 300 mg in 150 mL. Rate 10 mg/hr
• Intermittent IV infusion: dilute 100 mg in 50 mL and infuse over 15 min, 3 times daily

COMMENTS

• To maintain gastric pH $\geqslant$4, a continuous infusion of 10 mg/hr is recommended
• IV infusion: patients with moderate renal impairment (CrCl: 20–50 mL/min), dose should be reduced to 120–150 mg daily; patients with severe impairment (CrCl: <20 mL/min), dose should be reduced to 75 mg daily

Other information

• The effect of haemodialysis is unproven. It is not expected to be efficient since nizatidine has a large volume of distribution

Noradrenaline

Clinical use

Hypotension (sympathomimetic)

Dose in normal renal function

1–10 micrograms/min

Pharmacokinetics

Molecular weight (daltons)	169
% Protein binding	~ 50
% Excreted unchanged in urine	<10
Volume of distribution (L/kg)	0.09–0.4
Half-life – normal/ESRF (hrs)	0.01–0.05/ unchanged

Dose in renal impairment GFR (mL/min)

20–50	Dose as in normal renal function
10–20	Dose as in normal renal function
<10	Dose as in normal renal function

Dose in patients undergoing renal replacement therapies

CAPD	Not dialysed. Dose as in normal renal function
HD	Not dialysed. Dose as in normal renal function
CAV/VVHD	Not dialysed. Dose as in normal renal function

Important drug interactions

CYCLOSPORIN

–

POTENTIALLY HAZARDOUS INTERACTIONS WITH OTHER DRUGS

• Antidepressants: tricyclics may cause hypertension and arrhythmias; MAOIs may cause hypertensive crisis
• Beta-blockers: can cause severe hypertension
• Other sympathomimetics: dopexamine possibly potentiates effect of noradrenaline

Administration

RECONSTITUTION

• Dilute 1–4 mg in 100 mL glucose 5%. Can be given undiluted

ROUTE

• IV

RATE OF ADMINISTRATION

• According to response

COMMENTS

• Preferably give centrally (low pH)

Other information

• Do not mix with alkaline drugs/solutions
• The pharmacokinetics of noradrenaline are not significantly affected by renal or hepatic disease

Nortriptyline

Clinical use

Tricyclic antidepressant

Dose in normal renal function

Depression:

initially 25–50 mg daily, increased as necessary to 75–100 mg daily in a single dose or divided doses (maximum 150 mg daily in hospitalised patients)

Pharmacokinetics

Molecular weight (daltons)	263
% Protein binding	95
% Excreted unchanged in urine	<5
Volume of distribution (L/kg)	15–23
Half-life – normal/ESRF (hrs)	25–60/66–200

Dose in renal impairment GFR (mL/min)

20–50	Dose as in normal renal function
10–20	Dose as in normal renal function
<10	Dose as in normal renal function. Start with small dose

Dose in patients undergoing renal replacement therapies

CAPD	Not dialysed. Dose as in normal renal function
HD	Not dialysed. Dose as in normal renal function
CAV/VVHD	Not dialysed. Dose as in normal renal function

Important drug interactions

CYCLOSPORIN

–

POTENTIALLY HAZARDOUS INTERACTIONS WITH OTHER DRUGS

- Alcohol: increased sedative effect
- Anti-arrhythmics: increased risk of ventricular arrhythmias with drugs which prolong QT interval – amiodarone, disopyramide, procainamide and quinidine
- Other antidepressants: CNS excitation and hypertension with MAOIs. Do not start tricyclic until 2 weeks after stopping MAOI. Do not start MAOI until at least 1 week after stopping tricyclic
- Anti-epileptics: convulsive threshold lowered
- Antihistamines: increased antimuscarinic and sedative effects. Increased risk of ventricular arrhythmias with astemizole and terfenadine
- Antimalarials: increased risk of ventricular arrhythmias with halofantrine
- Antihypertensives: hypotensive effect increased. Antagonism of effect of adrenergic neurone blockers and of clonidine. Also increased risk of hypertension on clonidine withdrawal
- Beta-blockers: sotalol – increased risk of ventricular arrhythmias
- Sympathomimetics: hypertension and arrhythmias with adrenaline. Hypertension with noradrenaline

Administration

RECONSTITUTION

–

ROUTE

- Oral

RATE OF ADMINISTRATION

–

COMMENTS

–

Other information

- Optimal response to nortriptyline associated with plasma concentrations of 50–150 nanograms/mL
- Recommended to measure plasma levels at doses exceeding 100 mg daily
- All metabolites are highly lipophilic

Nystatin mouthwash (suspension) 100 000 u/mL

Clinical use

Antifungal agent

Dose in normal renal function

1–10 mL 4 times daily

Pharmacokinetics

Molecular weight (daltons)	926
% Protein binding	–
% Excreted unchanged in urine	–
Volume of distribution (L/kg)	–
Half-life – normal/ESRF (hrs)	–

Dose in renal impairment GFR (mL/min)

20–50	Dose as in normal renal function
10–20	Dose as in normal renal function
<10	Dose as in normal renal function

Dose in patients undergoing renal replacement therapies

CAPD	Not dialysed. Dose as in normal renal function
HD	Not dialysed. Dose as in normal renal function
CAV/VVHD	Not dialysed. Dose as in normal renal function

Important drug interactions

CYCLOSPORIN

–

POTENTIALLY HAZARDOUS INTERACTIONS WITH OTHER DRUGS

–

Administration

RECONSTITUTION

–

ROUTE

• Oral

RATE OF ADMINISTRATION

–

COMMENTS

–

Other information

• Not absorbed from intact skin or mucous membranes
• No significant gastrointestinal absorption

Octreotide

Clinical use

Relief of symptoms of gastroenteropancreatic endocrine tumours and acromegaly

Dose in normal renal function

50–600 micrograms daily

Pharmacokinetics

Molecular weight (daltons)	1019.3
% Protein binding	65
% Excreted unchanged in urine	10
Volume of distribution (L/kg)	0.27
Half-life – normal/ESRF (hrs)	1.25–2.0/ prolonged

Dose in renal impairment GFR (mL/min)

20–50	Dose as in normal renal function
10–20	Dose as in normal renal function
<10	Dose as in normal renal function

Dose in patients undergoing renal replacement therapies

CAPD	Unknown dialysability. Dose as in normal renal function
HD	Unknown dialysability. Dose as in normal renal function
CAV/VVHD	Unknown dialysability. Dose as in normal renal function

Important drug interactions

CYCLOSPORIN

• Absorption of cyclosporin may be reduced

POTENTIALLY HAZARDOUS INTERACTIONS WITH OTHER DRUGS

–

Administration

RECONSTITUTION

• IV: sodium chloride 0.9% to a ratio of not less than 1:1 and not more than 1:9

ROUTE

• SC, IV

RATE OF ADMINISTRATION

• IV bolus with ECG monitoring

COMMENTS

–

Other information

• SC: to reduce local discomfort, warm to room temperature before injection
• For multiple injections, use different sites
• Patients with reduced renal function have been shown to have a reduced clearance of the drug (75 mL/min vs. 175 mL/min)

Oestrogen, conjugated (unlicensed drug)

Clinical use

Second-line haemostatic agent for uraemic bleeding

Dose in normal renal function

0.6 mg/kg/day IV for 5 days

Pharmacokinetics

Molecular weight (daltons)	–
% Protein binding	–
% Excreted unchanged in urine	–
Volume of distribution (L/kg)	–
Half-life – normal/ESRF (hrs)	–

Dose in renal impairment GFR (mL/min)

20–50	Dose as in normal renal function
10–20	Dose as in normal renal function
<10	Dose as in normal renal function

Dose in patients undergoing renal replacement therapies

CAPD	Unknown dialysability. Dose as in normal renal function
HD	Unknown dialysability. Dose as in normal renal function
CAV/VVHD	Unknown dialysability. Dose as in normal renal function

Important drug interactions

CYCLOSPORIN

• Plasma concentration of cyclosporin increased

POTENTIALLY HAZARDOUS INTERACTIONS WITH OTHER DRUGS

• Anticoagulants: antagonism of anticoagulant effect of warfarin, nicoumalone and phenindione
• Anti-epileptics: accelerate metabolism

Administration

RECONSTITUTION

• To 50 mL with sodium chloride 0.9%

ROUTE

• IV

RATE OF ADMINISTRATION

• Over a minimum of 30 min

COMMENTS

–

Other information

• Duration of effect about 14 days
• Used in association with desmopressin (DDAVP) in intractable cases
• Orally 10–20 mg daily for 5–7 days
• Conjugated oestrogens are a mixture of sodium oestrone sulphate and sodium equilin sulphate and other oestrogenic substances of the type excreted by pregnant mares

Ofloxacin

Clinical use

Antibacterial agent

Dose in normal renal function

Oral:
200–400 mg daily, increased if necessary to 400 mg every 12 hrs
IV:
200 mg once or twice daily, increased if necessary to 400 mg every 12 hrs

Pharmacokinetics

Molecular weight (daltons)	361.4
% Protein binding	<20
% Excreted unchanged in urine	68–90
Volume of distribution (L/kg)	1.0–2.5
Half-life – normal/ESRF (hrs)	5–8/28–37

Dose in renal impairment GFR (mL/min)

20–50	Give normal loading dose, then reduce to 100–200 mg daily
10–20	Give normal loading dose, then reduce to 100 mg daily
<10	Give normal loading dose, then reduce to 100 mg daily

Dose in patients undergoing renal replacement therapies

CAPD	Not significantly dialysed. Dose as in GFR = <10 mL/min
HD	Dialysed. Dose as in GFR = <10 mL/min
CAV/VVHD	Dialysed. Dose as in GFR = 10–20 mL/min

Important drug interactions

CYCLOSPORIN

• Increased risk of nephrotoxicity

POTENTIALLY HAZARDOUS INTERACTIONS WITH OTHER DRUGS

• Anticoagulants: effect of nicoumalone and warfarin enhanced
• Antidiabetics: effect of sulphonylureas enhanced

Administration

RECONSTITUTION

–

ROUTE

• Oral, IV

RATE OF ADMINISTRATION

• IV: 200 mg over 30 min

COMMENTS

–

Other information

–

Olsalazine

Clinical use

Induction and maintenance of remission in ulcerative colitis

Dose in normal renal function

1–3 g daily

Pharmacokinetics

Molecular weight (daltons)	346.2
% Protein binding	99.8
% Excreted unchanged in urine	<10
Volume of distribution (L/kg)	0.1
Half-life – normal/ESRF (hrs)	1/unchanged

Dose in renal impairment GFR (mL/min)

20–50	Avoid – contraindicated
10–20	Avoid – contraindicated
<10	Avoid – contraindicated

Dose in patients undergoing renal replacement therapies

CAPD	Unknown dialysability. Avoid – contraindicated
HD	Unknown dialysability. Avoid – contraindicated
CAV/VVHD	Unknown dialysability. Avoid – contraindicated

Important drug interactions

CYCLOSPORIN

–

POTENTIALLY HAZARDOUS INTERACTIONS WITH OTHER DRUGS

–

Administration

RECONSTITUTION

–

ROUTE

• Oral, rectal

RATE OF ADMINISTRATION

–

COMMENTS

–

Other information

• Potential to be nephrotoxic due to 5-aminosalicylic acid (5-ASA) component. Both 5-ASA and its acetylated metabolite are rapidly excreted in the urine

• Less than 3% of an oral dose is absorbed before the drug reaches the colon

• It is unlikely that renal dysfunction will have any important effect on the kinetics of the drug

• The use of olsalazine in patients with significant renal impairment is contraindicated due to lack of experience of its use in this patient population

Omeprazole

Clinical use

Gastric acid suppression

Dose in normal renal function

10–120 mg daily

Pharmacokinetics

Molecular weight (daltons)	345
% Protein binding	95
% Excreted unchanged in urine	Minimal
Volume of distribution (L/kg)	0.3–0.4
Half-life – normal/ESRF (hrs)	1/unchanged

Dose in renal impairment GFR (mL/min)

20–50	Dose as in normal renal function
10–20	Dose as in normal renal function
<10	Dose as in normal renal function

Dose in patients undergoing renal replacement therapies

CAPD	Unknown dialysability. Dose as in normal renal function
HD	Not dialysed. Dose as in normal renal function
CAV/VVHD	Unknown dialysability. Dose as in normal renal function

Important drug interactions

CYCLOSPORIN

- Variable response. Mostly an increase in cyclosporin level

POTENTIALLY HAZARDOUS INTERACTIONS WITH OTHER DRUGS

- Warfarin: effects of warfarin enhanced
- Phenytoin: effects of phenytoin enhanced

Administration

RECONSTITUTION

- Reconstitute 40-mg vial with 10 mL water for injection. Add to 100 mL sodium chloride 0.9% or glucose 5%

ROUTE

- Oral, IV

RATE OF ADMINISTRATION

- IV: 40 mg over 20–30 min

COMMENTS

- IV dosage (unlicensed): 40 mg (single or divided dose) once or twice daily
- Use oral dose as soon as possible
- Stable for 12 hrs if sodium chloride 0.9% as infusion fluid, 6 hrs in glucose 5%

Other information

- Injection available on named patient basis only
- Capsules may be opened and contents flushed down nasogastric tube. If contents crushed, give with sodium bicarbonate solution 8.4% flush
- Omeprazole clearance is not limited by renal disease

Ondansetron

Clinical use

Anti-emetic

Dose in normal renal function

Oral:
4–24 mg daily
IV:
4–32 mg daily

Pharmacokinetics

Molecular weight (daltons)	365.9
% Protein binding	70–75
% Excreted unchanged in urine	<10
Volume of distribution (L/kg)	2.0–2.6
Half-life – normal/ESRF (hrs)	3.5/5–9

Dose in renal impairment GFR (mL/min)

20–50	Dose as in normal renal function
10–20	Dose as in normal renal function
<10	Dose as in normal renal function

Dose in patients undergoing renal replacement therapies

CAPD	Unknown dialysability. Dose as in normal renal function
HD	Not dialysed. Dose as in normal renal function
CAV/VVHD	Unknown dialysability. Dose as in normal renal function

Important drug interactions

CYCLOSPORIN

–

POTENTIALLY HAZARDOUS INTERACTIONS WITH OTHER DRUGS

–

Administration

RECONSTITUTION

–

ROUTE

• Oral, IV, IM, rectal

RATE OF ADMINISTRATION

• IV: bolus over 3–5 min; infusion not less than 15 min or 1 mg/hr

COMMENTS

• Compatible with sodium chloride 0.9% and glucose 5%

Other information

• Renal clearance of ondansetron is low

Orphenadrine

Clinical use

Antimuscarinic

Dose in normal renal function

150–400 mg daily

Pharmacokinetics

Molecular weight (daltons)	269.4
% Protein binding	95
% Excreted unchanged in urine	8
Volume of distribution (L/kg)	–
Half-life – normal/ESRF (hrs)	14/–

Dose in renal impairment GFR (mL/min)

20–50	Dose as in normal renal function
10–20	Dose as in normal renal function
<10	Dose as in normal renal function

Dose in patients undergoing renal replacement therapies

CAPD	Unknown dialysability. Dose as in normal renal function
HD	Unknown dialysability. Dose as in normal renal function
CAV/VVHD	Unknown dialysability. Dose as in normal renal function

Important drug interactions

CYCLOSPORIN

–

POTENTIALLY HAZARDOUS INTERACTIONS WITH OTHER DRUGS

–

Administration

RECONSTITUTION

–

ROUTE

• Oral

RATE OF ADMINISTRATION

–

COMMENTS

–

Other information

–

Oxazepam

Clinical use

Anxiolytic

Dose in normal renal function

15–30 mg 3 or 4 times a day

Pharmacokinetics

Molecular weight (daltons)	286.7
% Protein binding	97
% Excreted unchanged in urine	<1
Volume of distribution (L/kg)	0.6–1.6
Half-life – normal/ESRF (hrs)	6–25/25–90

Dose in renal impairment GFR (mL/min)

20–50	Dose as in normal renal function
10–20	Dose as in normal renal function
<10	10–20 mg 3 or 4 times a day

Dose in patients undergoing renal replacement therapies

CAPD	Not dialysed. Dose as in GFR = <10 mL/min
HD	Not dialysed. Dose as in GFR = <10 mL/min
CAV/VVHD	Unknown dialysability. Dose as in GFR = 10–20 mL/min

Important drug interactions

CYCLOSPORIN

–

POTENTIALLY HAZARDOUS INTERACTIONS WITH OTHER DRUGS

–

Administration

RECONSTITUTION

–

ROUTE

• Oral

RATE OF ADMINISTRATION

–

COMMENTS

–

Other information

• Protein binding decreased and volume of distribution increased in ESRD
• Glucuronide metabolite increases in ESRD. Significance of this unknown

Pamidronate disodium

Clinical use

Bisphosphonate, used for hypercalcaemia

Dose in normal renal function

Depends on serum calcium. These guidelines are based on data on uncorrected calcium levels, although corrected calcium values can also be used:

Serum calcium (uncorrected) (mmol/L)	Total dose (mg)
Up to 3.0	15–30
3.0–3.5	30–60
3.5–4.0	60–90
>4.0	90

Pharmacokinetics

Molecular weight (daltons)	279
% Protein binding	50
% Excreted unchanged in urine	50
Volume of distribution (L/kg)	0.5–0.6
Half-life – normal/ESRF (hrs)	2–5/unchanged

Dose in renal impairment GFR (mL/min)

20–50	Dose as in normal renal function
10–20	Dose as in normal renal function
<10	Serum calcium >4.0, give 60 mg. Serum calcium <4.0, give 30 mg

Dose in patients undergoing renal replacement therapies

CAPD	Unknown dialysability. Dose as in GFR = <10 mL/min
HD	Dialysed. Dose as in GFR = <10 mL/min
CAV/VVHD	Unknown dialysability. Dose as in normal renal function

Important drug interactions

CYCLOSPORIN

–

POTENTIALLY HAZARDOUS INTERACTIONS WITH OTHER DRUGS

–

Administration

RECONSTITUTION

• 15 mg in 5 mL water for injection
• 30 or 90 mg in 10 mL water for injection
• Final concentration should not exceed 30 mg per 125 mL sodium chloride 0.9%

ROUTE

• IV

RATE OF ADMINISTRATION

• Maximum 20 mg/hr in patients with impaired renal function

COMMENTS

–

Other information

• If pamidronate is not excreted adequately kidney stones may be formed
• In dialysis patients there is an increased risk of asymptomatic hypocalcaemia with 90-mg doses (anecdotal)

Pancuronium

Clinical use

Non-depolarising muscle relaxant of medium
duration

Dose in normal renal function

Initial dose:
20–100 micrograms/kg
Incremental dose:
10–20 micrograms/kg

Pharmacokinetics

Molecular weight (daltons)	732.7
% Protein binding	80–90
% Excreted unchanged in urine	40
Volume of distribution (L/kg)	0.23
Half-life – normal/ESRF (hrs)	1.5–2.2/4.3–8.2

Dose in renal impairment
GFR (mL/min)

20–50	Dose as in normal renal function
10–20	Initial dose: 10–50 micrograms/kg; incremental dose: 5–10 micrograms/kg
<10	Initial dose: 5–25 micrograms/kg; incremental dose: 2.5–5 micrograms/kg

Dose in patients undergoing renal replacement therapies

CAPD	Unknown dialysability. Dose as in GFR = <10 mL/min
HD	Unknown dialysability. Dose as in GFR = <10 mL/min
CAV/VVHD	Unknown dialysability. Dose as in GFR = 10–20 mL/min

Important drug interactions

CYCLOSPORIN

–

POTENTIALLY HAZARDOUS INTERACTIONS WITH
OTHER DRUGS

• Effects enhanced by aminoglycosides, azlocillin,
clindamycin, colistin and piperacillin

Administration

RECONSTITUTION

–

ROUTE

• IV

RATE OF ADMINISTRATION

• Bolus

COMMENTS

–

Other information

• Active metabolites accumulate in ESRD; duration
of action prolonged

Papaveretum

Higher strength (15.4 mg/mL): 1 mL contains 10 mg anhydrous morphine, 1.2 mg papaverine HCl and 1.04 mg codeine HCl

Clinical use

Opiate analgesia

Dose in normal renal function

0.5–1 mL every 4 hrs

Pharmacokinetics

	Papaverine	Morphine	Codeine
Molecular weight (daltons)	339	285	303
% Protein binding	87	25–35	7–25
% Excreted unchanged in urine	<1	Minor	6–20
Volume of distribution (L/kg)	0.99–1.52	3–5	3–4
Half-life – normal/ESRF (hrs)	1.5–2.2/–	1–7/15–66	2.5–3.5/19

Dose in renal impairment GFR (mL/min)

20–50	Dose as in normal renal function
10–20	0.4–0.75 mL every 6–8 hrs
<10	0.25–0.5 mL every 6–8 hrs. Avoid if possible

Dose in patients undergoing renal replacement therapies

CAPD	Unknown dialysability. Dose as in GFR = <10 mL/min
HD	Unknown dialysability. Dose as in GFR = <10 mL/min
CAV/VVHD	Unknown dialysability. Dose as in GFR = 10–20 mL/min

Important drug interactions

CYCLOSPORIN

–

POTENTIALLY HAZARDOUS INTERACTIONS WITH OTHER DRUGS

• Avoid use with MAOIs
• Hyperpyrexia and CNS toxicity reported with selegiline

Administration

RECONSTITUTION

–

ROUTE

• SC, IM, IV

RATE OF ADMINISTRATION

• IV bolus or continuous infusion (1 mg/mL)

COMMENTS

• In general IV dose should be ¼ to ½ that of corresponding SC or IM dose

Other information

• As with all opiates, use with extreme caution in patients with impaired renal function
• May cause excessive sedation and respiratory depression
• Contraindicated in women of child-bearing potential if preparation used contains noscopine (Omnopon®)
• Papaveretum 15.4 mg = 1 mL, providing the equivalent of 10 mg morphine
• Papaveretum paediatric 7.7 mg = 1 mL, providing the equivalent of 5 mg morphine

Paracetamol

Clinical use

Analgesic and antipyretic

Dose in normal renal function

500 mg–1 g every 4–6 hrs

Pharmacokinetics

Molecular weight (daltons)	151
% Protein binding	20–30
% Excreted unchanged in urine	1–4
Volume of distribution (L/kg)	0.9–1.0
Half-life – normal/ESRF (hrs)	2/unchanged

Dose in renal impairment GFR (mL/min)

20–50	Dose as in normal renal function
10–20	Dose as in normal renal function
<10	500 mg–1 g every 8 hrs

Dose in patients undergoing renal replacement therapies

CAPD	Not dialysed. Dose as in GFR = <10 mL/min
HD	Dialysed. Dose as in GFR = <10 mL/min
CAV/VVHD	Unknown dialysability. Dose as in normal renal function

Important drug interactions

CYCLOSPORIN

–

POTENTIALLY HAZARDOUS INTERACTIONS WITH OTHER DRUGS

–

Administration

RECONSTITUTION

–

ROUTE

• Oral, rectal

RATE OF ADMINISTRATION

–

COMMENTS

–

Other information

• Beware sodium content of soluble tablets (1 tablet ≈ 18.6 mmol sodium)
• Nephrotoxic in overdoses due to a reactive alkylating metabolite
• Metabolites may accumulate in ESRD. Normal doses are very often used in ESRD

Paroxetine

Clinical use

SSRI antidepressant, panic disorders

Dose in normal renal function

Initially 20 mg daily. May be increased by 10 mg increments to a maximum of 50 mg daily

Pharmacokinetics

Molecular weight (daltons)	365.8
% Protein binding	95
% Excreted unchanged in urine	<2
Volume of distribution (L/kg)	17.2
Half-life – normal/ESRF (hrs)	24/30

Dose in renal impairment GFR (mL/min)

10–30	20 mg daily
<10	20 mg daily

Dose in patients undergoing renal replacement therapies

CAPD	Unknown dialysability. Dose as in GFR = <10 mL/min
HD	Not dialysed. Dose as in GFR = <10 mL/min
CAV/VVHD	Unknown dialysability. Dose as in GFR = 10–30 mL/min

Important drug interactions

CYCLOSPORIN

–

POTENTIALLY HAZARDOUS INTERACTIONS WITH OTHER DRUGS

- Anticoagulants: effect of nicoumalone and warfarin possibly enhanced
- MAOIs: paroxetine should not be started until 2 weeks after stopping MAOI. Conversely, MAOI must not be started until 2 weeks after stopping paroxetine
- Phenytoin and possibly other anti-epileptics reduce plasma levels of paroxetine
- 5HT agonist: risk of CNS toxicity increased by sumatriptan (avoid concomitant use)
- Lithium: increased risk of CNS effects (monitor levels)

Administration

RECONSTITUTION

–

ROUTE

- Oral

RATE OF ADMINISTRATION

–

COMMENTS

–

Other information

- Incremental dosage, if required, should be restricted to lower end of range in patients with CrCl <30 mL/min

Penicillamine

Clinical use

Rheumatoid arthritis

Dose in normal renal function

125–250 mg daily for first month. Increase by the same amount every 4–12 weeks until remission occurs

Pharmacokinetics

Molecular weight (daltons)	149.2
% Protein binding	80
% Excreted unchanged in urine	10–40
Volume of distribution (L/kg)	0.8
Half-life – normal/ESRF (hrs)	1.5–3/–

Dose in renal impairment GFR (mL/min)

20–50	Avoid if possible or reduce dose. 50–125 mg for first 4–8 weeks. Increase by same amount every 4 weeks to a maximum of 1 g daily
10–20	Avoid – nephrotoxic
<10	Avoid – nephrotoxic

Dose in patients undergoing renal replacement therapies

CAPD	Unknown dialysability. Avoid – nephrotoxic
HD	Dialysed. 125–250 mg 3 times a week after HD
CAV/VVHD	Unknown dialysability. Avoid – nephrotoxic

Important drug interactions

CYCLOSPORIN

–

POTENTIALLY HAZARDOUS INTERACTIONS WITH OTHER DRUGS

–

Administration

RECONSTITUTION

–

ROUTE

• Oral

RATE OF ADMINISTRATION

–

COMMENTS

–

Other information

• Proteinuria occurs frequently and is partially dose related. In some patients it may progress to glomerulonephritis or nephrotic syndrome

• Urinalysis should be carried out weekly for the first 2 months of treatment, after any change in dosage and monthly thereafter. Increasing proteinuria may necessitate withdrawal of treatment

Pentamidine

Clinical use

Antibacterial agent, used for pneumocystis infection, treatment and prophylaxis

Dose in normal renal function

Nebuliser:
600 mg daily for 3 weeks, then 300 mg every 4 weeks
IV:
4 mg/kg/day for at least 14 days

Pharmacokinetics

Molecular weight (daltons)	340
% Protein binding	69
% Excreted unchanged in urine	<20
Volume of distribution (L/kg)	7–25
Half-life – normal/ESRF (hrs)	6–29/52–118

Dose in renal impairment GFR (mL/min)

20–50	Dose as in normal renal function
10–20	Dose as in normal renal function
<10	Depending on severity of infection: 4 mg/kg/day IV for 7–10 days, then on alternate days to complete minimum of 14 doses OR 4 mg/kg on alternate days to complete minimum of 14 doses

Dose in patients undergoing renal replacement therapies

CAPD	Not dialysed. Dose as in GFR = <10 mL/min
HD	Not dialysed. Dose as in GFR = <10 mL/min
CAV/VVHD	Unknown dialysability. Dose as in GFR = 10–20 mL/min

Important drug interactions

CYCLOSPORIN

–

POTENTIALLY HAZARDOUS INTERACTIONS WITH OTHER DRUGS

–

Administration

RECONSTITUTION

• IV: reconstitute 600 mg with 6 mL water for injection, then dilute calculated dose in 50–250 mL sodium chloride 0.9% or glucose 5%
• IM: dilute 300 mg with 3 mL water for injection

ROUTE

• IV, IM, nebulised

RATE OF ADMINISTRATION

• IV: 1 hr

COMMENTS

• Monitor patients closely

Other information

• Patient must be lying down when drug is administered
• If given by IV infusion, patient should be monitored closely: heart rate, blood pressure, blood glucose
• IV prophylaxis (unlicensed): 4–5 mg/kg over a minimum of 1 hr every 4 weeks
• Nebulise over 20 min using Respigard II or other suitable nebuliser, oxygen flow rate 6–10 mL/min
• 5 mg nebulised salbutamol may be given prior to pentamidine nebulisation to reduce risk of bronchospasm. Do not mix together in nebuliser
• May produce reversible impairment of renal function
• Renal clearance accounts for <5% of the plasma clearance of pentamidine

Perindopril

Clinical use

Angiotensin-converting enzyme inhibitor, used for hypertension, heart failure

Dose in normal renal function

2–8 mg daily

Pharmacokinetics

Molecular weight (daltons)	368.5
% Protein binding	10–20
% Excreted unchanged in urine	80–90
Volume of distribution (L/kg)	0.21
Half-life – normal/ESRF (hrs)	11/26–36

Dose in renal impairment GFR (mL/min)

30–60	2 mg daily
15–30	2 mg alternate days
<15	2 mg alternate days, adjust according to BP response

Dose in patients undergoing renal replacement therapies

CAPD	Unknown dialysability. Dose as in GFR = <15 mL/min
HD	Dialysed. Dose as in GFR = <15 mL/min
CAV/VVHD	Dialysed. Dose as in GFR = <15 mL/min

Important drug interactions

CYCLOSPORIN

• Increased risk of hyperkalaemia

POTENTIALLY HAZARDOUS INTERACTIONS WITH OTHER DRUGS

• NSAIDs: antagonism of hypotensive effect, increased risk of renal impairment and hyperkalaemia

• Epoetin: antagonism of hypotensive effect, increased risk of hyperkalaemia
• Lithium: increased lithium levels
• Potassium salts: increased risk of hyperkalaemia
• Anaesthetics: enhanced hypotensive effect
• Diuretics: enhanced hypotensive effect; increased risk of hyperkalaemia with potassium-sparing diuretics

Administration

RECONSTITUTION

–

ROUTE

• Oral

RATE OF ADMINISTRATION

–

COMMENTS

–

Other information

• Titrate dose according to response
• Small volume of distribution due to low lipophilicity
• Close monitoring of renal function during therapy is necessary in those with renal insufficiency
• Renal failure has been reported in association with ACE inhibitors in patients with renal artery stenosis, post renal transplant and those with severe congestive heart failure
• A high incidence of anaphylactoid reactions has been reported in patients dialysed with high-flux polyacrylonitrile membranes and treated concomitantly with an ACE inhibitor – this combination should therefore be avoided
• Hyperkalaemia and other side-effects are more common in patients with renal impairment

Pethidine

Clinical use

Opiate analgesia

Dose in normal renal function

IV:
25–50 mg every 4 hrs
Oral:
50–100 mg every 4 hrs
SC, IM:
25–100 mg every 4 hrs

Pharmacokinetics

Molecular weight (daltons)	284
% Protein binding	60–80
% Excreted unchanged in urine	0.6–27 depending on urinary pH
Volume of distribution (L/kg)	4–5
Half-life – normal/ESRF (hrs)	2–7/7–32

Dose in renal impairment GFR (mL/min)

20–50	Dose as in normal renal function
10–20	Use small doses. Increase dosing interval to 6 hrs and decrease dose by 25%
<10	Avoid if possible. If not, use small doses. Increase dosing interval to 8 hrs and decrease dose by 50%

Dose in patients undergoing renal replacement therapies

CAPD	Unknown dialysability. Dose as in GFR = <10 mL/min
HD	Unknown dialysability. Dose as in GFR = <10 mL/min
CAV/VVHD	Unknown dialysability. Dose as in GFR = 10–20 mL/min

Important drug interactions

CYCLOSPORIN

–

POTENTIALLY HAZARDOUS INTERACTIONS WITH OTHER DRUGS

- Avoid use with MAOIs
- Cimetidine: increases plasma concentrations
- Hyperpyrexia and CNS toxicity reported with selegiline

Administration

RECONSTITUTION

–

ROUTE

- Oral, IV, SC, IM

RATE OF ADMINISTRATION

- IV: bolus 3–4 min

COMMENTS

–

Other information

- Risk of CNS and respiratory depression or convulsions, particularly in ESRD patients receiving regular doses, due to accumulation of active metabolite norpethidine. Norpethidine levels can be measured

Phenelzine

Clinical use

Antidepressant (MAOI)

Dose in normal renal function

15 mg 3 times daily. Maximum 30 mg 3 times daily

Pharmacokinetics

Molecular weight (daltons)	136
% Protein binding	–
% Excreted unchanged in urine	0.25–1.1
Volume of distribution (L/kg)	–
Half-life – normal/ESRF (hrs)	1.5–4/–

Dose in renal impairment GFR (mL/min)

20–50	Dose as in normal renal function
10–20	Dose as in normal renal function
<10	Dose as in normal renal function

Dose in patients undergoing renal replacement therapies

CAPD	Unknown dialysability. Dose as in normal renal function
HD	Unknown dialysability. Dose as in normal renal function
CAV/VVHD	Unknown dialysability. Dose as in normal renal function

Important drug interactions

CYCLOSPORIN

–

POTENTIALLY HAZARDOUS INTERACTIONS WITH OTHER DRUGS

• Alcohol: some alcoholic and dealcoholised drinks contain tyramine which can cause hypertensive crisis

• Analgesics: CNS excitation or depression (hyper- or hypotension) with pethidine, other opioids and nefopam

• Other antidepressants: enhancement of CNS effects and toxicity. Care with all antidepressants including drug-free periods when changing therapies

• Anti-epileptics: antagonism of anticonvulsant effect (convulsive threshold lowered). Avoid carbamazepine with or within 2 weeks of MAOIs

• Antihypertensives: hypotensive effects enhanced. Avoid indoramin

• Antipsychotics: CNS excitation and hypertension with oxypertine and clozapine

• Dopaminergics: hypertensive crisis with levodopa (avoid for at least 2 weeks after stopping MAOI), hypotension with selegiline

• 5HT$_1$ agonist: risk of CNS toxicity (avoid sumatriptan for 2 weeks after MAOI)

• Sympathomimetics: hypertensive crisis with, for example, dexamphetamine, dexfenfluramine and other amphetamines, dopamine, dopexamine, ephedrine, phentermine, phenylephrine, propanolamine and pseudoephedrine

Administration

RECONSTITUTION

–

ROUTE

• Oral

RATE OF ADMINISTRATION

–

COMMENTS

–

Other information

–

Phenindione

Clinical use

Anticoagulant

Dose in normal renal function

Day 1: 200 mg; day 2: 100 mg; day 3 onwards: according to INR

Pharmacokinetics

Molecular weight (daltons)	222.2
% Protein binding	>97
% Excreted unchanged in urine	–
Volume of distribution (L/kg)	–
Half-life – normal/ESRF (hrs)	5–6/–

Dose in renal impairment GFR (mL/min)

20–50	Dose as in normal renal function
10–20	Dose as in normal renal function
<10	Dose as in normal renal function

Dose in patients undergoing renal replacement therapies

CAPD	Unknown dialysability. Dose as in normal renal function
HD	Unknown dialysability. Dose as in normal renal function
CAV/VVHD	Unknown dialysability. Dose as in normal renal function

Important drug interactions

CYCLOSPORIN

–

POTENTIALLY HAZARDOUS INTERACTIONS WITH OTHER DRUGS

- Analgesics: anticoagulant effect enhanced by aspirin; increased risk of haemorrhage with parenteral diclofenac and ketorolac (avoid concomitant use)
- Antiplatelets: anticoagulant effect enhanced by aspirin and dipyridamole
- Clofibrates: enhance anticoagulant effect
- Sex hormones: anticoagulant effect antagonised by oral contraceptives
- Thyroxine: enhanced anticoagulant effect
- Vitamin K: anticoagulant effect reduced

Administration

RECONSTITUTION

–

ROUTE

- Oral

RATE OF ADMINISTRATION

–

COMMENTS

–

Other information

- Titrate dose to end-point INR
- Enhanced anticoagulant effect in renal impairment, due to reduced protein binding
- Metabolites of phenindione often colour the urine pink or orange

Phenoxymethylpenicillin (penicillin V)

Clinical use

Antibacterial agent

Dose in normal renal function

500–750 mg every 6 hrs

Pharmacokinetics

Molecular weight (daltons)	350
% Protein binding	80
% Excreted unchanged in urine	60–90
Volume of distribution (L/kg)	0.2
Half-life – normal/ESRF (hrs)	0.5–1/4

Dose in renal impairment GFR (mL/min)

20–50	Dose as in normal renal function
10–20	Dose as in normal renal function
<10	Dose as in normal renal function

Dose in patients undergoing renal replacement therapies

CAPD	Dialysed. Dose as in normal renal function
HD	Dialysed. Dose as in normal renal function
CAV/VVHD	Dialysed. Dose as in normal renal function

Important drug interactions

CYCLOSPORIN

–

POTENTIALLY HAZARDOUS INTERACTIONS WITH OTHER DRUGS

• Reduces excretion of methotrexate

Administration

RECONSTITUTION

–

ROUTE

• Oral

RATE OF ADMINISTRATION

–

COMMENTS

–

Other information

• Potassium salt may produce hyperkalaemia. 250-mg tablet contains 0.68 mmol potassium

• Sodium salt may produce hypernatraemia. 2.8 mmol sodium per gram of salt

• Renal failure prolongs half-life of phenoxymethylpenicillin, but as it has a wide therapeutic index no dose adjustment is necessary

Phentolamine

Clinical use

Alpha-adrenoreceptor blocker, used for
hypertensive crisis

Dose in normal renal function

2–60 mg daily

Pharmacokinetics

Molecular weight (daltons)	281
% Protein binding	54
% Excreted unchanged in urine	13
Volume of distribution (L/kg)	–
Half-life – normal/ESRF (hrs)	1.5/–

Dose in renal impairment GFR (mL/min)

20–50	Dose as in normal renal function
10–20	Dose as in normal renal function
<10	Dose as in normal renal function. Titrate dose to end-point, i.e. lower BP

Dose in patients undergoing renal replacement therapies

CAPD	Unknown dialysability. Dose as in normal renal function
HD	Unknown dialysability. Dose as in normal renal function
CAV/VVHD	Unknown dialysability. Dose as in normal renal function

Important drug interactions

CYCLOSPORIN

–

POTENTIALLY HAZARDOUS INTERACTIONS WITH OTHER DRUGS

–

Administration

RECONSTITUTION

• Infusion fluid glucose 5% or sodium chloride 0.9%

ROUTE

• IV, IM

RATE OF ADMINISTRATION

• IV bolus: 2–5 mg, repeat if necessary
• IV infusion: 5–60 mg over 10–30 min (rate 0.2–2 mg/min)
• IM bolus: 5–10 mg

COMMENTS

–

Other information

• Titrate according to response
• May increase initial infusion dose to 5 mg/min for more rapid response

Phenytoin

Clinical use

Anti-epileptic agent

Dose in normal renal function

Oral:
150–600 mg/day or 3–4 mg/kg/day

Pharmacokinetics

Molecular weight (daltons)	252
% Protein binding	90
% Excreted unchanged in urine	Up to 5
Volume of distribution (L/kg)	0.7–1.0
Half-life – normal/ESRF (hrs)	10–40/unchanged

Dose in renal impairment GFR (mL/min)

20–50	Dose as in normal renal function
10–20	Dose as in normal renal function
<10	Dose as in normal renal function

Dose in patients undergoing renal replacement therapies

CAPD	Unknown dialysability. Dose as in normal renal function
HD	Unknown dialysability. Dose as in normal renal function
CAV/VVHD	Unknown dialysability. Dose as in normal renal function

Important drug interactions

CYCLOSPORIN

• Reduces cyclosporin blood levels

POTENTIALLY HAZARDOUS INTERACTIONS WITH OTHER DRUGS

• Analgesics: some NSAIDs increase phenytoin levels
• Anti-arrhythmics: amiodarone increases phenytoin levels. Phenytoin reduces levels of disopyramide, mexiletine and quinidine
• Antibacterials: level increased by chloramphenicol, isoniazid, metronidazole, co-trimoxazole and trimethoprim (+ antifolate effect), levels reduced by rifampicin

• Anticoagulants: increased metabolism (reduced effect)
• Antidepressants: antagonise anticonvulsant effect; fluoxetine, fluvoxamine and viloxazine increase phenytoin level
• Anti-epileptics: toxicity may be increased without enhanced effect
• Antifungals: levels increased by fluconazole and miconazole
• Antimalarials: antagonise anticonvulsant effect; increased antifolate effect with pyrimethamine
• Antipsychotics: antagonise anticonvulsant effect
• Calcium-channel blockers: levels increased by diltiazem and nifedipine
• Corticosteroids: metabolism accelerated (effect reduced)
• Disulfiram: levels of phenytoin increased
• Sex hormones: metabolism increased – reduced contraceptive effect
• Ulcer-healing drugs: cimetidine inhibits phenytoin metabolism; sucralfate reduces absorption; omeprazole enhances effect of phenytoin
• Uricosurics: sulphinpyrazone increases serum phenytoin levels

Administration

RECONSTITUTION

• Dilute in 50–100 mL sodium chloride 0.9%. Final concentration not exceeding 10 mg/mL

ROUTE

• Oral, IV

RATE OF ADMINISTRATION

• IV bolus: not greater than 50 mg/min
• IV infusion: 50–100 mL over 1 hr

COMMENTS

• Give by slow IV injection into large vein followed by sodium chloride 0.9% flush, to avoid irritation. Cardiac monitoring recommended
• With infusion a 0.22–0.5 micron in-line filter should be used

Other information

• Total phenytoin levels must be adjusted for hypoalbuminaemia and uraemia
• Decreased protein binding and volume of distribution in renal failure
• Free fraction of phenytoin is increased in uraemia to approximately 0.2

- Request free phenytoin serum levels, if possible
- Loading dose 15 mg/kg IV or oral, then 5 mg/kg/day. Steady state reached in 3–5 days if loading dose given
- Increase dose gradually (25–50 mg/day at weekly intervals). Demonstrates saturation kinetics
- Phenytoin absorption is markedly reduced by concurrent nasogastric enteral nutrition administration. Avoid concomitant administration with divalent cations
- May cause folate deficiency

Phosphate supplements

Clinical use

Hypophosphataemia

Dose in normal renal function

Oral:

according to response. Maximum oral dose 100 mmol in 24 hrs

IV:

10–50 mmol/day

Pharmacokinetics

Molecular weight (daltons)	94–97 (phosphate)
% Protein binding	–
% Excreted unchanged in urine	High
Volume of distribution (L/kg)	–
Half-life – normal/ESRF (hrs)	–

Dose in renal impairment GFR (mL/min)

20–50	Dose as in normal renal function
10–20	Dose as in normal renal function
<10	Start at ⅓ of normal dose

Dose in patients undergoing renal replacement therapies

CAPD	Unknown dialysability. Dose as in GFR = <10 mL/min
HD	Not dialysed. Dose as in GFR = <10 mL/min
CAV/VVHD	Dialysed. Dose as in GFR = 10–20 mL/min

Important drug interactions

CYCLOSPORIN

–

POTENTIALLY HAZARDOUS INTERACTIONS WITH OTHER DRUGS

• Avoid insoluble incompatibilities, e.g. calcium salts

Administration

RECONSTITUTION

• Phosphate polyfusor: give undiluted over 24 hrs peripherally

• Addiphos: give each vial (20 mL) diluted to 250–500 mL with glucose 5% over 6–12 hrs peripherally; 20-mL vial made up to 60 mL with glucose 5% centrally over 6–8 hrs via syringe driver

• Potassium phosphate: each 5-mL ampoule should be diluted to at least 100 mL with glucose 5% and given over at least 1 hr

ROUTE

• IV, Oral

RATE OF ADMINISTRATION

• See under reconstitution

COMMENTS

–

Other information

• Oral dosing: maximum oral dose 100 mmol phosphate in 24 hrs. (i) Slow Phosphate tablet (unlicensed product from Ciba) – 3.16 mmol phosphate/tablet; (ii) Phosphate-Sandoz – 16.1 mmol phosphate, 20.4 mmol sodium, 3 mmol potassium/tablet

• IV dosing: (i) Phosphate Polyfusor (500 mL) – 50 mmol phosphate, 81 mmol sodium, 9.5 mmol potassium; (ii) Addiphos (20 mL) – 40 mmol phosphate, 30 mmol sodium, 30 mmol potassium; (iii) Potassium Phosphate 17.42% (5 mL) – 10 mmol potassium, 5 mmol phosphate. This preparation should only be used for patients with a high sodium level. Available from Martindale Pharmaceuticals

• HD patients usually need 15–20 mmol/day in TPN

• CAV/VVHD patients usually need 30–40 mmol/day

• During IV phosphate replacement, serum calcium, potassium and phosphate should be monitored 6–12-hourly to determine the duration of the infusion. Repeat the dose within 24 hrs if an adequate level has not been achieved. Urinary output should also be monitored. Excessive doses of phosphates may cause hypocalcaemia and metastatic calcification

• Optimum IV infusion rate is 18 mmol phosphate over 24 hrs

• There is experience of giving 15 mmol over 2 hrs up to 3 times a day

Phytomenadione (vitamin K)

Clinical use

Vitamin K deficiency, antidote to oral anticoagulants

Dose in normal renal function

Oral:

10–20 mg daily

IV:

10–40 mg daily

Pharmacokinetics

Molecular weight (daltons)	451
% Protein binding	90
% Excreted unchanged in urine	<10
Volume of distribution (L/kg)	0.05–0.13
Half-life – normal/ESRF (hrs)	1.5–3/unchanged

Dose in renal impairment GFR (mL/min)

20–50	Dose as in normal renal function
10–20	Dose as in normal renal function
<10	Dose as in normal renal function

Dose in patients undergoing renal replacement therapies

CAPD	Unlikely to be dialysed. Dose as in normal renal function
HD	Unlikely to be dialysed. Dose as in normal renal function
CAV/VVHD	Unlikely to be dialysed. Dose as in normal renal function

Important drug interactions

CYCLOSPORIN

–

POTENTIALLY HAZARDOUS INTERACTIONS WITH OTHER DRUGS

• Antagonises effect of warfarin, nicoumalone and phenindione

Administration

RECONSTITUTION

–

ROUTE

• IV, Oral

RATE OF ADMINISTRATION

• Konakion® – very slow injection (1 mg/min)
• Konakion MM® – dilute each 10 mg with 55 mL of glucose 5% and give by slow infusion over 15–30 min

COMMENTS

• Dissolve oral tablets in mouth
• Risk of anaphylaxis if IV injected too rapidly
• Protect infusion from light
• Konakion® should not be diluted (non-micellar)
• Only Konakion® can be given IM

Other information

• Konakion MM® recommended for severe haemorrhage
• Anticoagulation antidote: retest prothrombin time 8–12 hrs after Konakion®, 3 hrs after Konakion MM®. Repeat dose if inadequate
• Patients with obstructive jaundice requiring oral phytomenadione should be prescribed the water-soluble preparation menadiol sodium diphosphate – the dosage range is similar

Pimozide

Clinical use

Antipsychotic

Dose in normal renal function

2–20 mg daily

Pharmacokinetics

Molecular weight (daltons)	461.6
% Protein binding	99
% Excreted unchanged in urine	<1
Volume of distribution (L/kg)	–
Half-life – normal/ESRF (hrs)	55–150/–

Dose in renal impairment GFR (mL/min)

20–50	Dose as in normal renal function
10–20	Dose as in normal renal function
<10	Start with 50% of normal dose

Dose in patients undergoing renal replacement therapies

CAPD	Unknown dialysability. Dose as in GFR = <10 mL/min
HD	Unknown dialysability. Dose as in GFR = <10 mL/min
CAV/VVHD	Unknown dialysability. Dose as in normal renal function

Important drug interactions

CYCLOSPORIN

–

POTENTIALLY HAZARDOUS INTERACTIONS WITH OTHER DRUGS

• Do not give with other antipsychotic drugs (including depots) or tricyclic antidepressants which can prolong the QT interval
• Risk of arrhythmias if clarithromycin and possibly erythromycin co-administered
• Do not give with drugs which can cause electrolyte disturbances (especially diuretics)
• Concurrent use of drugs which can prolong the QT interval is not recommended: quinine, mefloquine, amiodarone, bretylium, disopyramide, procainamide, quinidine, sotalol, terfenadine and astemizole

Administration

RECONSTITUTION

–

ROUTE

• Oral

RATE OF ADMINISTRATION

–

COMMENTS

–

Other information

• ECG required before treatment. To be repeated annually

Pindolol

Clinical use

Hypertension, angina (beta-blocker)

Dose in normal renal function

7.5–45 mg daily

Pharmacokinetics

Molecular weight (daltons)	248.3
% Protein binding	50
% Excreted unchanged in urine	40
Volume of distribution (L/kg)	1.2
Half-life – normal/ESRF (hrs)	2.5–4/unchanged

Dose in renal impairment GFR (mL/min)

20–50	Dose as in normal renal function
10–20	Dose as in normal renal function
<10	Dose as in normal renal function

Dose in patients undergoing renal replacement therapies

CAPD	Not dialysed. Dose as in normal renal function
HD	Not dialysed. Dose as in normal renal function
CAV/VVHD	Not dialysed. Dose as in normal renal function

Important drug interactions

CYCLOSPORIN

–

POTENTIALLY HAZARDOUS INTERACTIONS WITH OTHER DRUGS

• Concurrent use with sympathomimetics may result in severe hypertension
• Care with diltiazem, nifedipine and verapamil because of potential effects on cardiac conduction system and contractility

Administration

RECONSTITUTION

–

ROUTE

• Oral

RATE OF ADMINISTRATION

–

COMMENTS

–

Other information

• The fate of metabolites, even if they are inactive, is unknown
• For dialysis patients and when GFR <10 mL/min, start with smallest possible dose and titrate to response

Piperacillin

Clinical use

Antibacterial agent

Dose in normal renal function

Serious infection:

200–300 mg/kg/day (usually 4 g every 6–8 hrs)

Mild infection:

100–150 mg/kg/day (usually 2 g every 6–8 hrs or 4 g every 12 hrs)

Pharmacokinetics

Molecular weight (daltons)	517.6
% Protein binding	30
% Excreted unchanged in urine	75–90
Volume of distribution (L/kg)	0.18–0.3
Half-life – normal/ESRF (hrs)	0.8–1.5/3.3–5.1

Dose in renal impairment GFR (mL/min)

20–50	4 g every 8 hrs
10–20	4 g every 8–12 hrs
<10	4 g every 12 hrs

Dose in patients undergoing renal replacement therapies

CAPD	Dialysed. Dose as in GFR = <10 mL/min
HD	Dialysed. 2 g every 8 hrs
CAV/VVHD	Dialysed. Dose as in GFR = 10–20 mL/min

Important drug interactions

CYCLOSPORIN

–

POTENTIALLY HAZARDOUS INTERACTIONS WITH OTHER DRUGS

• Reduced excretion of methotrexate
• Prolonged action of vecuronium and similar neuromuscular blocking agents

Administration

RECONSTITUTION

• IM: each 1 g in 2 mL water for injection
• IV: each 1 g in 5 mL water for injection

ROUTE

• IM, IV

RATE OF ADMINISTRATION

• IV: in at least 50 mL glucose 5% or sodium chloride 0.9% over at least 20–40 min
• Bolus: over 3–5 min

COMMENTS

–

Other information

• Each 1 g of Pipril contains 1.85 mmol of sodium
• Single IM dose should not exceed 2 g
• Haemodialysis removes 30–50% in 4 hrs

Piperacillin/tazobactam

Clinical use

Antibacterial agent

Dose in normal renal function

4.5 g every 8 hrs

Pharmacokinetics

Molecular weight (daltons)	861.8
% Protein binding	30 (piperacillin)
% Excreted unchanged in urine	75–90 (piperacillin)
Volume of distribution (L/kg)	0.18–0.3 (piperacillin)
Half-life – normal/ESRF (hrs)	0.8–1.5/3.3–5.1 (piperacillin)

Dose in renal impairment GFR (mL/min)

20–50	4.5 g every 8 hrs
10–20	4.5 g every 12 hrs
<10	4.5 g every 12 hrs

Dose in patients undergoing renal replacement therapies

CAPD	Dialysed. Dose as in GFR = <10 mL/min
HD	Dialysed. Dose as in GFR = <10 mL/min
CAV/VVHD	Dialysed. Dose as in GFR = 10–20 mL/min

Important drug interactions

CYCLOSPORIN

–

POTENTIALLY HAZARDOUS INTERACTIONS WITH OTHER DRUGS

- Reduced excretion of methotrexate
- Prolonged action of vecuronium and similar neuromuscular blocking agents

Administration

RECONSTITUTION

- Reconstitute each 4.5 g with 20 mL water for injection

ROUTE

- IV

RATE OF ADMINISTRATION

- IV: bolus over 3–5 min

COMMENTS

- May be given as an infusion (20–30 min) in glucose 5% or sodium chloride 0.9%

Other information

- Each 4.5-g vial contains 9.37 mmol sodium

Piracetam

Clinical use

Myoclonus

Dose in normal renal function

7.2 g daily titrated to a maximum of 20 g

Pharmacokinetics

Molecular weight (daltons)	142.2
% Protein binding	15
% Excreted unchanged in urine	>90
Volume of distribution (L/kg)	0.4
Half-life – normal/ESRF (hrs)	5/–

Dose in renal impairment GFR (mL/min)

40–60	3.6 g daily titrated to a maximum of 10 g
20–40	1.8 g daily titrated to a maximum of 5 g
10–20	Contraindicated
<10	Contraindicated

Dose in patients undergoing renal replacement therapies

CAPD	Unknown dialysability. Avoid – contraindicated
HD	Dialysed. Avoid – contraindicated
CAV/VVHD	Unknown dialysability. Avoid – contraindicated

Important drug interactions

CYCLOSPORIN

–

POTENTIALLY HAZARDOUS INTERACTIONS WITH OTHER DRUGS

–

Administration

RECONSTITUTION

–

ROUTE

• Oral

RATE OF ADMINISTRATION

–

COMMENTS

–

Other information

–

Piroxicam

Clinical use

NSAID, anti-inflammatory analgesic

Dose in normal renal function

20 mg daily

Pharmacokinetics

Molecular weight (daltons)	331.4
% Protein binding	98
% Excreted unchanged in urine	10
Volume of distribution (L/kg)	1.12–0.15
Half-life – normal/ESRF (hrs)	41/unchanged

Dose in renal impairment GFR (mL/min)

20–50	Dose as in normal renal function, but avoid if possible
10–20	Dose as in normal renal function, but avoid if possible
<10	Only use if ESRD on dialysis, then use normal dose

Dose in patients undergoing renal replacement therapies

CAPD	Not dialysed. Dose as in GFR = <10 mL/min
HD	Not dialysed. Dose as in GFR = <10 mL/min
CAV/VVHD	Not dialysed. Dose as in GFR = 10–20 mL/min

Important drug interactions

CYCLOSPORIN

• Increased risk of nephrotoxicity

POTENTIALLY HAZARDOUS INTERACTIONS WITH OTHER DRUGS

• Reduced excretion of lithium
• Cytotoxic agents: reduced excretion of methotrexate
• Anticoagulants: effects of warfarin and nicoumalone enhanced
• Antidiabetic agents: effects of sulphonylureas enhanced
• Anti-epileptic agents: effects of phenytoin enhanced
• ACE inhibitors: antagonism of hypotensive effects. Increased risk of hyperkalaemia and renal damage
• Probenecid delays excretion of NSAIDs

Administration

RECONSTITUTION

–

ROUTE

• Oral

RATE OF ADMINISTRATION

–

COMMENTS

–

Other information

• Inhibition of renal prostaglandin synthesis by NSAIDs may interfere with renal function, especially in the presence of existing renal disease. Avoid if possible. If not, check serum creatinine 48–72 hrs after starting NSAID. If serum creatinine is increased, stop NSAID
• Use normal doses in patients with ESRD on dialysis
• Use with caution in renal transplant recipients – can reduce intra-renal autocoid synthesis
• Water-soluble inactive metabolites may be removed by HD and CAPD

Pivampicillin

Clinical use

Antibacterial agent

Dose in normal renal function

Mild/moderate infections:
500 mg every 12 hrs
Severe infections:
1 g every 12 hrs

Pharmacokinetics

Molecular weight (daltons)	464
% Protein binding	<20
% Excreted unchanged in urine	30–90
Volume of distribution (L/kg)	0.3
Half-life – normal/ESRF (hrs)	0.8–1.5/20

Dose in renal impairment GFR (mL/min)

20–50	Dose as in normal renal function
10–20	Dose as in normal renal function
<10	Dose as in normal renal function

Dose in patients undergoing renal replacement therapies

CAPD	Dialysed. Dose as in normal renal function
HD	Dialysed. Dose as in normal renal function
CAV/VVHD	Dialysed. Dose as in normal renal function

Important drug interactions

CYCLOSPORIN

–

POTENTIALLY HAZARDOUS INTERACTIONS WITH OTHER DRUGS

• Reduced excretion of methotrexate
• Antacids reduce absorption
• Avoid concurrent treatment with valproic acid, valproate

Administration

RECONSTITUTION

–

ROUTE

• Oral

RATE OF ADMINISTRATION

–

COMMENTS

–

Other information

• Rash more common in severe renal impairment
• Normal doses can be used in ESRD as ampicillin (pivampicillin) has a wide therapeutic index
• Pivampicillin is well absorbed and completely hydrolysed to ampicillin

Potassium chloride

Clinical use

Hypokalaemia

Dose in normal renal function

2–4 g (25–50 mmol) daily

Pharmacokinetics

Molecular weight (daltons)	75
% Protein binding	N/A
% Excreted unchanged in urine	N/A
Volume of distribution (L/kg)	N/A
Half-life – normal/ESRF (hrs)	N/A

Dose in renal impairment GFR (mL/min)

20–50	According to response
10–20	According to response
<10	According to response

Dose in patients undergoing renal replacement therapies

CAPD	Dose according to response
HD	Dose according to response
CAV/VVHD	Dose according to response

Important drug interactions

CYCLOSPORIN

• Cyclosporin: hyperkalaemia

POTENTIALLY HAZARDOUS INTERACTIONS WITH OTHER DRUGS

• ACE inhibitors: hyperkalaemia
• Potassium-sparing diuretics: hyperkalaemia

Administration

RECONSTITUTION

• Give IV solution well diluted not exceeding 40 mmol/500 mL for peripheral administration. Mix IV solutions thoroughly to avoid layering effect

ROUTE

• Oral, IV peripherally

RATE OF ADMINISTRATION

• Infusion up to 20 mmol potassium/hr except in extreme hypokalaemic emergency where some units give up to 40 mmol/hr with cardiac monitoring

COMMENTS

• Some units give more concentrated solution centrally, 100–200 mmol/100 mL sodium chloride 0.9% or glucose 5%, but at a rate no more than 20 mmol/hr. Cardiac monitoring is mandatory

Other information

• Potassium chloride injection MUST NOT be injected undiluted
• Monitor potassium levels
• Sando-K: 12 mmol potassium per tablet
• Slow-K: 8 mmol potassium per tablet
• Potassium chloride strong 15% injection: 20 mmol potassium/10 mL

Pravastatin

Clinical use

HMG CoA reductase inhibitor, used for
hyperlipidaemia

Dose in normal renal function

10–40 mg daily

Pharmacokinetics

Molecular weight (daltons)	446.5
% Protein binding	45
% Excreted unchanged in urine	47
Volume of distribution (L/kg)	0.9
Half-life – normal/ESRF (hrs)	0.8–3.2/unchanged

Dose in renal impairment
GFR (mL/min)

20–50	Dose as in normal renal function
10–20	Dose as in normal renal function
<10	Dose as in normal renal function

Dose in patients undergoing renal replacement therapies

CAPD	Unknown dialysability. Dose as in normal renal function
HD	Unknown dialysability. Dose as in normal renal function
CAV/VVHD	Unknown dialysability. Dose as in normal renal function

Important drug interactions

CYCLOSPORIN

• Statins and cyclosporin can cause myalgia, myositis
and myopathy. Different statins are reported to be
associated with a reduced incidence of this adverse
effect. Until further information is available, it is
prudent to advise all patients taking pravastatin and
cyclosporin to report any muscle pain or weakness

POTENTIALLY HAZARDOUS INTERACTIONS WITH
OTHER DRUGS

• Increased incidence of myopathy if a statin is
co-prescribed with a fibrate

Administration

RECONSTITUTION

–

ROUTE

• Oral

RATE OF ADMINISTRATION

–

COMMENTS

–

Other information

• Rhabdomyolysis with acute renal failure secondary
to statin-induced myoglobinaemia has been
reported

Prazosin

Clinical use

Alpha-adrenoreceptor blocker, used for
hypertension

Dose in normal renal function

500 micrograms–20 mg daily

Pharmacokinetics

Molecular weight (daltons)	419.9
% Protein binding	97
% Excreted unchanged in urine	<5
Volume of distribution (L/kg)	0.6–1.1
Half-life – normal/ESRF (hrs)	2.9/unchanged

Dose in renal impairment
GFR (mL/min)

20–50	Dose as in normal renal function
10–20	Dose as in normal renal function
<10	Dose as in normal renal function

Dose in patients undergoing renal replacement therapies

CAPD	Not dialysed. Dose as in normal renal function
HD	Not dialysed. Dose as in normal renal function
CAV/VVHD	Not dialysed. Dose as in normal renal function

Important drug interactions

CYCLOSPORIN

–

POTENTIALLY HAZARDOUS INTERACTIONS WITH
OTHER DRUGS

• Anaesthetics: enhanced hypotensive effects
• NSAIDs: antagonism of hypotensive effect
• Antidepressants: enhanced hypotensive effect,
  especially with MAOIs
• Beta-blockers: increased risk of first-dose
  hypotensive effect
• Calcium-channel blockers: increased risk of first-
  dose hypotensive effect
• Diuretics: enhanced hypotensive effect

Administration

RECONSTITUTION

–

ROUTE

• Oral

RATE OF ADMINISTRATION

–

COMMENTS

–

Other information

–

Prednisolone

Clinical use

Corticosteroid, used for immunosuppression, inflammation

Dose in normal renal function

Variable

Pharmacokinetics

Molecular weight (daltons)	361
% Protein binding	70–95 saturable
% Excreted unchanged in urine	7–34
Volume of distribution (L/kg)	0.3–0.7
Half-life – normal/ESRF (hrs)	2.2–3.5/unchanged

Dose in renal impairment GFR (mL/min)

20–50	Dose as in normal renal function
10–20	Dose as in normal renal function
<10	Dose as in normal renal function

Dose in patients undergoing renal replacement therapies

CAPD	Not dialysed. Dose as in normal renal function
HD	Not dialysed. Dose as in normal renal function. Give dose after HD
CAV/VVHD	Unknown dialysability. Dose as in normal renal function

Important drug interactions

CYCLOSPORIN

- Cyclosporin increases plasma levels of prednisolone; decreased cyclosporin levels reported with prednisolone

POTENTIALLY HAZARDOUS INTERACTIONS WITH OTHER DRUGS

- Metabolism accelerated by rifampicin, phenytoin, carbamazepine, phenobarbitone and primidone
- Antagonises effects of hypoglycaemic agents
- Increased risk of hypokalaemia with amphotericin

Administration

RECONSTITUTION

–

ROUTE

- Oral, IV

RATE OF ADMINISTRATION

–

COMMENTS

–

Other information

- Evidence of unpredictable bioavailability from enteric coated tablets. Avoid if possible
- Methylprednisolone anecdotally exhibits less mineralocorticoid activity compared with prednisolone in equipotent glucocorticoid activity doses

Prochlorperazine

Clinical use

Nausea and vomiting, labyrinthine disorders

Dose in normal renal function

Oral:
5–10 mg 2–3 times daily
IM/IV:
12.5 mg (unlicensed IV)
PR:
25 mg, or migraine 5 mg 3 times daily

Pharmacokinetics

Molecular weight (daltons)	373.9
% Protein binding	96
% Excreted unchanged in urine	0.005–0.04
Volume of distribution (L/kg)	23
Half-life – normal/ESRF (hrs)	3–13/–

Dose in renal impairment GFR (mL/min)

20–50	Dose as in normal renal function
10–20	Dose as in normal renal function
<10	Start with small doses, i.e. 6.25 mg IM or 5 mg orally

Dose in patients undergoing renal replacement therapies

CAPD	Unknown dialysability. Dose as in GFR = <10 mL/min
HD	Unknown dialysability. Dose as in GFR = <10 mL/min
CAV/VVHD	Unknown dialysability. Dose as in GFR = 10–20 mL/min

Important drug interactions

CYCLOSPORIN

–

POTENTIALLY HAZARDOUS INTERACTIONS WITH OTHER DRUGS

• Anaesthetics: enhanced hypotensive effect
• Anti-arrhythmics: increased risk of ventricular arrhythmias with drugs which prolong QT interval, e.g. quinidine, procainamide, disopyramide, amiodarone and sotalol
• Antidepressants: increase plasma concentrations and additive antimuscarinic effects, notably with tricyclics
• Anti-epileptics: antagonised
• Astemizole/terfenadine: increased risk of arrhythmias
• Avoid desferrioxamine
• Possible severe postural hypotension with ACE inhibitors

Administration

RECONSTITUTION

–

ROUTE

• IM or IV (unlicensed), PO, PR

RATE OF ADMINISTRATION

• IM or IV over 3–4 min

COMMENTS

• **Unlicensed** IV administration methods: either dilute injection to give in 5 times its own volume with water for injection and administer slowly over not less than 5 min, or dilute to 1 mg/mL and administer at a rate not greater than 1 mg/min

Other information

• Increased CNS sensitivity in severe renal impairment

Procyclidine

Clinical use

Control of extrapyramidal symptoms

Dose in normal renal function

2.5–10 mg 3 times a day

Pharmacokinetics

Molecular weight (daltons)	323.9
% Protein binding	–
% Excreted unchanged in urine	<5
Volume of distribution (L/kg)	1.0
Half-life – normal/ESRF (hrs)	12/–

Dose in renal impairment GFR (mL/min)

20–50	Dose as in normal renal function
10–20	Dose as in normal renal function
<10	Dose as in normal renal function

Dose in patients undergoing renal replacement therapies

CAPD	Unknown dialysability. Dose as in normal renal function
HD	Not dialysed. Dose as in normal renal function
CAV/VVHD	Unknown dialysability. Dose as in normal renal function

Important drug interactions

CYCLOSPORIN

–

POTENTIALLY HAZARDOUS INTERACTIONS WITH OTHER DRUGS

–

Administration

RECONSTITUTION

• N/A

ROUTE

• IV

RATE OF ADMINISTRATION

• Bolus over 3–5 min

COMMENTS

–

Other information

–

Promethazine

Clinical use

Antihistamine

Dose in normal renal function

12.5–25 mg 4 times daily

Pharmacokinetics

Molecular weight (daltons)	320.9
% Protein binding	93
% Excreted unchanged in urine	0
Volume of distribution (L/kg)	13.5
Half-life – normal/ESRF (hrs)	12/–

Dose in renal impairment GFR (mL/min)

20–50	Dose as in normal renal function
10–20	Dose as in normal renal function
<10	Dose as in normal renal function

Dose in patients undergoing renal replacement therapies

CAPD	Unknown dialysability. Dose as in normal renal function
HD	Unknown dialysability. Dose as in normal renal function
CAV/VVHD	Unknown dialysability. Dose as in normal renal function

Important drug interactions

CYCLOSPORIN

–

POTENTIALLY HAZARDOUS INTERACTIONS WITH OTHER DRUGS

–

Administration

RECONSTITUTION

• In 10 mL water for injection

ROUTE

• IV, (IM)

RATE OF ADMINISTRATION

• Bolus over 3–5 min

COMMENTS

–

Other information

–

Propofol

Clinical use

Induction and maintenance of general anaesthesia; sedation of ventilated patients for up to 3 days

Dose in normal renal function

Induction:
2–2.5 mg/kg
Maintenance:
4–12 mg/kg/hr
Sedation:
1–4 mg/kg/hr

Pharmacokinetics

Molecular weight (daltons)	178.3
% Protein binding	>95
% Excreted unchanged in urine	<0.3
Volume of distribution (L/kg)	3.0–14.4
Half-life – normal/ESRF (hrs)	3–4.5/unchanged

Dose in renal impairment GFR (mL/min)

20–50	Dose as in normal renal function
10–20	Dose as in normal renal function
<10	Dose as in normal renal function

Dose in patients undergoing renal replacement therapies

CAPD	Unknown dialysability. Dose as in normal renal function
HD	Unknown dialysability. Dose as in normal renal function
CAV/VVHD	Unknown dialysability. Dose as in normal renal function

Important drug interactions

CYCLOSPORIN

–

POTENTIALLY HAZARDOUS INTERACTIONS WITH OTHER DRUGS

- ACE inhibitors: enhanced hypotensive effect
- Calcium-channel blockers: enhanced hypotensive effect
- Beta-blockers: enhanced hypotensive effect

Administration

RECONSTITUTION

–

ROUTE

- IV

RATE OF ADMINISTRATION

- See local protocols

COMMENTS

–

Other information

–

Propranolol

Clinical use

Beta-adrenoreceptor blocker, used for
hypertension, angina, arrhythmias, anxiety, migraine
prophylaxis

Dose in normal renal function

30–320 mg daily

Pharmacokinetics

Molecular weight (daltons)	259
% Protein binding	80–95
% Excreted unchanged in urine	1–4
Volume of distribution (L/kg)	2.3–5.5
Half-life – normal/ESRF (hrs)	2–6/unchanged

Dose in renal impairment
GFR (mL/min)

20–50	Dose as in normal renal function
10–20	Start with small doses
<10	Start with small doses

Dose in patients undergoing renal replacement therapies

CAPD	Unknown dialysability. Dose as in GFR = <10 mL/min
HD	Not dialysed. Dose as in GFR = <10 mL/min
CAV/VVHD	Unknown dialysability. Dose as in GFR = 10–20 mL/min

Important drug interactions

CYCLOSPORIN

–

POTENTIALLY HAZARDOUS INTERACTIONS WITH
OTHER DRUGS

- Anaesthetics: enhanced hypotensive effect, risk of
  bupivacaine toxicity increased
- Anti-arrhythmics: increased risk of myocardial
  depression and bradycardia, risk of lignocaine
  toxicity increased
- Amiodarone: increased risk of bradycardia and
  AV block
- Antihypertensives: enhanced effect
- Calcium-channel blockers: increased risk of
  bradycardia and AV block with diltiazem
- Chlorpromazine: plasma concentration increased
- Sympathomimetics: severe hypertension

Administration

RECONSTITUTION

–

ROUTE

- Oral

RATE OF ADMINISTRATION

–

COMMENTS

–

Other information

- Avoid use. Non-selective. Active metabolites
  accumulate in renal impairment. Consider
  metoprolol or atenolol
- May reduce renal blood flow in severe impairment

Propylthiouracil

Clinical use

Hyperthyroidism

Dose in normal renal function

Maintenance dose:
50–150 mg daily, oral

Pharmacokinetics

Molecular weight (daltons)	170.2
% Protein binding	80
% Excreted unchanged in urine	<10
Volume of distribution (L/kg)	0.3–0.4
Half-life – normal/ESRF (hrs)	1.2/8.5

Dose in renal impairment GFR (mL/min)

20–50	Dose as in normal renal function
10–20	75% of normal dose
<10	50% of normal dose

Dose in patients undergoing renal replacement therapies

CAPD	Unknown dialysability. Dose as in GFR = <10 mL/min
HD	Unknown dialysability. Dose as in GFR = <10 mL/min
CAV/VVHD	Unknown dialysability. Dose as in GFR = 10–20 mL/min

Important drug interactions

CYCLOSPORIN

–

POTENTIALLY HAZARDOUS INTERACTIONS WITH OTHER DRUGS

–

Administration

RECONSTITUTION

–

ROUTE

• Oral

RATE OF ADMINISTRATION

–

COMMENTS

–

Other information

• Renally impaired patients are at greater risk of cardiotoxicity and leucopenia

Protamine

Clinical use

Counteracts anticoagulant effect of heparin

Dose in normal renal function

Depends on time since stopping IV/SC heparin and dose of heparin

Pharmacokinetics

Molecular weight (daltons)	–
% Protein binding	I
% Excreted unchanged in urine	–
Volume of distribution (L/kg)	–
Half-life – normal/ESRF (hrs)	–

Dose in renal impairment GFR (mL/min)

20–50	Dose as in normal renal function
10–20	Dose as in normal renal function
<10	Dose as in normal renal function

Dose in patients undergoing renal replacement therapies

CAPD	Unknown dialysability. Dose as in normal renal function
HD	Unknown dialysability. Dose as in normal renal function
CAV/VVHD	Unknown dialysability. Dose as in normal renal function

Important drug interactions

CYCLOSPORIN

–

POTENTIALLY HAZARDOUS INTERACTIONS WITH OTHER DRUGS

–

Administration

RECONSTITUTION

–

ROUTE

–

RATE OF ADMINISTRATION

• Slow IV injection over 10 min

COMMENTS

–

Other information

• In general, Img of protamine sulphate will neutralise approximately 90 units of heparin sodium derived from bovine lung tissue, and 100 units of heparin calcium or 115 units of heparin sodium derived from porcine intestinal mucosa

• Most clinicians recommend a dose of 1.0–1.5 mg protamine sulphate for each 100 units of heparin given

Protriptyline

Clinical use

Tricyclic antidepressant

Dose in normal renal function

15–60 mg daily

Pharmacokinetics

Molecular weight (daltons)	299.8
% Protein binding	92
% Excreted unchanged in urine	<5
Volume of distribution (L/kg)	15–31
Half-life – normal/ESRF (hrs)	55–198/–

Dose in renal impairment GFR (mL/min)

20–50	Dose as in normal renal function
10–20	Dose as in normal renal function
<10	Dose as in normal renal function

Dose in patients undergoing renal replacement therapies

CAPD	Not dialysed. Dose as in normal renal function
HD	Not dialysed. Dose as in normal renal function
CAV/VVHD	Unknown dialysability. Dose as in normal renal function

Important drug interactions

CYCLOSPORIN

–

POTENTIALLY HAZARDOUS INTERACTIONS WITH OTHER DRUGS

–

Administration

RECONSTITUTION

–

ROUTE

• Oral

RATE OF ADMINISTRATION

–

COMMENTS

–

Other information

–

Pseudoephedrine

Clinical use

Decongestant (nasal)

Dose in normal renal function

60 mg 4 times a day

Pharmacokinetics

Molecular weight (daltons)	201.7
% Protein binding	–
% Excreted unchanged in urine	90–98
Volume of distribution (L/kg)	2.7
Half-life – normal/ESRF (hrs)	5.5 (depends on pH of urine)

Dose in renal impairment GFR (mL/min)

20–50	Dose as in normal renal function
10–20	Dose as in normal renal function
<10	Dose as in normal renal function

Dose in patients undergoing renal replacement therapies

CAPD	Unknown dialysability. Dose as in normal renal function
HD	5–20% removed. Dose as in normal renal function
CAV/VVHD	Unknown dialysability. Dose as in normal renal function

Important drug interactions

CYCLOSPORIN

–

POTENTIALLY HAZARDOUS INTERACTIONS WITH OTHER DRUGS

• MAOIs: risk of hypertensive crisis
• Beta-blockers: risk of severe hypertension

Administration

RECONSTITUTION

–

ROUTE

• Oral

RATE OF ADMINISTRATION

–

COMMENTS

–

Other information

–

Pyrazinamide

Clinical use

Antimicrobial agent for tuberculosis

Dose in normal renal function

20–35 mg/kg/day (usually 1.5–2.0 g day)

Pharmacokinetics

Molecular weight (daltons)	123.1
% Protein binding	5
% Excreted unchanged in urine	1–3
Volume of distribution (L/kg)	0.75–1.3
Half-life – normal/ESRF (hrs)	9/26

Dose in renal impairment GFR (mL/min)

20–50	Dose as in normal renal function
10–20	Dose as in normal renal function
<10	Dose as in normal renal function

Dose in patients undergoing renal replacement therapies

CAPD	Unknown dialysability. Dose as in normal renal function
HD	50–100% dialysed. Dose as in normal renal function
CAV/VVHD	Unknown dialysability. Dose as in normal renal function

Important drug interactions

CYCLOSPORIN

• On limited evidence, pyrazinamide appears to reduce cyclosporin levels

POTENTIALLY HAZARDOUS INTERACTIONS WITH OTHER DRUGS

–

Administration

RECONSTITUTION

–

ROUTE

• Oral

RATE OF ADMINISTRATION

–

COMMENTS

–

Other information

–

Pyridostigmine

Clinical use

Myasthenia gravis

Dose in normal renal function

60 mg–1.5 g daily in divided doses

Pharmacokinetics

Molecular weight (daltons)	261.1
% Protein binding	–
% Excreted unchanged in urine	80–90
Volume of distribution (L/kg)	0.8–1.4
Half-life – normal/ESRF (hrs)	1.5–2/6

Dose in renal impairment GFR (mL/min)

20–30	35% of daily dose
10–20	35% of daily dose
<10	20% of daily dose

Dose in patients undergoing renal replacement therapies

CAPD	Unknown dialysability. Dose as in GFR = <10 mL/min
HD	Unknown dialysability. Dose as in GFR = <10 mL/min
CAV/VVHD	Unknown dialysability. Dose as in GFR = 10–20 mL/min

Important drug interactions

CYCLOSPORIN

–

POTENTIALLY HAZARDOUS INTERACTIONS WITH OTHER DRUGS

• Aminoglycosides, clindamycin and colistin antagonise effects of pyridostigmine

Administration

RECONSTITUTION

–

ROUTE

• Oral

RATE OF ADMINISTRATION

–

COMMENTS

–

Other information

–

Pyridoxine

Clinical use

Vitamin B$_6$

Dose in normal renal function

10–150 mg daily

Pharmacokinetics

Molecular weight (daltons)	205.6
% Protein binding	High (as pyridoxal and pyridoxal phosphate)
% Excreted unchanged in urine	–
Volume of distribution (L/kg)	–
Half-life – normal/ESRF	15–20 days

Dose in renal impairment GFR (mL/min)

20–50	Dose as in normal renal function
10–20	Dose as in normal renal function
<10	Dose as in normal renal function

Dose in patients undergoing renal replacement therapies

CAPD	Unknown dialysability. Dose as in normal renal function
HD	Unknown dialysability. Dose as in normal renal function
CAV/VVHD	Unknown dialysability. Dose as in normal renal function

Important drug interactions

CYCLOSPORIN

–

POTENTIALLY HAZARDOUS INTERACTIONS WITH OTHER DRUGS

–

Administration

RECONSTITUTION

–

ROUTE

• Oral

RATE OF ADMINISTRATION

–

COMMENTS

–

Other information

–

Pyrimethamine

Clinical use

Antiprotozoal agent

Dose in normal renal function

50–75 mg daily

Pharmacokinetics

Molecular weight (daltons)	248.7
% Protein binding	80–90
% Excreted unchanged in urine	16–30
Volume of distribution (L/kg)	2.9
Half-life – normal/ESRF (hrs)	80/unchanged

Dose in renal impairment GFR (mL/min)

20–50	Dose as in normal renal function
10–20	Dose as in normal renal function
<10	Dose as in normal renal function

Dose in patients undergoing renal replacement therapies

CAPD	Not dialysed. Dose as in normal renal function
HD	Not dialysed. Dose as in normal renal function
CAV/VVHD	Not dialysed. Dose as in normal renal function

Important drug interactions

CYCLOSPORIN

–

POTENTIALLY HAZARDOUS INTERACTIONS WITH OTHER DRUGS

• Increased antifolate effect with cotrimoxazole, trimethoprim and methotrexate

Administration

RECONSTITUTION

–

ROUTE

• Oral

RATE OF ADMINISTRATION

–

COMMENTS

–

Other information

–

Quinapril

Clinical use

Angiotensin-converting enzyme inhibitor – used for hypertension, heart failure

Dose in normal renal function

10–20 mg daily

Pharmacokinetics

Molecular weight (daltons)	475
% Protein binding	97
% Excreted unchanged in urine	30
Volume of distribution (L/kg)	1.5
Half-life – normal/ESRF (hrs)	1–2/6–15

Dose in renal impairment GFR (mL/min)

20–50	75–100% of normal dose
10–20	75–100% of normal dose
<10	50% of normal dose

Dose in patients undergoing renal replacement therapies

CAPD	Not dialysed. Dose as in GFR = <10 mL/min
HD	25% dialysed. Dose as in GFR = 10–20 mL/min
CAV/VVHD	Unknown dialysability. Dose as in GFR = 10–20 mL/min

Important drug interactions

CYCLOSPORIN

• Increased risk of hyperkalaemia

POTENTIALLY HAZARDOUS INTERACTIONS WITH OTHER DRUGS

• Anaesthetics: enhanced hypotensive effect
• NSAIDs: antagonism of hypotensive effects, hyperkalaemia, risk of renal impairment
• Diuretics: enhanced hypotensive effects, increased risk of hyperkalaemia with potassium-sparing diuretics
• Epoetin: increased risk of hyperkalaemia
• Lithium: reduced excretion of lithium and increased plasma levels
• Potassium salts: increased risk of hyperkalaemia

Administration

RECONSTITUTION

–

ROUTE

• Oral

RATE OF ADMINISTRATION

–

COMMENTS

–

Other information

• Renal failure has been reported with ACE inhibitors mainly in patients with renal artery stenosis, post renal transplant or those with severe congestive heart failure
• A high incidence of anaphylactoid reactions has been reported in patients dialysed with high-flux polyacrylonitrile membranes and treated concomitantly with an ACE inhibitor – this combination should therefore be avoided
• Hyperkalaemia and other side-effects are more common in patients with renal impairment
• Close monitoring of renal function during therapy is necessary in those patients with known renal insufficiency

Quinidine bisulphate

Clinical use

Supraventricular tachycardias and ventricular arrhythmias

Dose in normal renal function

500 mg 12-hourly

Pharmacokinetics

Molecular weight (daltons)	422.5
% Protein binding	70–95
% Excreted unchanged in urine	20
Volume of distribution (L/kg)	2–3.5
Half-life – normal/ESRF (hrs)	6/4–14

Dose in renal impairment GFR (mL/min)

20–50	Dose as in normal renal function
10–20	Dose as in normal renal function
<10	Dose as in normal renal function

Dose in patients undergoing renal replacement therapies

CAPD	Not dialysed. Dose as in normal renal function
HD	Dialysed. Dose as in normal renal function
CAV/VVHD	Dialysed. Dose as in normal renal function

Important drug interactions

CYCLOSPORIN

–

POTENTIALLY HAZARDOUS INTERACTIONS WITH OTHER DRUGS

• Increased risk of myocardial depression with anti-arrhythmics. Amiodarone increases plasma levels of quinidine – increased risk of ventricular arrhythmias
• Increased risk of ventricular arrhythmias with tricyclic antidepressants
• Terfenadine and astemizole: increased risk of ventricular arrhythmias
• Halofantrine and mefloquine: increased risk of ventricular arrhythmias
• Phenothiazines: increased risk of ventricular arrhythmias
• Sotalol: increased risk of ventricular arrhythmias – avoid concomitant use
• Calcium-channel blockers: nifedipine decreases plasma levels of quinidine; verapamil increases plasma levels of quinidine
• Plasma levels of digoxin increased – halve dose of digoxin
• Diuretics: quinidine toxicity is enhanced by hypokalaemia, e.g. with acetazolamide, loop and thiazide diuretics
• Muscle relaxants: effects enhanced by quinidine
• Cimetidine: inhibits metabolism of quinidine, hence increases plasma levels

Administration

RECONSTITUTION

–

ROUTE

• Oral

RATE OF ADMINISTRATION

–

COMMENTS

–

Other information

–

Quinine dihydrochloride injection
300 mg in 1 mL, 600 mg in 2 mL

Clinical use

Treatment of severe and complicated falciparum malaria

Dose in normal renal function

Quinine salt (not bisulphate):

loading dose 20 mg/kg to maximum 1.4 g, then after 8–12 hrs; maintenance 10 mg/kg (up to maximum 700 mg) 8–12-hourly, reduced to 5–7 mg/kg if parenteral treatment required for more than 48 hrs

Pharmacokinetics

Molecular weight (daltons)	379
% Protein binding	70–90
% Excreted unchanged in urine	<20
Volume of distribution (L/kg)	1.5 (healthy subjects), 1.2 (severe malaria)
Half-life – normal/ESRF (hrs)	9 (healthy), 18 (malaria)/ unchanged

Dose in renal impairment GFR (mL/min)

20–50	5–10 mg/kg every 8 hrs
10–20	5–10 mg/kg every 8–12 hrs
<10	5–10 mg/kg every 24 hrs

Dose in patients undergoing renal replacement therapies

CAPD	Unknown dialysability. Dose as in GFR = <10 mL/min
HD	Unknown dialysability. Dose as in GFR = <10 mL/min
CAV/VVHD	Unknown dialysability. Dose as in GFR = 10–20 mL/min

Important drug interactions

CYCLOSPORIN

• Decreased cyclosporin levels reported

POTENTIALLY HAZARDOUS INTERACTIONS WITH OTHER DRUGS

• Digoxin: plasma levels of digoxin increased (halve maintenance dose)
• Cimetidine: may increase plasma levels of quinine
• Halofantrine: do not give halofantrine with quinine or other drugs which may induce arrhythmias (CSM advice)
• Astemizole and terfenadine: increased risk of ventricular arrhythmias
• Rifampicin: may decrease quinine levels
• Warfarin: effect may be increased

Administration

RECONSTITUTION

• Add to sodium chloride 0.9% or glucose 5% for infusion

ROUTE

• IV infusion

RATE OF ADMINISTRATION

• 4 hrs

COMMENTS

• Loading dose of 20 mg/kg may be required in some cases (refer to specialist treatment). Not to be given if patient has had quinine, quinidine or mefloquine in previous 24 hrs

Other information

• Quinine dihydrochloride injection is available as a special order
• Monitor for signs of cardiotoxicity
• Give doses after haemodialysis

Quinine sulphate, bisulphate or hydrochloride

Clinical use

Nocturnal cramp

Dose in normal renal function

200–300 mg at night

Pharmacokinetics

Molecular weight (daltons)	379
% Protein binding	70–90
% Excreted unchanged in urine	5–20
Volume of distribution (L/kg)	1.5
Half-life – normal/ESRF (hrs)	7–11/unchanged

Dose in renal impairment GFR (mL/min)

20–50	Dose as in normal renal function
10–20	Dose as in normal renal function
<10	Dose as in normal renal function

Dose in patients undergoing renal replacement therapies

CAPD	Unknown dialysability. Dose as in normal renal function
HD	Dialysed. Dose as in normal renal function
CAV/VVHD	Dialysed. Dose as in normal renal function

Important drug interactions

CYCLOSPORIN

• Decreased cyclosporin levels reported

POTENTIALLY HAZARDOUS INTERACTIONS WITH OTHER DRUGS

• Halofantrine: do not give with quinine (CSM advice) – serious risk of cardiac arrhythmias
• Cimetidine: increased quinine levels
• Increases digoxin plasma levels. Use small quinine dose and monitor digoxin levels. Halve digoxin maintenance dose
• Astemizole and terfenadine: increased risk of ventricular arrhythmias

Administration

RECONSTITUTION

–

ROUTE

• Oral

RATE OF ADMINISTRATION

–

COMMENTS

–

Other information

• Monitor quinine levels if patient exhibits any symptoms of toxicity
• Give dose after haemodialysis

Ramipril

Clinical use

Angiotensin-converting enzyme inhibitor, used for hypertension, secondary prevention of myocardial infarction, congestive heart failure

Dose in normal renal function

1.25–10 mg once a day

Pharmacokinetics

Molecular weight (daltons)	388*
% Protein binding	50–60*
% Excreted unchanged in urine	10–21
Volume of distribution (L/kg)	430*
Half-life – normal/ESRF (hrs)	3/15*

Dose in renal impairment GFR (mL/min)

20–50	Dose as in normal renal function
10–20	1.25–5 mg daily
<10	1.25–2.5 mg daily

Dose in patients undergoing renal replacement therapies

CAPD	Unknown dialysability. Dose as in GFR = <10 mL/min
HD	Dialysed. Dose as in GFR = <10 mL/min
CAV/VVHD	Dialysed. Dose as in GFR = 10–20 mL/min

Important drug interactions

CYCLOSPORIN

• Increased risk of hyperkalaemia

POTENTIALLY HAZARDOUS INTERACTIONS WITH OTHER DRUGS

• Potassium supplements: increased risk of hyperkalaemia
• Lithium levels may be increased
• NSAIDs: risk of renal impairment, antagonism of hypotensive effects, increased risk of hyperkalaemia
• Anaesthetics: enhanced hypotensive effect
• Diuretics: enhanced hypotensive effect, increased risk of hyperkalaemia with potassium-sparing diuretics
• Epoetin: increased risk of hyperkalaemia

Administration

RECONSTITUTION

–

ROUTE

• Oral

RATE OF ADMINISTRATION

–

COMMENTS

–

Other information

* Refers to active metabolite ramiprilat
• Renal failure has been reported in association with ACE inhibitors in patients with renal artery stenosis, post renal transplant, or those with congestive heart failure
• A high incidence of anaphylactoid reactions has been reported in patients dialysed with high-flux polyacrylonitrile membranes and treated concomitantly with an ACE inhibitor – this combination should therefore be avoided
• Hyperkalaemia and other side-effects are more common in patients with impaired renal function
• Close monitoring of renal function during therapy is necessary in those patients with known renal insufficiency

Ranitidine

Clinical use

H_2 antagonist, used for conditions associated with hyperacidity

Dose in normal renal function

Oral:

150–300 mg once or twice daily

Zollinger Ellison:

150 mg 3 times daily up to 6 g/day

IM/slow IV injection:

50 mg every 6–8 hrs

IV infusion:

25 mg/hr for 2 hrs, 6–8-hourly; or for stress ulceration prophylaxis 125–250 mg/kg/hr

Pharmacokinetics

Molecular weight (daltons)	314
% Protein binding	15
% Excreted unchanged in urine	oral: 30–70; IV: 70–80
Volume of distribution (L/kg)	1–2
Half-life – normal/ESRF (hrs)	2–3/6–9

Dose in renal impairment GFR (mL/min)

20–50	Dose as in normal renal function
10–20	Dose as in normal renal function
<10	50–100% of normal dose

Dose in patients undergoing renal replacement therapies

CAPD	Unknown dialysability. Dose as in GFR = <10 mL/min
HD	Dialysed. Dose as in GFR = <10mL/min
CAV/VVHD	Probably dialysed. Dose as in GFR = 10–20 mL/min

Important drug interactions

CYCLOSPORIN

- May increase or not change cyclosporin levels
- Nephrotoxicity, additive hepatotoxicity and thrombocytopenia reported

POTENTIALLY HAZARDOUS INTERACTIONS WITH OTHER DRUGS

–

Administration

RECONSTITUTION

- Compatible with sodium chloride 0.9%, glucose 5% and other fluids

ROUTE

- Oral, IV peripherally, IM (undiluted)

RATE OF ADMINISTRATION

- Bolus: 50 mg made up to 20 mL over at least 2 min
- Intermittent infusion: 50 mg to 100 mL of appropriate intravenous solution run over 2 hrs
- Continuous infusion: required dose in 250 mL of intravenous fluid over 24 hrs

COMMENTS

- Admixtures stable for 24 hrs

Other information

- Use in preference to cimetidine in elderly patients, those who have side-effects to cimetidine and those in whom drug interactions may be a problem

Ribavirin (tribavirin)

Clinical use

Antiviral agent for treatment of severe respiratory syncytial virus bronchiolitis

Dose in normal renal function

6 g nebulised daily for 3–7 days

Pharmacokinetics

Molecular weight (daltons)	244
% Protein binding	0
% Excreted unchanged in urine	10–40
Volume of distribution (L/kg)	647
Half-life – normal/ESRF (hrs)	9/–

Dose in renal impairment GFR (mL/min)

20–50	Dose as in normal renal function
10–20	Dose as in normal renal function
<10	Dose as in normal renal function

Dose in patients undergoing renal replacement therapies

CAPD	Unknown dialysability. Dose as in normal renal function
HD	Unknown dialysability. Dose as in normal renal function
CAV/VVHD	Unknown dialysability. Dose as in normal renal function

Important drug interactions

CYCLOSPORIN

–

POTENTIALLY HAZARDOUS INTERACTIONS WITH OTHER DRUGS

• Ribavirin may antagonise the effects of zidovudine

Administration

RECONSTITUTION

• Dissolve contents of one vial in water for injection and further dilute to a volume of 300 mL

ROUTE

• Nebulised

RATE OF ADMINISTRATION

• Administer over 12–18 hrs per day

COMMENTS

• Treatment should be carried out for at least 3 days and no more than 7 days

Other information

• Refer to literature for information on the administration of ribavirin
• Ribavirin is also available as an intravenous infusion (named patient basis). Refer to product literature for dosage reduction in renal failure

Rifampicin

Clinical use

Antibacterial agent for tuberculosis and staphylococcal infection

Dose in normal renal function

Oral or IV:
450–1200 mg daily

Pharmacokinetics

Molecular weight (daltons)	823
% Protein binding	60–90
% Excreted unchanged in urine	15–30
Volume of distribution (L/kg)	0.9
Half-life – normal/ESRF (hrs)	1.5–5/1.8–11

Dose in renal impairment GFR (mL/min)

20–50	Dose as in normal renal function
10–20	Dose as in normal renal function
<10	50–100% of normal dose

Dose in patients undergoing renal replacement therapies

CAPD	Not dialysed. Dose as in GFR = <10 mL/min
HD	Not dialysed. Dose as in GFR = <10 mL/min
CAV/VVHD	Unknown dialysability. Dose as in normal renal function

Important drug interactions

CYCLOSPORIN

- Markedly reduced plasma levels (danger of transplant rejection); cyclosporin dose may need to be increased 5-fold or more

POTENTIALLY HAZARDOUS INTERACTIONS WITH OTHER DRUGS

- Drugs metabolised by the cytochrome p450 IIIa system
- Double steroid dose. Give as twice-daily dosage
- Reduced plasma concentration of chloramphenicol and dapsone
- Reduced anticoagulant effect of warfarin
- Reduced antidiabetic effect of chlorpropamide and tolbutamide
- Reduced plasma concentration of phenytoin
- Reduced plasma concentration of fluconazole, itraconazole, ketoconazole and terbinafine
- Reduced plasma level of corticosteroids
- Increased metabolism of azathioprine – reduced plasma levels
- Reduced plasma levels of combined and progestogen-only oral contraceptive
- Rifampicin also accelerates the metabolism of the following drugs (possible reduced effect): methadone, antacids, disopyramide, mexiletine, propafenone, quinidine, tricyclic antidepressants, haloperidol, benzodiazepines, bisoprolol, propranolol, diltiazem, verapamil, isradipine, nifedipine, digitoxin, fluvastatin

Administration

RECONSTITUTION

- Use solvent provided. Dilute in 500 mL glucose 5% or sodium chloride 0.9%

ROUTE

- IV peripherally (or orally)

RATE OF ADMINISTRATION

- 2–3 hrs

COMMENTS

- For central administration, 600 mg in 100 mL glucose 5% over 0.5–2 hrs has been used (unlicensed). Stable for up to 24 hrs at room temperature

Other information

- Some units give dose in concentrations up to 60 mg/mL over 10 min in its own solvent on prescriber's responsibility
- May cause acute interstitial nephritis, potassium wasting or renal tubular defects
- Reduce dose if LFT abnormal or patient <45 kg
- Absorption from gastrointestinal tract can be reduced by up to 80% by the presence of food in the gastrointestinal tract
- CAPD exit site infections: 300 mg twice daily for 4 weeks has been used
- Rifampicin is excreted into CAPD fluid causing an orange/yellow colour
- Monitor rifampicin levels if necessary

Rocuronium bromide

Clinical use

Muscle relaxant in general anaesthesia

Dose in normal renal function

IV injection:

intubation dose = 0.6 mg/kg;
maintenance = 0.15 mg/kg

IV infusion:

0.6 mg/kg loading dose, followed by
0.3–0.6 mg/kg/hr

Pharmacokinetics

Molecular weight (daltons)	610
% Protein binding	25–30
% Excreted unchanged in urine	13–30
Volume of distribution (L/kg)	0.21
Half-life – normal/ESRF (hrs)	1.5/2

Dose in renal impairment GFR (mL/min)

20–50	Dose as in normal renal function
10–20	Dose as in normal renal function
<10	Dose as in normal renal function

Dose in patients undergoing renal replacement therapies

CAPD	Unknown dialysability. Dose as in normal renal function
HD	Unknown dialysability. Dose as in normal renal function
CAV/VVHD	Unknown dialysability. Dose as in normal renal function

Important drug interactions

CYCLOSPORIN

–

POTENTIALLY HAZARDOUS INTERACTIONS WITH OTHER DRUGS

• Effects of rocuronium enhanced by quinidine and aminoglycoside and polypeptide antibiotics

Administration

RECONSTITUTION

• Compatible with sodium chloride 0.9% and glucose 5%

ROUTE

• IV

RATE OF ADMINISTRATION

• Slow bolus or continuous infusion

COMMENTS

–

Other information

• Use with caution in renal failure. Prolongation of action may be seen
• There are no clinically active metabolites of rocuronium

Salbutamol

Clinical use

Beta$_2$-adrenoreceptor agonist, used for reversible airways disease

Dose in normal renal function

Oral:

4 mg 3–4 times daily

SC/IM:

500 micrograms repeated 4-hourly if necessary

IV:

250 micrograms/5 mL slow bolus

Infusion:

start with 5 micrograms/min, adjust according to response, usually 3–20 micrograms/min

Aerosol:

100–200 micrograms (1–2 puffs) 4 times daily

Powder:

200–400 micrograms 4 times daily

Nebulisation:

2.5–5 mg 4 times daily or more frequently

Pharmacokinetics

Molecular weight (daltons)	239.3
% Protein binding	10
% Excreted unchanged in urine	50–64
Volume of distribution (L/kg)	2.8–4.0
Half-life – normal/ESRF (hrs)	2.7–5/unchanged

Dose in renal impairment GFR (mL/min)

20–50	Dose as in normal renal function
10–20	Dose as in normal renal function
<10	Dose as in normal renal function

Dose in patients undergoing renal replacement therapies

CAPD	Unknown dialysability. Dose as in normal renal function
HD	Unknown dialysability. Dose as in normal renal function
CAV/VVHD	Unknown dialysability. Dose as in normal renal function

Important drug interactions

CYCLOSPORIN

–

POTENTIALLY HAZARDOUS INTERACTIONS WITH OTHER DRUGS

• Increased risk of hypokalaemia when diuretics, theophylline or large doses of corticosteroids are given with high doses of salbutamol

Administration

RECONSTITUTION

• Infusion: dilute 10mL to 500mL sodium chloride 0.9% or glucose 5% (20 micrograms/mL)
• Via syringe pump: dilute 10mL to 50mL sodium chloride 0.9% or glucose 5% (200 micrograms/mL)

ROUTE

• IV

RATE OF ADMINISTRATION

• IV slow bolus; IV infusion 3–20 micrograms/min

COMMENTS

–

Other information

• Monitor ECG/BP/pulse
• Nebulised salbutamol may be prescribed for hypokalaemic effect in acute hyperkalaemia (unlicensed)

Senna (Sennoside B)

Clinical use

Constipation

Dose in normal renal function

15–30 mg (2–4 tablets) at night

Pharmacokinetics

Molecular weight (daltons)	862.7
% Protein binding	Systemic bioavailability less than 5%
% Excreted unchanged in urine	–
Volume of distribution (L/kg)	–
Half-life – normal/ESRF (hrs)	–

Dose in renal impairment GFR (mL/min)

20–50	Dose as in normal renal function
10–20	Dose as in normal renal function
<10	Dose as in normal renal function

Dose in patients undergoing renal replacement therapies

CAPD	Unknown dialysability. Dose as in normal renal function
HD	Unknown dialysability. Dose as in normal renal function
CAV/VVHD	Unknown dialysability. Dose as in normal renal function

Important drug interactions

CYCLOSPORIN

–

POTENTIALLY HAZARDOUS INTERACTIONS WITH OTHER DRUGS

–

Administration

RECONSTITUTION

–

ROUTE

• Oral

RATE OF ADMINISTRATION

–

COMMENTS

–

Other information

• Acts in 8–12 hrs
• Syrup available, 1 tablet = 5 mL; granules available, 1 x 5-mL spoonful = 2 tablets
• Diabetic patients should use the tablets as these have a negligible sugar content

Sertraline

Clinical use

SSRI antidepressant

Dose in normal renal function

50 mg daily (maximum 200 mg for 8 weeks only)

Pharmacokinetics

Molecular weight (daltons)	342.7
% Protein binding	>98
% Excreted unchanged in urine	0
Volume of distribution (L/kg)	>20
Half-life – normal/ESRF (hrs)	26/probably unchanged

Dose in renal impairment GFR (mL/min)

20–50	Dose as in normal renal function
10–20	Dose as in normal renal function
<10	Dose as in normal renal function

Dose in patients undergoing renal replacement therapies

CAPD	Unknown dialysability. Dose as in normal renal function
HD	Unknown dialysability. Dose as in normal renal function
CAV/VVHD	Unknown dialysability. Dose as in normal renal function

Important drug interactions

CYCLOSPORIN

–

POTENTIALLY HAZARDOUS INTERACTIONS WITH OTHER DRUGS

• Effect of warfarin possibly enhanced
• Increased risk of toxic CNS effects of MAOIs; sertraline and MAOIs should not be prescribed within a 2-week period of each other
• Lithium: increased risk of CNS effects – lithium toxicity reported

Administration

RECONSTITUTION

–

ROUTE

• Oral

RATE OF ADMINISTRATION

–

COMMENTS

–

Other information

• Sertraline is extensively metabolised by the liver. It can be used in renal failure at normal doses with caution

Simple linctus

Clinical use

Relief of dry, irritating coughs

Dose in normal renal function

5–10 mL 3–4 times daily

Pharmacokinetics

Molecular weight (daltons)	210.1 (citric acid monohydrate)
% Protein binding	–
% Excreted unchanged in urine	–
Volume of distribution (L/kg)	–
Half-life – normal/ESRF (hrs)	–

Dose in renal impairment GFR (mL/min)

20–50	Dose as in normal renal function
10–20	Dose as in normal renal function
<10	Dose as in normal renal function

Dose in patients undergoing renal replacement therapies

CAPD	Unknown dialysability. Dose as in normal renal function
HD	Unknown dialysability. Dose as in normal renal function
CAV/VVHD	Unknown dialysability. Dose as in normal renal function

Important drug interactions

CYCLOSPORIN

–

POTENTIALLY HAZARDOUS INTERACTIONS WITH OTHER DRUGS

–

Administration

RECONSTITUTION

–

ROUTE

• Oral

RATE OF ADMINISTRATION

–

COMMENTS

–

Other information

• Avoid in diabetic patients
• Sugar content has not been found to alter diabetics' insulin requirements. Use diabetic cough preparations

Simvastatin

Clinical use

HMG CoA reductase inhibitor, used for primary hypercholesterolaemia

Dose in normal renal function

10–40 mg at night

Pharmacokinetics

Molecular weight (daltons)	418
% Protein binding	>94
% Excreted unchanged in urine	13
Volume of distribution (L/kg)	54
Half-life – normal/ESRF (hrs)	1.9/–

Dose in renal impairment GFR (mL/min)

20–50	Dose as in normal renal function
10–20	Dose as in normal renal function
<10	10 mg daily*

Dose in patients undergoing renal replacement therapies

CAPD	Unknown dialysability. Dose as in GFR = <10 mL/min
HD	Unknown dialysability. Dose as in GFR = <10 mL/min
CAV/VVHD	Unknown dialysability. Dose as in normal renal function

Important drug interactions

CYCLOSPORIN

• Increased risk of myopathy. Maximum recommended dosage of simvastatin is 10 mg/day

POTENTIALLY HAZARDOUS INTERACTIONS WITH OTHER DRUGS

• Warfarin effect potentiated
• Increased risk of myopathy if prescribed concomitantly with fibrates

Administration

RECONSTITUTION

–

ROUTE

–

RATE OF ADMINISTRATION

–

COMMENTS

–

Other information

* In severe renal impairment doses above 10 mg should be used with caution

Sodium bicarbonate

Clinical use

Metabolic acidosis, alkalinisation of urine

Dose in normal renal function

Oral:
600 mg–1.8 g 3 times daily (or more may be required)
IV:
8.4%: 60–120 mL/hr; 4.2%: up to 120 mL/hr

Pharmacokinetics

Molecular weight (daltons)	84
% Protein binding	0
% Excreted unchanged in urine	–
Volume of distribution (L/kg)	Dependent on the physical state of the patient at the time
Half-life – normal/ESRF (hrs)	–

Dose in renal impairment GFR (mL/min)

20–50	Dose as in normal renal function
10–20	Dose as in normal renal function
<10	Use with caution

Dose in patients undergoing renal replacement therapies

CAPD	Dialysed. Dose as in GFR = <10 mL/min
HD	Dialysed. Dose as in GFR = <10 mL/min
CAV/VVHD	Dialysed. Dose as in normal renal function

Important drug interactions

CYCLOSPORIN

–

POTENTIALLY HAZARDOUS INTERACTIONS WITH OTHER DRUGS

• Increases lithium excretion

Administration

RECONSTITUTION

–

ROUTE

• IV, central administration for undiluted infusion

RATE OF ADMINISTRATION

–

COMMENTS

–

Other information

• **Caution** – may result in sodium retention and oedema
• 8.4% ≡ 1 mmol bicarbonate/mL + 1 mmol sodium/mL
• 600 mg sodium bicarbonate ≡ 7 mmol sodium + 7 mmol bicarbonate
• Sodium bicarbonate reduces serum potassium concentrations by inducing a shift of potassium ions into the cell

Sodium chloride

Clinical use

Treatment and prophylaxis of sodium chloride
deficiency

Dose in normal renal function

Oral:

prophylaxis: 40–80 mmol sodium daily, up to a
maximum of 200 mmol sodium daily

100–160 mmol sodium after haemodialysis

Pharmacokinetics

Molecular weight (daltons)	58.5
% Protein binding	0
% Excreted unchanged in urine	–
Volume of distribution (L/kg)	Dependent on the physiological state of the patient at the time
Half-life – normal/ESRF (hrs)	–

Dose in renal impairment GFR (mL/min)

20–50	Dose as in normal renal function
10–20	Dose as in normal renal function
<10	Dose as in normal renal function

Dose in patients undergoing renal replacement therapies

CAPD	Dialysed. Dose as in normal renal function
HD	Dialysed. Dose as in normal renal function
CAV/VVHD	Dialysed. Dose as in normal renal function

Important drug interactions

CYCLOSPORIN

–

POTENTIALLY HAZARDOUS INTERACTIONS WITH
OTHER DRUGS

• May impair the efficacy of antihypertensive drugs
in chronic renal failure

Administration

RECONSTITUTION

–

ROUTE

• Oral, IV

RATE OF ADMINISTRATION

–

COMMENTS

–

Other information

• Other regimens: for acute muscular cramps
post haemodialysis 10 mL sodium chloride
30% injection diluted in 100 mL sodium chloride
0.9% and infused over 30 min or in dialysis
washback

• Sodium salts should be administered with
caution to patients with congestive heart failure,
peripheral or pulmonary oedema, or impaired
renal function

Sodium nitroprusside

Clinical use

Hypertensive crisis, cardiac failure

Dose in normal renal function

IV:

0.3–8.0 micrograms/kg/min. Range 10–400 micrograms/min

Pharmacokinetics

Molecular weight (daltons)	298
% Protein binding	0
% Excreted unchanged in urine	<10
Volume of distribution (L/kg)	0.2
Half-life – normal/ESRF	2–10 min/unchanged

Dose in renal impairment GFR (mL/min)

20–50	Dose as in normal renal function
10–20	Dose as in normal renal function. Avoid prolonged use
<10	Dose as in normal renal function. Avoid prolonged use

Dose in patients undergoing renal replacement therapies

CAPD	Dialysed. Dose as in GFR = <10 mL/min
HD	Dialysed. Dose as in GFR = <10 mL/min
CAV/VVHD	Unknown dialysability. Dose as in GFR = 10–20 mL/min

Important drug interactions

CYCLOSPORIN

–

POTENTIALLY HAZARDOUS INTERACTIONS WITH OTHER DRUGS

• Anaesthetics: enhanced hypotensive effect

Administration

RECONSTITUTION

• 2 mL glucose 5%, then dilute 50 mg to 50 mL with glucose 5%

ROUTE

• IV

RATE OF ADMINISTRATION

• 10–400 micrograms/min adjusted according to response

COMMENTS

• Wrap syringes and lines in foil to protect from light
• For peripheral use dilute 50 mg to 250 mL (200 micrograms/mL)

Other information

• Sodium nitroprusside is rapidly metabolised to cyanogen which is converted to thiocyanate
• Avoid prolonged use in renal impairment. Accumulation of thiocyanate (toxic), which is dialysable
• Monitor thiocyanate and cyanide levels
• Do not stop infusion abruptly – tail off over 10–30 min

Sodium valproate

Clinical use

All forms of epilepsy

Dose in normal renal function

Oral:

600 mg–2.5 g daily in divided doses

IV:

for continuation of therapy give existing oral dose. Initiation: 400–800 mg (up to 10 mg/kg), then further doses up to 2.5 g daily

Pharmacokinetics

Molecular weight (daltons)	166
% Protein binding	90
% Excreted unchanged in urine	3–7
Volume of distribution (L/kg)	0.1–0.4
Half-life – normal/ESRF (hrs)	6–15/unchanged

Dose in renal impairment GFR (mL/min)

20–50	Dose as in normal renal function
10–20	Dose as in normal renal function
<10	Dose as in normal renal function

Dose in patients undergoing renal replacement therapies

CAPD	Unknown dialysability. Dose as in normal renal function
HD	Not dialysed. Dose as in normal renal function
CAV/VVHD	Unknown dialysability. Dose as in normal renal function

Important drug interactions

CYCLOSPORIN

• Variable cyclosporin blood level response

POTENTIALLY HAZARDOUS INTERACTIONS WITH OTHER DRUGS

• Antidepressants, antipsychotics and antimalarials: antagonise anticonvulsant effect
• Other anti-epileptics: enhance toxicity and possibly reduce plasma concentrations

Administration

RECONSTITUTION

• IV: use solvent provided

ROUTE

• IV

RATE OF ADMINISTRATION

• 3–5 min bolus, or continuous infusion

COMMENTS

Other information

• Available as enteric-coated controlled-release, crushable tablets, liquid and syrup
• Increases ketones in urine. May give false-positive urine tests for ketones
• Sodium valproate serum levels do not correlate with anti-epileptic activity
• Monitor serum levels to ensure not greater than 100 micrograms/mL, or if non-compliance is suspected
• In severe renal insufficiency it may be necessary to alter doses according to free serum levels

Sotalol

Clinical use

Beta-adrenoreceptor blocker, used for treatment of ventricular arrhythmias; prophylaxis of supra-ventricular tachycardia

Dose in normal renal function

Oral:
80–640 mg per day in single or divided doses
IV:
0.5–1.5 mg/kg every 6 hrs

Pharmacokinetics

Molecular weight (daltons)	309
% Protein binding	0
% Excreted unchanged in urine	>90%
Volume of distribution (L/kg)	1–2
Half-life – normal/ESRF (hrs)	7–15/56

Dose in renal impairment GFR (mL/min)

20–50	50% of normal dose
10–20	25% of normal dose
<10	Avoid or use with caution

Dose in patients undergoing renal replacement therapies

CAPD	Unknown dialysability. Dose as in GFR = <10 mL/min
HD	Unknown dialysability. Dose as in GFR = <10 mL/min
CAV/VVHD	Unknown dialysability. Dose as in GFR = 10–20 mL/min

Important drug interactions

CYCLOSPORIN

–

POTENTIALLY HAZARDOUS INTERACTIONS WITH OTHER DRUGS

- Anti-arrhythmics: increased risk of bradycardia and AV block with amiodarone
- Calcium-channel blockers: increased risk of bradycardia and AV block with diltiazem and verapamil
- Mefloquine may increase risk of bradycardia
- Risk of ventricular arrhythmias associated with sotalol increased by halofantrine, tricyclic antidepressants, astemizole, terfenadine and erythromycin

Administration

RECONSTITUTION

–

ROUTE

- IV

RATE OF ADMINISTRATION

- Slow IV bolus with ECG monitoring. Give doses of 60–100 mg over 3 min

COMMENTS

–

Other information

- Sotalol prolongs the QT interval, which predisposes to the development of torsades de pointes
- If used in haemodialysis, give lowest possible dose, after dialysis

Spectinomycin

Clinical use

Antibacterial agent

Dose in normal renal function

IM:

single dose of 2 g (maximum 4 g)

Pharmacokinetics

Molecular weight (daltons)	495.4
% Protein binding	5–20
% Excreted unchanged in urine	35–90
Volume of distribution (L/kg)	0.25
Half-life – normal/ESRF (hrs)	2/16–29

Dose in renal impairment GFR (mL/min)

20–50	Dose as in normal renal function
10–20	Dose as in normal renal function
<10	Dose as in normal renal function

Dose in patients undergoing renal replacement therapies

CAPD	Probably dialysed. Dose as in normal renal function
HD	Probably dialysed. Dose as in normal renal function. Give post-dialysis
CAV/VVHD	Probably dialysed. Dose as in normal renal function

Important drug interactions

CYCLOSPORIN

–

POTENTIALLY HAZARDOUS INTERACTIONS WITH OTHER DRUGS

• Increased lithium effect and toxicity

Administration

RECONSTITUTION

• Add 3.2 mL of diluent to a 2-g vial

ROUTE

• IM (deep intragluteal)

RATE OF ADMINISTRATION

–

COMMENTS

–

Other information

• A standard single dose may be given in all degrees of renal insufficiency. If multiple doses are required, give at intervals of 48 hrs. In haemodialysis no further doses are required in the interdialytic period

• Give IM injection after haemodialysis

Streptokinase

Clinical use

Fibrinolytic, used for thrombolysis in deep vein thrombosis, pulmonary embolism, acute arterial thromboembolism, acute myocardial infarction, thrombosed A-V shunts

Dose in normal renal function

Loading dose:

600 000 iu followed by 100 000 iu/hr for 72 hrs

MI:

1.5 M iu followed by aspirin

Thrombolysed HD shunts:

10–25 000 iu sealed in shunt and repeated after 30–45 min

Pharmacokinetics

Molecular weight (daltons)	47 408
% Protein binding	–
% Excreted unchanged in urine	0
Volume of distribution (L/kg)	–
Half-life – normal/ESRF	18–20 min/–

Dose in renal impairment GFR (mL/min)

20–50	Dose as in normal renal function
10–20	Dose as in normal renal function
<10	Dose as in normal renal function

Dose in patients undergoing renal replacement therapies

CAPD	Not dialysed. Dose as in normal renal function
HD	Not dialysed. Dose as in normal renal function
CAV/VVHD	Not dialysed. Dose as in normal renal function

Important drug interactions

CYCLOSPORIN

–

POTENTIALLY HAZARDOUS INTERACTIONS WITH OTHER DRUGS

• Anticoagulants should not be given with streptokinase

• Heparin infusions should be stopped 4 hrs before streptokinase infusion. If this is not possible, protamine sulphate should be used to neutralise the heparin

• Heparin infusions can be restarted 4 hrs post streptokinase infusion, followed by oral anticoagulants

Administration

RECONSTITUTION

• See manufacturer's literature

ROUTE

• IV

RATE OF ADMINISTRATION

• Give loading dose of 600 000 iu in 100 mL fluid over 30 min, followed by an appropriate volume for the maintenance dose

• Give 1.5 M iu for acute MI in 100 mL fluid over 1 hr

COMMENTS

• For occluded HD shunts, add 100 000 iu to 100 mL sodium chloride 0.9% and put 10–25 mL into the clotted portion of the shunt

Other information

• There are no significant changes in pharmacokinetics in patients with renal insufficiency. Dosage reduction is therefore not necessary

Sucralfate (aluminium sucrose sulphate)

Clinical use

Treatment of peptic ulcer and chronic gastritis; prophylaxis of stress ulceration in seriously ill patients

Dose in normal renal function

4 g daily in 2–4 divided doses. Maximum 8 g daily
Prophylaxis of stress ulceration: 1 g 6 times daily

Pharmacokinetics

Molecular weight (daltons)	2087
% Protein binding	–
% Excreted unchanged in urine	3–5
Volume of distribution (L/kg)	–
Half-life – normal/ESRF (hrs)	–

Dose in renal impairment GFR (mL/min)

20–50	4 g daily
10–20	2–4 g daily
<10	2–4 g daily

Dose in patients undergoing renal replacement therapies

CAPD	Not dialysed. Dose as in GFR = <10 mL/min
HD	Not dialysed. Dose as in GFR = <10 mL/min
CAV/VVHD	Not dialysed. Dose as in GFR = 10–20 ml/min

Important drug interactions

CYCLOSPORIN

–

POTENTIALLY HAZARDOUS INTERACTIONS WITH OTHER DRUGS

• Absorption of digoxin, tetracyclines, ciprofloxacin, warfarin and phenytoin reduced – give 2 hrs after sucralfate

Administration

RECONSTITUTION

• Tablets may be dispersed in 10–15 mL of water

ROUTE

• Oral

RATE OF ADMINISTRATION

–

COMMENTS

• Sucralfate exerts its action at the site of the ulcer and is minimally absorbed (3–5%) from the gastrointestinal tract as sucrose sulphate
• In normal renal function any aluminium which is absorbed is excreted in the urine

Other information

• Sucralfate should be used with caution in renal impairment as aluminium may be absorbed and accumulate
• In severe renal impairment and patients receiving dialysis, sucralfate should be used with extreme caution and only for short periods
• Absorbed aluminium is bound to plasma proteins and is not dialysable
• Use of other aluminium-containing products with sucralfate can increase the total body burden of aluminium

Sulindac

Clinical use

NSAID, used for pain and inflammation in musculoskeletal disorders and acute gout

Dose in normal renal function

200 mg twice daily

Pharmacokinetics

Molecular weight (daltons)	356
% Protein binding	93
% Excreted unchanged in urine	–
Volume of distribution (L/kg)	–
Half-life – normal/ESRF (hrs)	8/17 (metabolite)

Dose in renal impairment GFR (mL/min)

20–50	Dose as in normal renal function. Avoid if possible
10–20	Give 50–100% of normal dose. Avoid if possible
<10	Give 50–100% of normal dose. Avoid if possible

Dose in patients undergoing renal replacement therapies

CAPD	Unknown dialysability. Dose as in GFR = <10 mL/min
HD	Unknown dialysability. Dose as in GFR = <10 mL/min
CAV/VVHD	Unknown dialysability. Dose as in GFR = 10–20 mL/min

Important drug interactions

CYCLOSPORIN

• Increased risk of nephrotoxicity

POTENTIALLY HAZARDOUS INTERACTIONS WITH OTHER DRUGS

• Excretion of lithium reduced
• Cytotoxic agents: reduced excretion of methotrexate
• Anticoagulants: effects of nicoumalone and warfarin enhanced
• Antidiabetic agents: effects of sulphonylureas enhanced
• Anti-epileptic agents: effects of phenytoin enhanced
• ACE inhibitors: antagonism of hypotensive effect; increased risk of hyperkalaemia and renal damage
• Uricosurics: probenecid delays excretion of NSAIDs

Administration

RECONSTITUTION

–

ROUTE

• Oral

RATE OF ADMINISTRATION

–

COMMENTS

–

Other information

• Sulindac has become the NSAID of choice in some centres for patients with renal impairment. This is due to reports of renal sparing effects. There is evidence that this sparing effect is dose related and is lost if doses above 100 mg twice daily are used
• Inhibition of renal prostaglandin synthesis by NSAIDs may interfere with renal function, especially in the presence of existing renal disease. Avoid NSAIDs if possible; if not, check serum creatinine 48–72 hrs after starting NSAID. If increased, discontinue therapy
• Use normal doses in patients with ESRD on dialysis

Sulphasalazine

Clinical use

Ulcerative colitis, Crohn's disease, rheumatoid
arthritis

Dose in normal renal function

1–2 g 4 times daily reduced to 0.5 g 4 times daily
Rheumatoid arthritis:
0.5 g daily increased to 1.5 g twice daily

Pharmacokinetics

Molecular weight (daltons)	398.4
% Protein binding	95–99
% Excreted unchanged in urine	10–15
Volume of distribution (L/kg)	–
Half-life – normal/ESRF (hrs)	6–17/–

Dose in renal impairment
GFR (mL/min)

20–50	Dose as in normal renal function. Use with caution
10–20	Dose as in normal renal function. Use with caution
<10	Avoid

Dose in patients undergoing renal replacement therapies

CAPD	Unknown dialysability. Dose as in GFR = <10 mL/min
HD	Unknown dialysability. Dose as in GFR = <10 mL/min
CAV/VVHD	Unknown dialysability. Dose as in GFR = 10–20 mL/min

Important drug interactions

CYCLOSPORIN

–

POTENTIALLY HAZARDOUS INTERACTIONS WITH
OTHER DRUGS

–

Administration

RECONSTITUTION

–

ROUTE

• Oral

RATE OF ADMINISTRATION

–

COMMENTS

–

Other information

• 20–30% of a dose of sulphasalazine is absorbed in
the small intestine and becomes highly bound to
plasma proteins. The remainder is split into
sulphapyridine and 5-ASA by colonic bacteria.
Sulphapyridine is rapidly absorbed from the colon,
whereas 5-ASA is poorly absorbed

• Most of a dose of sulphasalazine is excreted in
the urine. Unchanged sulphasalazine accounts for
15% of the original dose, sulphapyridine and its
metabolites 60% and 5-ASA and its metabolites
20–33%

• Up to 5% of a dose is excreted in the faeces,
mainly as sulphapyridine metabolites

Sulpiride

Clinical use

Antipsychotic, used for acute and chronic
schizophrenia

Dose in normal renal function

400–800 mg daily increasing to a maximum of 1.2 g
twice daily

Pharmacokinetics

Molecular weight (daltons)	341.4
% Protein binding	14–40
% Excreted unchanged in urine	90–95
Volume of distribution (L/kg)	0.65–1.4
Half-life – normal/ESRF (hrs)	6–8/26

Dose in renal impairment GFR (mL/min)

20–50	Give 70% of normal dose, or increase dosing interval by factor of 1.5
10–20	Give 50% of normal dose, or increase dosing interval by factor of 2
<10	Give 30% of normal dose, or increase dosing interval by factor of 3

Dose in patients undergoing renal replacement therapies

CAPD	Unknown dialysability. Dose as in GFR = <10 mL/min
HD	Unknown dialysability. Dose as in GFR = <10 mL/min
CAV/VVHD	Unknown dialysability. Dose as in GFR = 10–20 mL/min

Important drug interactions

CYCLOSPORIN

–

POTENTIALLY HAZARDOUS INTERACTIONS WITH
OTHER DRUGS

–

Administration

RECONSTITUTION

–

ROUTE

• Oral

RATE OF ADMINISTRATION

–

COMMENTS

–

Other information

• Sulpiride is almost entirely excreted in the urine
  as unchanged drug. Administer with caution and
  decrease the dose in renal impairment

Sumatriptan

Clinical use

Acute relief of migraine

Dose in normal renal function

Oral:
50–100 mg, maximum 300 mg in 24 hrs
SC:
6 mg, maximum 12 mg in 24 hrs

Pharmacokinetics

Molecular weight (daltons)	413.5
% Protein binding	14–21
% Excreted unchanged in urine	<20
Volume of distribution (L/kg)	170
Half-life – normal/ESRF (hrs)	2/probably unchanged

Dose in renal impairment GFR (mL/min)

20–50	Dose as in normal renal function
10–20	Dose as in normal renal function. Use with caution
<10	Dose as in normal renal function. Use with caution

Dose in patients undergoing renal replacement therapies

CAPD	Unknown dialysability. Dose as in normal renal function. Use with caution
HD	Unknown dialysability. Dose as in normal renal function. Use with caution
CAV/VVHD	Unknown dialysability. Dose as in normal renal function. Use with caution

Important drug interactions

CYCLOSPORIN

–

POTENTIALLY HAZARDOUS INTERACTIONS WITH OTHER DRUGS

• MAOIs, SSRIs and lithium: risk of CNS toxicity
• Ergotamine: increased risk of vasospasm

Administration

RECONSTITUTION

• Injection is pre-filled into syringes ready for administration

ROUTE

–

RATE OF ADMINISTRATION

–

COMMENTS

–

Other information

• Non-renal clearance accounts for about 80% of the total clearance. The remaining 20% is excreted in urine, mainly as metabolites and involving active renal tubular secretion

Suxamethonium

Clinical use

Depolarising muscle relaxant used in short procedures and ECT

Dose in normal renal function

0.3–1.1 mg/kg
IV infusion:
2–5 mg/min

Pharmacokinetics

Molecular weight (daltons)	361
% Protein binding	70%
% Excreted unchanged in urine	≥10%
Volume of distribution (L/kg)	–
Half-life – normal/ESRF	3 min/–

Dose in renal impairment GFR (mL/min)

20–50	Dose as in normal renal function
10–20	Dose as in normal renal function
<10	Dose as in normal renal function. Use with caution. See 'Other information'

Dose in patients undergoing renal replacement therapies

CAPD	Unknown dialysability. Dose as in GFR = <10 mL/min
HD	Unknown dialysability. Dose as in GFR = <10 mL/min
CAV/VVHD	Dose as in normal renal function

Important drug interactions

CYCLOSPORIN

–

POTENTIALLY HAZARDOUS INTERACTIONS WITH OTHER DRUGS

• Neuromuscular blockade may be enhanced by certain antibiotics, local anaesthetics, quinidine, calcium-channel blockers and lithium cimetidine
• Procainamide, quinidine, lithium, cyclophosphamide and thiotepa enhance muscle relaxant effect
• Increased risk of cardiac arrhythmias if suxamethonium is given with digoxin

Administration

RECONSTITUTION

• For continuous infusion add 10 mL to 500 mL glucose 5% or sodium chloride 0.9% = 0.1% solution

ROUTE

• IV

RATE OF ADMINISTRATION

• Over 10–30 sec

COMMENTS

–

Other information

• Suxamethonium is predominantly excreted in the urine as active and inactive metabolites. Patients on dialysis may require a dose at the lower end of the range due to reduced plasma cholinesterase activity
• Use with caution in hyperkalaemia as potassium is released from depolarised muscle
• Hyperkalaemia may occur when suxamethonium is used in ESRF

Tacrolimus

Clinical use

Immunosuppressive agent, used for prophylaxis and treatment of acute rejection in liver and kidney transplantation

Dose in normal renal function

Oral:

liver transplantation: 0.1–0.2 mg/kg/day in 2 divided doses. Maximum 0.3 mg/kg/day

kidney transplantation: 0.15–0.3 mg/kg/day in 2 divided doses

IV:

liver transplantation: 0.01–0.05 mg/kg as a continuous 24-hr infusion, starting 6 hrs post surgery

kidney transplantation: 0.05–0.10 mg/kg as a continuous 24-hr infusion, starting within 24 hrs of surgery

Pharmacokinetics

Molecular weight (daltons)	822
% Protein binding	>98
% Excreted unchanged in urine	<1
Volume of distribution	1300 L
Half-life – normal/ESRF (hrs)	12–16/probably unchanged

Dose in renal impairment GFR (mL/min)

20–50	Dose as in normal renal function
10–20	Dose as in normal renal function
<10	Dose as in normal renal function

Dose in patients undergoing renal replacement therapies

CAPD	Not dialysed. Dose as in normal renal function
HD	Not dialysed. Dose as in normal renal function
CAV/VVHD	Not dialysed. Dose as in normal renal function

Important drug interactions

CYCLOSPORIN

- Tacrolimus may increase the half-life of cyclosporin and exacerbate any toxic effects. The two should not be prescribed concomitantly. Care should be taken when converting from cyclosporin to tacrolimus

POTENTIALLY HAZARDOUS INTERACTIONS WITH OTHER DRUGS

- Data is limited, but it can be assumed that tacrolimus will be subject to many of the drug interactions that are associated with cyclosporin
- Tacrolimus levels are increased by imidazole antifungals, macrolides, danazol, omeprazole, bromocriptine, cortisone, dapsone, ethinyloestradiol, gestodene, lignocaine, nicardipine, nifedipine, quinidine and verapamil
- Tacrolimus levels are decreased by rifampicin, phenytoin, phenobarbitone, carbamazepine and isoniazid
- Increased nephrotoxicity with amphotericin, ibuprofen, aminoglycosides, vancomycin, cotrimoxazole, NSAIDs, ganciclovir and aciclovir
- Increased risk of hyperkalaemia with potassium-sparing diuretics
- Tacrolimus potentiates the effects of oral anticoagulants and antidiabetic drugs

Administation

RECONSTITUTION

- Dilute in glucose 5% to a concentration of 4–20 micrograms/mL, i.e. 5 mg in 250–1000 mL

ROUTE

- IV

RATE OF ADMINISTRATION

- Continuous infusion over 24 hrs

COMMENTS

- Incompatible with PVC. Reconstitute in either glucose 5% in polyethylene or glass containers or in sodium chloride 0.9% in polyethylene containers
- Contains polyethoxylated castor oil which has been associated with anaphylaxis

Other information

–

Tamoxifen

Clinical use

Treatment of breast cancer and anovulatory fertility

Dose in normal renal function

Oral:
10–40 mg daily

Pharmacokinetics

Molecular weight (daltons)	372
% Protein binding	>99
% Excreted unchanged in urine	<10
Volume of distribution (L/kg)	20
Half-life – normal/ESRF	7 days/probably unchanged

Dose in renal impairment GFR (mL/min)

20–50	Dose as in normal renal function
10–20	Dose as in normal renal function
<10	Dose as in normal renal function

Dose in patients undergoing renal replacement therapies

CAPD	Unknown dialysability. Dose as in normal renal function
HD	Unknown dialysability. Dose as in normal renal function
CAV/VVHD	Unknown dialysability. Dose as in normal renal function

Important drug interactions

CYCLOSPORIN

–

POTENTIALLY HAZARDOUS INTERACTIONS WITH OTHER DRUGS

• Warfarin: effects enhanced

Administration

RECONSTITUTION

–

ROUTE

• Oral

RATE OF ADMINISTRATION

–

COMMENTS

–

Other information

–

Teicoplanin

Clinical use

Antibacterial agent

Dose in normal renal function

IM/IV:
3–6 mg/kg/day to 12 mg/kg/day (higher in some
reports) in life-threatening infections

Pharmacokinetics

Molecular weight (daltons)	1993
% Protein binding	90–95
% Excreted unchanged in urine	>97
Volume of distribution (L/kg)	0.94–1.4
Half-life – normal/ESRF (hrs)	150/270–490

Dose in renal impairment GFR (mL/min)

20–50	Give 50% of normal dose daily or 100% every 48 hrs
10–20	Give 30% of normal dose daily or 100% every 72 hrs
<10	Give 30% of normal dose daily or 100% every 72 hrs

Dose in patients undergoing renal replacement therapies

CAPD	Unknown dialysability. Dose as in GFR = <10 mL/min
HD	Not dialysed. Dose as in GFR = <10 mL/min
CAV/VVHD	Unknown dialysability. Dose as in GFR = 10–20 mL/min

Important drug interactions

CYCLOSPORIN

–

POTENTIALLY HAZARDOUS INTERACTIONS WITH
OTHER DRUGS

–

Administration

RECONSTITUTION

• Use water for injection provided

ROUTE

• IV bolus, IM

RATE OF ADMINISTRATION

• IV bolus: 2–3 min; IV infusion: 30 min

COMMENTS

• Use in CAPD. Give 400 mg IV stat dose
then 20 mg/L/bag IP for 7 days, then
20 mg/L/**alternate** bags for 7 days,
20 mg/L/**night** bag only for 7 days

Other information

• TDM optimises therapy, but is not essential.
Troughs not less than 10 mg/L. Peaks 1 hr after
400 mg IV dose 20–50 mg/L

• Relationship between blood level and toxicity
not established

• For patients with impaired renal function a
reduction in dose is not required until day 4 of
therapy. Measurement of serum levels may help

Temazepam

Clinical use

Benzodiazepine, used for insomnia (short-term use), pre-med anxiolytic prior to minor procedures

Dose in normal renal function

Insomnia:

at night, up to 40 mg in severe cases

Oral:

5–20 mg/day

Premedication:

20–40 mg, 30–60 min prior to procedure

Pharmacokinetics

Molecular weight (daltons)	300.7
% Protein binding	96–98
% Excreted unchanged in urine	1
Volume of distribution (L/kg)	1.3–1.5
Half-life – normal/ESRF (hrs)	2–4/unchanged

Dose in renal impairment GFR (mL/min)

20–50	Dose as in normal renal function
10–20	Dose as in normal renal function. Start with small doses. Up to 20 mg daily
<10	Dose as in normal renal function. Start with small doses. Up to 10 mg daily (20 mg if single dose)

Dose in patients undergoing renal replacement therapies

CAPD	Unknown dialysability. Dose as in GFR = <10 mL/min
HD	Not dialysed. Dose as in GFR = <10 mL/min
CAV/VVHD	Unknown dialysability. Dose as in GFR = 10–20 mL/min

Important drug interactions

CYCLOSPORIN

–

POTENTIALLY HAZARDOUS INTERACTIONS WITH OTHER DRUGS

• Temazepam toxicity reported with disulfiram

Administration

RECONSTITUTION

–

ROUTE

• Oral

RATE OF ADMINISTRATION

–

COMMENTS

–

Other information

• Liquid available
• Increased CNS sensitivity in renal impairment
• Long-term use may lead to dependence and withdrawal symptoms in certain patients
• 80% of metabolites excreted in the urine

Terazosin

Clinical use

Alpha-adrenoreceptor blocker, used for
hypertension and benign prostatic hyperplasia

Dose in normal renal function

Oral:
2–10 mg daily (hypertension); 5–10 mg daily
(benign prostatic hyperplasia)

Pharmacokinetics

Molecular weight (daltons)	459.9
% Protein binding	90–94
% Excreted unchanged in urine	10
Volume of distribution (L/kg)	0.5–0.9
Half-life – normal/ESRF (hrs)	9–12/unchanged

Dose in renal impairment
GFR (mL/min)

20–50	Dose as in normal renal function
10–20	Dose as in normal renal function
<10	Dose as in normal renal function

Dose in patients undergoing renal replacement therapies

CAPD	Unknown dialysability. Dose as in normal renal function
HD	Unknown dialysability. Dose as in normal renal function
CAV/VVHD	Unknown dialysability. Dose as in normal renal function

Important drug interactions

CYCLOSPORIN

–

POTENTIALLY HAZARDOUS INTERACTIONS WITH
OTHER DRUGS

• Increased hypotensive effect with beta-blockers,
calcium-channel blockers, diuretics, general
anaesthetics and antidepressants

Administration

RECONSTITUTION

–

ROUTE

• Oral

RATE OF ADMINISTRATION

–

COMMENTS

–

Other information

• Therapy should be initiated with a single dose of
1 mg given at bedtime
• In severe renal impairment use doses above 5 mg
with caution

Terbinafine

Clinical use

Antifungal agent, used for fungal infections of the skin and nails

Dose in normal renal function

250 mg daily

Pharmacokinetics

Molecular weight (daltons)	327.9
% Protein binding	99
% Excreted unchanged in urine	0
Volume of distribution	1000 L
Half-life – normal/ESRF (hrs)	17/24

Dose in renal impairment GFR (mL/min)

20–50	50% of normal dose or 100% on alternate days
10–20	50% of normal dose or 100% on alternate days
<10	50% of normal dose or 100% on alternate days

Dose in patients undergoing renal replacement therapies

CAPD	Unknown dialysability. Dose as in GFR = <10 mL/min
HD	Unknown dialysability. Dose as in GFR = <10 mL/min
CAV/VVHD	Unknown dialysability. Dose as in GFR = 10–20 mL/min

Important drug interactions

CYCLOSPORIN

–

POTENTIALLY HAZARDOUS INTERACTIONS WITH OTHER DRUGS

–

Administration

RECONSTITUTION

–

ROUTE

• Oral

RATE OF ADMINISTRATION

–

COMMENTS

–

Other information

• Terbinafine is hepatically metabolised to two major metabolites, 80% of which are renally excreted

• Little information is available regarding the handling of terbinafine in renal failure

• In ESRF use with caution and monitor for side-effects

Terbutaline

Clinical use

Beta$_2$-adrenoreceptor agonist, used for reversible airways obstruction

Dose in normal renal function

Oral:

2.5–5 mg 3 times daily

SC/IM:

250–500 micrograms up to 4 times daily

IV:

Slow injection, 250–500 micrograms up to 4 times daily; infusion, 1.5–5 micrograms/min for 8–10 hrs

Aerosol:

250–500 micrograms (1–2 puffs) up to 3–4 times daily

Powder:

500 micrograms (1 inhalation) up to 4 times daily

Nebulisation:

5–10 mg 2–4 times daily or more frequently

Pharmacokinetics

Molecular weight (daltons)	274.3
% Protein binding	15–25
% Excreted unchanged in urine	90
Volume of distribution (L/kg)	1.6
Half-life – normal/ESRF (hrs)	3/–

Dose in renal impairment GFR (mL/min)

20–50	50% of normal parenteral dose. Other routes dose as in normal renal function
10–20	50% of normal parenteral dose. Other routes dose as in normal renal function
<10	Avoid parenteral dose. Other routes dose as in normal renal function

Dose in patients undergoing renal replacement therapies

CAPD	Likely to be dialysed. Dose as in GFR = <10 mL/min
HD	Likely to be dialysed. Dose as in GFR = <10 mL/min
CAV/VVHD	Likely to be dialysed. Dose as in GFR = 10–20 mL/min

Important drug interactions

CYCLOSPORIN

–

POTENTIALLY HAZARDOUS INTERACTIONS WITH OTHER DRUGS

• Effect may be diminished by beta-blockers

• Theophylline: increased risk of hyperkalaemia

Administration

RECONSTITUTION

• For IV infusion add 3–5 mL to 500 mL glucose 5% or sodium chloride 0.9% (3–5 micrograms/mL)

ROUTE

• IV

RATE OF ADMINISTRATION

• Asthma: 0.5–1 mL/min

COMMENTS

–

Other information

–

Terfenadine

Clinical use

Antihistamine, used for symptomatic relief of allergy and pruritus

Dose in normal renal function

Oral:
60–120 mg daily

Pharmacokinetics

Molecular weight (daltons)	471.7
% Protein binding	97
% Excreted unchanged in urine	0
Volume of distribution (L/kg)	–
Half-life – normal/ESRF (hrs)	16–23/probably unchanged

Dose in renal impairment GFR (mL/min)

20–50	Dose as in normal renal function
10–20	Dose as in normal renal function
<10	Dose as in normal renal function

Dose in patients undergoing renal replacement therapies

CAPD	Not dialysed. Dose as in normal renal function
HD	Not dialysed. Dose as in normal renal function
CAV/VVHD	Not dialysed. Dose as in normal renal function

Important drug interactions

CYCLOSPORIN

–

POTENTIALLY HAZARDOUS INTERACTIONS WITH OTHER DRUGS

• Increased risk of ventricular arrhythmias with amiodarone, disopyramide, procainamide, quinidine, erythromycin, clarithromycin, tricyclic antidepressants, fluvoxamine, imidazole antifungals, mibefradil, cisapride, antipsychotics, sotalol, halofantrine, quinine and diuretics

• Metabolism inhibited by erythromycin and other macrolides, imidazoles (and possibly thiazides)

• Concomitant use with astemizole is not recommended

Administration

RECONSTITUTION

–

ROUTE

• Oral

RATE OF ADMINISTRATION

–

COMMENTS

–

Other information

• Hypokalaemia increases the risk of ventricular arrhythmias

• Rare hazardous arrhythmias are associated with terfenadine, particularly with increased blood concentrations. Do not exceed the recommended dose. Terfenadine is not recommended for patients in whom electrolyte imbalance or prolonged QT interval are known or suspected

Thioridazine

Clinical use

Schizophrenia; psychomotor agitation; severe
anxiety agitation and restlessness in elderly patients

Dose in normal renal function

Schizophrenia:

150–600 mg daily (maximum 800 mg in hospitalised
patients)

Psychomotor agitation:

75–200 mg daily

Severe anxiety agitation:

30–100 mg daily

Pharmacokinetics

Molecular weight (daltons)	407
% Protein binding	97–99
% Excreted unchanged in urine	<1
Volume of distribution (L/kg)	10
Half-life – normal/ESRF (hrs)	16–36/probably unchanged

Dose in renal impairment GFR (mL/min)

20–50	Dose as in normal renal function. Use lower initial doses and increase more gradually
10–20	Dose as in normal renal function. Use lower initial doses and increase more gradually
<10	Dose as in normal renal function. Use lower initial doses and increase more gradually

Dose in patients undergoing renal replacement therapies

CAPD	Unlikely to be dialysed. Dose as in normal renal function
HD	Unlikely to be dialysed. Dose as in normal renal function
CAV/VVHD	Unlikely to be dialysed. Dose as in normal renal function

Important drug interactions

CYCLOSPORIN

–

POTENTIALLY HAZARDOUS INTERACTIONS WITH
OTHER DRUGS

- Increased risk of ventricular arrhythmias with anti-arrhythmics, astemizole, halofantrine, sotalol and terfenadine
- Plasma concentrations of tricyclic antidepressants may be increased
- Increased cardiac depressant effects with quinidine
- Antagonises effect of anti-epileptics (reduced convulsive threshold)

Administration

RECONSTITUTION

–

ROUTE

- Oral

RATE OF ADMINISTRATION

–

COMMENTS

–

Other information

- Elimination of metabolites is mainly via the bile, with <10% of the dose appearing in the urine

Thyroxine

Clinical use

Hypothyroidism

Dose in normal renal function

Oral:
25–200 micrograms daily

Pharmacokinetics

Molecular weight (daltons)	798.9
% Protein binding	99.97
% Excreted unchanged in urine	–
Volume of distribution (L/kg)	8.7–9.7
Half-life – normal/ESRF	6–7 days/–

Dose in renal impairment GFR (mL/min)

20–50	Dose as in normal renal function
10–20	Dose as in normal renal function
<10	Dose as in normal renal function

Dose in patients undergoing renal replacement therapies

CAPD	Not dialysed. Dose as in normal renal function
HD	Not dialysed. Dose as in normal renal function
CAV/VVHD	Not dialysed. Dose as in normal renal function

Important drug interactions

CYCLOSPORIN

–

POTENTIALLY HAZARDOUS INTERACTIONS WITH OTHER DRUGS

• Effect of warfarin enhanced

Administration

RECONSTITUTION

–

ROUTE

• Oral

RATE OF ADMINISTRATION

–

COMMENTS

–

Other information

• Uraemic toxins may result in inhibition of the enzyme associated with conversion of L-thyroxine to liothyronine

Ticarcillin

Clinical use

Antibacterial agent

Dose in normal renal function

IV:

15–20 g daily in divided doses at 4–8-hourly intervals, 3–4 g daily in divided doses for uncomplicated UTI

Pharmacokinetics

Molecular weight (daltons)	428
% Protein binding	45–60
% Excreted unchanged in urine	85–90
Volume of distribution (L/kg)	0.14–0.21
Half-life – normal/ESRF (hrs)	1.2/11–16

Dose in renal impairment GFR (mL/min)

20–50	2 g every 4–6 hrs
10–20	2 g every 8 hrs
<10	2 g every 12 hrs

Dose in patients undergoing renal replacement therapies

CAPD	Unknown dialysability, but likely. Dose as in GFR = <10 mL/min
HD	Unknown dialysability, but likely. Dose as in GFR = <10 mL/min
CAV/VVHD	Unknown dialysability, but likely. Dose as in GFR = 10–20 mL/min

Important drug interactions

CYCLOSPORIN

–

POTENTIALLY HAZARDOUS INTERACTIONS WITH OTHER DRUGS

• Methotrexate: excretion reduced, increasing the risk of toxicity

Administration

RECONSTITUTION

• With water for injection to 20 mL for slow IV bolus. Add to 100 mL glucose 5% or water for injection for IV infusion

ROUTE

• IV

RATE OF ADMINISTRATION

• 30–40 min

COMMENTS

–

Other information

• Each 1 g of ticarcillin contains 5.3 mmol of sodium

Ticarcillin/clavulanic acid

Clinical use

Antibacterial agent

Dose in normal renal function

3.2 g every 6–8 hrs. Maximum every 4 hrs

Pharmacokinetics

Molecular weight (daltons)	ticarcillin 428; clavulanic acid 199
% Protein binding	ticarcillin 45–60; clavulanic acid 22–30
% Excreted unchanged in urine	ticarcillin 85–90; clavulanic acid 60
Volume of distribution (L/kg)	ticarcillin 0.14–0.21; clavulanic acid 0.3
Half-life – normal/ESRF (hrs)	ticarcillin 1.2/11–16; clavulanic acid 15/3–4

Dose in renal impairment GFR (mL/min)

>30	3.2 g every 8 hrs
10–30	1.6 g every 8 hrs
<10	1.6 g every 12 hrs

Dose in patients undergoing renal replacement therapies

CAPD	Unknown dialysability. Dose as in GFR = <10 mL/min
HD	Dialysed. Dose as in GFR = <10 mL/min
CAV/VVHD	Unknown dialysability. Dose as in GFR = 10–30 mL/min

Important drug interactions

CYCLOSPORIN

–

POTENTIALLY HAZARDOUS INTERACTIONS WITH OTHER DRUGS

–

Administration

RECONSTITUTION

• With 10 mL water for injection and add to 100 mL glucose 5%

ROUTE

• IV

RATE OF ADMINISTRATION

• 30–40 min

COMMENTS

• Each 3.2 g of ticarcillin/clavulanic acid contains 17 mmol of sodium and 1 mmol of potassium

Other information

–

Timolol

Clinical use

Beta-adrenoreceptor blocker, used for
hypertension, angina and migraine prophylaxis

Dose in normal renal function

Oral:
10–60 mg daily

Pharmacokinetics

Molecular weight (daltons)	317
% Protein binding	60
% Excreted unchanged in urine	5–20
Volume of distribution (L/kg)	1–3.5
Half-life – normal/ESRF (hrs)	3–5/unchanged

Dose in renal impairment GFR (mL/min)

20–50	Dose as in normal renal function
10–20	Dose as in normal renal function. Start with lowest dose and titrate according to response
<10	Dose as in normal renal function. Start with lowest dose and titrate according to response

Dose in patients undergoing renal replacement therapies

CAPD	Unknown dialysability. Dose as in GFR = <10 mL/min
HD	Unknown dialysability. Dose as in GFR = <10 mL/min
CAV/VVHD	Unknown dialysability. Dose as in GFR = 10–20 mL/min

Important drug interactions

CYCLOSPORIN

–

POTENTIALLY HAZARDOUS INTERACTIONS WITH OTHER DRUGS

• Anti-arrhythmics: increased risk of myocardial depression and bradycardia
• Calcium-channel blockers: increased risk of bradycardia and AV block with diltiazem, and severe hypotension, asystole and heart failure with verapamil

Administration

RECONSTITUTION

–

ROUTE

• Oral

RATE OF ADMINISTRATION

–

COMMENTS

–

Other information

• Timolol is more hydrophilic than lipophilic

Tinidazole

Clinical use

Antibacterial agent

Dose in normal renal function

Oral:
1–4 g daily

Pharmacokinetics

Molecular weight (daltons)	247
% Protein binding	8–12
% Excreted unchanged in urine	25
Volume of distribution (L/kg)	0.7
Half-life – normal/ESRF (hrs)	12–14/unchanged

Dose in renal impairment GFR (mL/min)

20–50	Dose as in normal renal function
10–20	Dose as in normal renal function
<10	Dose as in normal renal function

Dose in patients undergoing renal replacement therapies

CAPD	Unknown dialysability, but likely to be dialysed. Dose as in normal renal function
HD	Dialysed. Dose as in normal renal function
CAV/VVHD	Unknown dialysability. Dose as in normal renal function

Important drug interactions

CYCLOSPORIN

–

POTENTIALLY HAZARDOUS INTERACTIONS WITH OTHER DRUGS

–

Administration

RECONSTITUTION

–

ROUTE

• Oral

RATE OF ADMINISTRATION

–

COMMENTS

–

Other information

• Dosage adjustment in renal failure is not necessary, as a decrease in renal clearance is compensated for by increased faecal excretion of tinidazole

Tobramycin

Clinical use

Antibacterial agent

Dose in normal renal function

IM/IV:

3 mg/kg/day in 3 divided doses.
Maximum 5 mg/kg/day in 3–4 divided doses

Pharmacokinetics

Molecular weight (daltons)	468
% Protein binding	<10
% Excreted unchanged in urine	90
Volume of distribution (L/kg)	0.25
Half-life – normal/ESRF (hrs)	2–3/≥70

Dose in renal impairment
GFR (mL/min)

20–50	Give 1 mg/kg, then dose according to serum levels
10–20	Give 1 mg/kg, then dose according to serum levels
<10	Give 1 mg/kg, then dose according to serum levels

Dose in patients undergoing renal replacement therapies

CAPD	Unlikely to be dialysed. Dose as in GFR = <10 mL/min
HD	Dialysed. Dose as in GFR = <10 mL/min
CAV/VVHD	Dialysed. Dose as in GFR = 10–20 mL/min

Important drug interactions

CYCLOSPORIN

• Increased risk of nephrotoxicity

POTENTIALLY HAZARDOUS INTERACTIONS WITH OTHER DRUGS

• Loop diuretics: increased risk of ototoxicity
• Botulinum toxin: neuromuscular block enhanced
• Neostigmine and pyridostigmine: antagonism of effects
• Cisplatin: increased risk of nephrotoxicity and possibly ototoxicity
• Non-depolarising muscle relaxants: effects enhanced

Administration

RECONSTITUTION

• Add to 50–100 mL sodium chloride 0.9% or glucose 5% for IV infusion

ROUTE

• IV, IM

RATE OF ADMINISTRATION

• 20–60 min

COMMENTS

• Plasma concentrations should be measured frequently. Trough ≤2 mg/L. Peak 60 min post-dose IM ≤10 mg/L. Avoid prolonged peaks above 12 mg/L

Other information

• Dosing nomograms (patient's weight and renal function) are available which detail either reduced dose administered every 8 hrs or normal dose (1 mg/kg) given at an increased interval. Doses must be adjusted according to serum levels
• As a rough guide, to calculate the reduced dose given every 8 hrs, divide the normal dose by serum creatinine (mg/dL). An extended dosage interval in hours can be calculated by multiplying the serum creatinine (mg/dL) by 6. NB: mg/dL x 88.4 = micromol/L

Tolbutamide

Clinical use

Hypoglycaemic agent for non-insulin-dependent
diabetes

Dose in normal renal function

0.5–2 g daily

Pharmacokinetics

Molecular weight (daltons)	270
% Protein binding	95
% Excreted unchanged in urine	<10
Volume of distribution (L/kg)	0.1–0.15
Half-life – normal/ESRF (hrs)	5–11/prolonged

Dose in renal impairment
GFR (mL/min)

20–50	Dose as in normal renal function. Use with caution
10–20	Dose as in normal renal function. Use with caution
<10	Dose as in normal renal function. Use with caution

Dose in patients undergoing renal replacement therapies

CAPD	Insignificantly dialysed. Dose as in GFR = <10 mL/min
HD	Insignificantly dialysed. Dose as in GFR = <10 mL/min
CAV/VVHD	Unknown dialysability. Dose as in GFR = 10–20 mL/min

Important drug interactions

CYCLOSPORIN

–

POTENTIALLY HAZARDOUS INTERACTIONS WITH
OTHER DRUGS

• Enhanced effect with phenylbutazone,
azapropazone, chloramphenicol, sulphonamides,
sulphinpyrazone, 4-quinolones, trimethoprim and
co-trimoxazole
• Decreased effect with rifampicin

Administration

RECONSTITUTION

–

ROUTE

• Oral

RATE OF ADMINISTRATION

–

COMMENTS

–

Other information

• Tolbutamide is contraindicated in severe renal
impairment. It is not removed by dialysis and
should be used with great caution in mild to
moderate renal impairment because of the risk
of hypoglycaemia

Tramadol

Clinical use

Analgesic

Dose in normal renal function

Oral:

50–100 mg up to 4-hourly

IM/IV:

50–100 mg hourly. Total daily dose 600 mg

Pharmacokinetics

Molecular weight (daltons)	300
% Protein binding	4
% Excreted unchanged in urine	30
Volume of distribution (L/kg)	–
Half-life – normal/ESRF (hrs)	6/11

Dose in renal impairment (GFR (mL/min)

20–50	Dose as in normal renal function
10–20	50–100 mg every 12 hrs
<10	50 mg every 12 hrs

Dose in patients undergoing renal replacement therapies

CAPD	Unknown dialysability. Dose as in GFR = <10 mL/min
HD	Dialysed. Dose as in GFR = <10 mL/min
CAV/VVHD	Dialysed. Dose as in GFR = 10–20 mL/min

Important drug interactions

CYCLOSPORIN

–

POTENTIALLY HAZARDOUS INTERACTIONS WITH OTHER DRUGS

• Carbamazepine: tramadol metabolism increased

Administration

RECONSTITUTION

–

ROUTE

• Oral, IV, IM

RATE OF ADMINISTRATION

• Slow bolus or continuous IV infusion/patient-controlled analgesia

COMMENTS

–

Other information

• Tramadol is a centrally acting opioid agonist which also acts on inhibitory pain pathways

• It should be used with caution in moderate renal impairment and is not recommended in severe impairment

Trandolapril

Clinical use

Angiotensin-converting enzyme inhibitor, used for hypertension

Dose in normal renal function

0.5 mg once daily increased to 1–2 mg once daily (maximum 4 mg daily)

Pharmacokinetics

Molecular weight (daltons)	430
% Protein binding	>80
% Excreted unchanged in urine	10–15
Volume of distribution (L/kg)	–
Half-life – normal/ESRF (hrs)	16–24/–

Dose in renal impairment GFR (mL/min)

20–50	Dose as in normal renal function
10–20	Dose as in normal renal function
<10	Maximum 2 mg daily

Dose in patients undergoing renal replacement therapies

CAPD	Unknown dialysability. Dose as in GFR = <10 mL/min
HD	Unknown dialysability. Dose as in GFR = <10 mL/min
CAV/VVHD	Unknown dialysability. Dose as in GFR = 10–20 mL/min

Important drug interactions

CYCLOSPORIN

• Increased risk of hyperkalaemia

POTENTIALLY HAZARDOUS INTERACTIONS WITH OTHER DRUGS

• Potassium supplements: risk of hyperkalaemia
• Epoetin: risk of hyperkalaemia
• Lithium levels may be increased
• NSAIDs: antagonism of hypotensive effect; increased risk of renal damage and hyperkalaemia
• Diuretics: enhanced hypotensive effect. Increased risk of hyperkalaemia with potassium-sparing diuretics
• Anaesthetics: enhanced hypotensive effect

Administration

RECONSTITUTION

–

ROUTE

• Oral

RATE OF ADMINISTRATION

–

COMMENTS

–

Other information

• Hyperkalaemia and other side-effects are more common in patients with impaired renal function
• Close monitoring of renal function during therapy is necessary in those patients with renal insufficiency
• Renal failure has been reported in association with ACE inhibitors in patients with renal artery stenosis, post renal transplant and those with congestive heart failure
• A high incidence of anaphylactoid reactions has been reported in patients dialysed with high-flux polyacrylonitrile membranes and treated concomitantly with an ACE inhibitor – this combination should therefore be avoided

Tranexamic acid

Clinical use

Haemostatic agent

Dose in normal renal function

Oral:
1–1.5 g every 6–12 hrs (15–25 mg/kg every 6–12 hrs)
IV:
0.5–1 g every 8 hrs (7.5–15 mg/kg every 8 hrs)

Pharmacokinetics

Molecular weight (daltons)	157
% Protein binding	3
% Excreted unchanged in urine	90
Volume of distribution (L/kg)	1
Half-life – normal/ESRF (hrs)	1.5/–

Dose in renal impairment GFR (mL/min)

20–50	IV: 10 mg/kg 12-hourly; PO: 25 mg/kg 12-hourly
10–20	IV: 10 mg/kg 24-hourly; PO: 25 mg/kg 24-hourly
<10	IV: 5 mg/kg 24-hourly; PO: 12.5 mg/kg 24-hourly

Dose in patients undergoing renal replacement therapies

CAPD	Unknown dialysability. Dose as in GFR = <10 mL/min
HD	Unknown dialysability. Dose as in GFR = <10 mL/min
CAV/VVHD	Unknown dialysability. Dose as in GFR = 10–20 mL/min

Important drug interactions

CYCLOSPORIN

–

POTENTIALLY HAZARDOUS INTERACTIONS WITH OTHER DRUGS

–

Administration

RECONSTITUTION

–

ROUTE

• IV

RATE OF ADMINISTRATION

• Slow bolus: 100 mg/min or continuous IV infusion in glucose 5% or sodium chloride 0.9%

COMMENTS

–

Other information

–

Trazodone

Clinical use

Antidepressant

Dose in normal renal function

Oral:
150–300 mg daily. Maximum 600 mg for hospital
patients

Pharmacokinetics

Molecular weight (daltons)	372
% Protein binding	89–95
% Excreted unchanged in urine	<5
Volume of distribution (L/kg)	0.8–1.3
Half-life – normal/ESRF (hrs)	6–14/–

Dose in renal impairment (GFR (mL/min)

20–50	Dose as in normal renal function
10–20	Dose as in normal renal function. Start with small doses and increase gradually
<10	Avoid or use half the dose or half the frequency

Dose in patients undergoing renal replacement therapies

CAPD	Unknown dialysability. Dose as in GFR = <10 mL/min
HD	Unknown dialysability. Dose as in GFR = <10 mL/min
CAV/VVHD	Unknown dialysability. Dose as in GFR = 10–20 mL/min

Important drug interactions

CYCLOSPORIN

–

POTENTIALLY HAZARDOUS INTERACTIONS WITH
OTHER DRUGS

• Anti-epileptics: antagonism of anticonvulsant effect

Administration

RECONSTITUTION

–

ROUTE

• Oral

RATE OF ADMINISTRATION

–

COMMENTS

–

Other information

• Use lower doses in elderly patients
• The majority of a dose (75%) is excreted by the kidney, mainly as metabolites

Triamcinolone

Clinical use

Corticosteroid

Dose in normal renal function

Oral:

2–24 mg daily

IM:

40 mg of acetonide, maximum single dose 100 mg

Intra-articular:

5–40 mg of acetonide

Pharmacokinetics

Molecular weight (daltons)	394 [acetonide (Kenalog) = 435, hexacetonide (Lederspan) = 533]
% Protein binding	Low
% Excreted unchanged in urine	<1
Volume of distribution (L/kg)	99.5–148
Half-life – normal/ESRF (hrs)	1.5–5/unchanged

Dose in renal impairment GFR (mL/min)

20–50	Dose as in normal renal function
10–20	Dose as in normal renal function
<10	Dose as in normal renal function

Dose in patients undergoing renal replacement therapies

CAPD	Unknown dialysability. Dose as in normal renal function
HD	Unknown dialysability. Dose as in normal renal function
CAV/VVHD	Unknown dialysability. Dose as in normal renal function

Important drug interactions

CYCLOSPORIN

–

POTENTIALLY HAZARDOUS INTERACTIONS WITH OTHER DRUGS

• Metabolism increased by rifampicin, carbamazepine, phenytoin and primidone

Administration

RECONSTITUTION

–

ROUTE

• Oral, IM, intra-articular

RATE OF ADMINISTRATION

–

COMMENTS

–

Other information

• Use with caution in severe renal impairment as sodium retention may occur

Triamterene

Clinical use

Diuretic

Dose in normal renal function

Oral:

150–200 mg daily in divided doses. Reduce to alternate days after 1 week

Pharmacokinetics

Molecular weight (daltons)	253
% Protein binding	45–70
% Excreted unchanged in urine	5–10
Volume of distribution (L/kg)	2.2–3.7
Half-life – normal/ESRF (hrs)	2/10

Dose in renal impairment GFR (mL/min)

20–50	Dose as in normal renal function
10–20	Avoid
<10	Avoid

Dose in patients undergoing renal replacement therapies

CAPD	Unknown dialysability. Avoid
HD	Unknown dialysability. Avoid
CAV/VVHD	Unknown dialysability. Avoid

Important drug interactions

CYCLOSPORIN

• Increased risk of hyperkalaemia

POTENTIALLY HAZARDOUS INTERACTIONS WITH OTHER DRUGS

• Risk of hyperkalaemia with ACE inhibitors, indomethacin and possibly other NSAIDs, potassium salts, losartan and valsartan
• Lithium: excretion reduced

Administration

RECONSTITUTION

–

ROUTE

• Oral

RATE OF ADMINISTRATION

–

COMMENTS

–

Other information

• Hyperkalaemia is common when GFR = <30 mL/min. May cause acute renal failure
• Potassium-sparing diuretics are weak diuretics and are ineffective in moderate to severe renal failure

Trifluoperazine

Clinical use

Schizophrenia and other psychoses, anxiety, severe
nausea and vomiting

Dose in normal renal function

Oral:

schizophrenia: initially 5 mg twice daily, increased by
5 mg after 1 week, then at intervals of 3 days
according to response

Anxiolytic and anti-emetic:

2–4 mg daily in divided doses (maximum 6 mg)

IM:

1–3 mg/day (maximum 6 mg)

Pharmacokinetics

Molecular weight (daltons)	408
% Protein binding	>99
% Excreted unchanged in urine	<1
Volume of distribution (L/kg)	160
Half-life – normal/ESRF (hrs)	7–18 /–

Dose in renal impairment GFR (mL/min)

20–50	Dose as in normal renal function
10–20	Dose as in normal renal function
<10	Dose as in normal renal function

Dose in patients undergoing renal replacement therapies

CAPD	Unlikely to be dialysed. Dose as in normal renal function
HD	Unlikely to be dialysed. Dose as in normal renal function
CAV/VVHD	Unlikely to be dialysed. Dose as in normal renal function

Important drug interactions

CYCLOSPORIN

–

POTENTIALLY HAZARDOUS INTERACTIONS WITH
OTHER DRUGS

• Anaesthetics: enhanced hypotensive effect
• Antidepressants: increased plasma concentrations
  and increased antimuscarinic effects with tricyclics
• Anti-epileptics: antagonism (convulsive threshold
  lowered)
• Antihistamines: increased risk of ventricular
  arrhythmias with astemizole and terfenadine
• Antimalarials: increased risk of ventricular
  arrhythmias with halofantrine
• Beta-blockers: increased risk of ventricular
  arrhythmias with sotalol

Administration

RECONSTITUTION

–

ROUTE

• Oral, IM

RATE OF ADMINISTRATION

–

COMMENTS

–

Other information

• Reduce starting dose in elderly or frail patients by
  at least half

Trimeprazine

Clinical use

Urticaria and pruritus, pre-med in children

Dose in normal renal function

10 mg every 8–12 hrs (maximum 100 mg/day);
elderly patients 10 mg once or twice daily
Pre-med:
child 2–7 years. Maximum 2 mg/kg

Pharmacokinetics

Molecular weight (daltons)	298
% Protein binding	>90
% Excreted unchanged in urine	20
Volume of distribution (L/kg)	–
Half-life – normal/ESRF (hrs)	4–8/–

Dose in renal impairment GFR (mL/min)

20–50	Dose as in normal renal function
10–20	Use with caution
<10	Use with caution

Dose in patients undergoing renal replacement therapies

CAPD	Unlikely to be dialysed. Dose as in GFR = <10 mL/min
HD	Unlikely to be dialysed. Dose as in GFR = <10 mL/min
CAV/VVHD	Unlikely to be dialysed. Dose as in GFR = 10–20 mL/min

Important drug interactions

CYCLOSPORIN

–

POTENTIALLY HAZARDOUS INTERACTIONS WITH OTHER DRUGS

• Antidepressants: MAOIs and tricyclics increase antimuscarinic and sedative effects

Administration

RECONSTITUTION

–

ROUTE

–

RATE OF ADMINISTRATION

–

COMMENTS

–

Other information

• Significant amounts of trimeprazine are excreted in urine. It is therefore contraindicated in renal failure; reduced clearance and elevated serum levels will occur in patients with impaired renal function. The dose should be reduced appropriately or an alternative phenothiazine that undergoes hepatic clearance used instead

Trimethoprim

Clinical use

Antibacterial agent

Dose in normal renal function

Oral:

treatment: 200 mg every 12 hrs; prophylaxis:
100 mg at night

IV:

150–250 mg every 12 hrs

Pharmacokinetics

Molecular weight (daltons)	290
% Protein binding	45
% Excreted unchanged in urine	40–80
Volume of distribution (L/kg)	1–2.2
Half-life – normal/ESRF (hrs)	9–13/20–49

Dose in renal impairment GFR (mL/min)

>25	Dose as in normal renal function
15–25	Dose as in normal renal function for 3 days then 50% of dose every 18 hrs
<15	Give 50% of normal dose every 24 hrs

Dose in patients undergoing renal replacement therapies

CAPD	Not dialysed. Dose as in GFR = <15 mL/min
HD	Dialysed. Dose as in GFR = <15 mL/min
CAV/VVHD	Probably dialysed. Dose as in GFR = 15–25 mL/min

Important drug interactions

CYCLOSPORIN

• IV trimethoprim lowers cyclosporin blood levels
• Increased risk of nephrotoxicity

POTENTIALLY HAZARDOUS INTERACTIONS WITH OTHER DRUGS

• Antimalarials: increased risk of antifolate effect with pyrimethamine

Administration

RECONSTITUTION

–

ROUTE

• IV injection

RATE OF ADMINISTRATION

• 3–4 min (infusion over 15 min)

COMMENTS

–

Other information

• Serum creatinine may rise due to competition for renal secretion
• Monitor trimethoprim serum levels in patients with reduced renal function requiring chronic therapy or high doses of trimethoprim

Triprolidine

Clinical use

Antihistamine, used for allergic disease and urticaria

Dose in normal renal function

2.5–15 mg daily

Pharmacokinetics

Molecular weight (daltons)	278
% Protein binding	90
% Excreted unchanged in urine	1
Volume of distribution (L/kg)	8.7
Half-life – normal/ESRF (hrs)	5/–

Dose in renal impairment GFR (mL/min)

<50   Start with lowest dose and increase according to response

Dose in patients undergoing renal replacement therapies

CAPD   Unlikely to be dialysed. Dose as in normal renal function

HD   Unlikely to be dialysed. Dose as in normal renal function

CAV/VVHD   Unlikely to be dialysed. Dose as in normal renal function

Important drug interactions

CYCLOSPORIN

–

POTENTIALLY HAZARDOUS INTERACTIONS WITH OTHER DRUGS

–

Administration

RECONSTITUTION

–

ROUTE

–

RATE OF ADMINISTRATION

–

COMMENTS

–

Other information

• In severe renal dysfunction triprolidine should be given initially at a reduced dose and the response to it used as a guide to the patient's requirements for further administration

• Increased sensitivity to CNS effects is seen in patients with renal failure

Tubocurarine

Clinical use

Non-depolarising muscle relaxant

Dose in normal renal function

Initially 10–30 mg, followed by 5–10 mg as required

Pharmacokinetics

Molecular weight (daltons)	772
% Protein binding	30–50
% Excreted unchanged in urine	40–60
Volume of distribution (L/kg)	0.22–0.39
Half-life – normal/ESRF (hrs)	0.5–4/5.5

Dose in renal impairment GFR (mL/min)

20–50	Give 75% of normal dose
10–20	Give 50% of normal dose
<10	Avoid/use with caution

Dose in patients undergoing renal replacement therapies

CAPD	Unknown dialysability. Dose as in GFR = <10 mL/min
HD	Unknown dialysability. Dose as in GFR = <10 mL/min
CAV/VVHD	Unknown dialysability. Dose as in GFR = 10–20 mL/min

Important drug interactions

CYCLOSPORIN

–

POTENTIALLY HAZARDOUS INTERACTIONS WITH OTHER DRUGS

• Effects enhanced by aminoglycosides, clindamycin and colistin

Administration

RECONSTITUTION

–

ROUTE

• IV

RATE OF ADMINISTRATION

–

COMMENTS

–

Other information

• Tubocurarine is contraindicated in renal failure. However, metabolism and excretion via bile compensates for partly decreased renal clearance. It has been suggested that normal doses may be given in renal failure, but use with caution

Urokinase

Clinical use

Fibrinolytic agent, used for thrombosed
arteriovenous shunts and intravenous cannulas

Dose in normal renal function

Instillation:
5000–25 000 iu in 2–3 mL sodium chloride 0.9%

Pharmacokinetics

Molecular weight (daltons)	33 000–54 000
% Protein binding	–
% Excreted unchanged in urine	Low
Volume of distribution (L/kg)	–
Half-life – normal/ESRF	11–16 min/–

Dose in renal impairment GFR (mL/min)

20–50	Dose as in normal renal function
10–20	Dose as in normal renal function
<10	Dose as in normal renal function

Dose in patients undergoing renal replacement therapies

CAPD	Not dialysed. Dose as in normal renal function
HD	Not dialysed. Dose as in normal renal function
CAV/VVHD	Not dialysed. Dose as in normal renal function

Important drug interactions

CYCLOSPORIN

–

POTENTIALLY HAZARDOUS INTERACTIONS WITH
OTHER DRUGS

–

Administration

RECONSTITUTION

• 2–3 mL of sodium chloride 0.9% to 5000 u

ROUTE

–

RATE OF ADMINISTRATION

–

COMMENTS

• Use 2500 iu up each side of shunt and leave for
  2–4 hrs
• Venous side 5000 iu in 200 mL run in over
  30 min – less satisfactory than more concentrated
  solution

Other information

• Care is needed in patients with uraemic
  coagulopathies or bleeding diatheses
• Some units mix 5000 iu with 1.5 mL heparin
  1000 u/mL

Ursodeoxycholic acid

Clinical use

Dissolution of radiolucent cholesterol gallstones

Dose in normal renal function

8–12 mg/kg/day in 2–3 divided doses

Pharmacokinetics

Molecular weight (daltons)	393
% Protein binding	96–99
% Excreted unchanged in urine	–
Volume of distribution (L/kg)	–
Half-life – normal/ESRF (hrs)	–

Dose in renal impairment GFR (mL/min)

20–50	Dose as in normal renal function
10–20	Dose as in normal renal function
<10	Dose as in normal renal function

Dose in patients undergoing renal replacement therapies

CAPD	Unknown dialysability. Dose as in normal renal function
HD	Unknown dialysability. Dose as in normal renal function
CAV/VVHD	Unknown dialysability. Dose as in normal renal function

Important drug interactions

CYCLOSPORIN

–

POTENTIALLY HAZARDOUS INTERACTIONS WITH OTHER DRUGS

–

Administration

RECONSTITUTION

–

ROUTE

• Oral

RATE OF ADMINISTRATION

–

COMMENTS

–

Other information

• Completely metabolised in the liver and excreted via the faecal route

Vancomycin

Clinical use

Antibacterial agent

Dose in normal renal function

IV:

1 g every 12 hrs

Oral:

125–250 mg 4 times daily (not significantly absorbed by this route)

Pharmacokinetics

Molecular weight (daltons)	1486
% Protein binding	10–50 (19 ESRF)
% Excreted unchanged in urine	90–100
Volume of distribution (L/kg)	0.47–1.1 (0.88 ESRF)
Half-life – normal/ESRF (hrs)	6/200–250

Dose in renal impairment GFR (mL/min)

	See 'Other information' for alternative method in moderate and severe renal impairment
20–50	500 mg every 12 hrs
10–20	500 mg every 24–48 hrs
<10	500 mg every 48–96 hrs

Dose in patients undergoing renal replacement therapies

CAPD	Not dialysed. Dose as in GFR = <10 mL/min
HD	Not dialysed. Dose as in GFR = <10 mL/min
CAV/VVHD	Unknown dialysability. Dose as in GFR = 10–20 mL/min

Important drug interactions

CYCLOSPORIN

• Variable response

POTENTIALLY HAZARDOUS INTERACTIONS WITH OTHER DRUGS

–

Administration

RECONSTITUTION

• 10 mL water for injection then dilute to 100 mL (1 g) with sodium chloride 0.9% (50 mL if giving centrally)

ROUTE

• IV peripherally or centrally

RATE OF ADMINISTRATION

• Not faster than 10 mg/min

COMMENTS

• Use in CAPD peritonitis: 12.5–25 mg/L per bag (see local protocol)

• Various other regimens used in CAPD ranging from IV dosing to high-dose-stat IP use

• Some units use the following: patient's weight >60 kg – stat dose of 2 g IP on days 1 and 7 in one bag 6-hr dwell; patient's weight <60 kg, 1.5 g IP on days 1 and 7

Other information

• Second line to metronidazole in treatment of pseudomonas colitis

• Not absorbed via oral route

• Injection solution may be given orally. However, oral capsules are available

• Alternative dosage adjustment in moderate and severe renal impairment: give 1-g loading dose and monitor serum levels at 24-hr intervals. When level is <10 mg/L give another 1-g dose. Peak levels, 2 hrs after dose, should be in range 18–26 mg/L. Some units use a 500-mg loading dose

• Anephric/dialysis patients usually need 1 g once or twice weekly

Vecuronium

Clinical use

Non-depolarising muscle relaxant

Dose in normal renal function

Intubation:
80–100 micrograms/kg, with maintenance of
20–30 micrograms/kg
IV infusion:
40–100 micrograms/kg bolus followed by
50–80 micrograms/kg/hr

Pharmacokinetics

Molecular weight (daltons)	638
% Protein binding	30
% Excreted unchanged in urine	25
Volume of distribution (L/kg)	0.18–0.27
Half-life – normal/ESRF (hrs)	0.5–1.2/unchanged

Dose in renal impairment
GFR (mL/min)

20–50	Dose as in normal renal function
10–20	Dose as in normal renal function
<10	Dose as in normal renal function

Dose in patients undergoing renal replacement therapies

CAPD	Unknown dialysability. Dose as in normal renal function
HD	Unknown dialysability. Dose as in normal renal function
CAV/VVHD	Unknown dialysability. Dose as in normal renal function

Important drug interactions

CYCLOSPORIN

–

POTENTIALLY HAZARDOUS INTERACTIONS WITH OTHER DRUGS

• Enhances neuromuscular block of botulinum toxin
• Effects increased by aminoglycosides, azlocillin, clindamycin, colistin, quinidine, procainamide and piperacillin

Administration

RECONSTITUTION

• 5 mL water for injection to reconstitute 10-mg vial. Up to 10 mL sodium chloride 0.9% or glucose 5% may be used
• May be added to sodium chloride 0.9%, glucose 5% or Ringer's solution to give a final concentration of 40 mg/L

ROUTE

• IV

RATE OF ADMINISTRATION

• See dose

COMMENTS

–

Other information

• Vecuronium is largely excreted via the liver. Use normal doses with caution in renal failure

Verapamil

Clinical use

Calcium-channel blocker, used for supraventricular arrhythmias, angina and hypertension

Dose in normal renal function

Oral:
120–480 mg daily in 2–3 divided doses
IV:
5–10 mg followed by 5 mg 5–10 min later if required

Pharmacokinetics

Molecular weight (daltons)	454.6
% Protein binding	83–93
% Excreted unchanged in urine	<10
Volume of distribution (L/kg)	4–7
Half-life – normal/ESRF (hrs)	2–7/ 2.4–4

Dose in renal impairment
GFR (mL/min)

20–50	Dose as in normal renal function. Monitor carefully
10–20	Dose as in normal renal function. Monitor carefully
<10	Dose as in normal renal function. Monitor carefully

Dose in patients undergoing renal replacement therapies

CAPD	Dialysability minimal. Dose as in GFR = <10 mL/min
HD	Dialysability minimal. Dose as in GFR = <10 mL/min
CAV/VVHD	Dialysability minimal. Dose as in GFR = 10–20 mL/min

Important drug interactions

CYCLOSPORIN

• Variable reports of decreased nephrotoxicity and potentiated effect

POTENTIALLY HAZARDOUS INTERACTIONS WITH OTHER DRUGS

• Anaesthetics: increased hypotensive effect
• Anti-arrhythmics: increased risk of amiodarone-induced bradycardia, AV block and myocardial depression. Increased risk of myocardial depression and asystole with disopyramide and flecainide. Plasma levels of quinidine raised
• Anti-epileptics: enhanced effect of carbamazepine. Effect of verapamil reduced by phenobarbitone and phenytoin
• Beta-blockers: asystole, severe hypotension and heart failure
• Cardiac glycosides: increased levels of digoxin. Increased AV block and bradycardia
• Theophylline: enhanced effect

Administration

RECONSTITUTION

–

ROUTE

• Oral, IV

RATE OF ADMINISTRATION

• 5–10 mg over 2 min (3 min in elderly patients)

COMMENTS

–

Other information

• Monitor BP and ECG
• Active metabolites may accumulate in renal impairment

Vigabatrin

Clinical use

Epilepsy

Dose in normal renal function

Oral:

2 g daily in 1 or 2 doses. Maximum 4 g daily, unless exceptional circumstances

Pharmacokinetics

Molecular weight (daltons)	130
% Protein binding	Negligible
% Excreted unchanged in urine	50–80
Volume of distribution (L/kg)	0.8
Half-life – normal/ESRF (hrs)	7–8/13–15

Dose in renal impairment GFR (mL/min)

20–50	Give 50% of normal dose
10–20	Give 50% of normal dose
<10	Give 25% of normal dose

Dose in patients undergoing renal replacement therapies

CAPD	Unknown dialysability. Dose as in GFR = <10 mL/min
HD	Unknown dialysability. Dose as in GFR = <10 mL/min. Give post dialysis
CAV/VVHD	Unknown dialysability. Dose as in GFR = 10–20 mL/min

Important drug interactions

CYCLOSPORIN

–

POTENTIALLY HAZARDOUS INTERACTIONS WITH OTHER DRUGS

• Other anti-epileptics: risk of enhanced toxicity and may reduce plasma concentrations of phenytoin, phenobarbitone and primidone

Administration

RECONSTITUTION

–

ROUTE

• Oral

RATE OF ADMINISTRATION

–

COMMENTS

–

Other information

–

Vinblastine

Clinical use

Antineoplastic agent

Dose in normal renal function

6 mg/m^2 (maximum of once a week) or up to
0.2 mg/kg. Consult relevant local protocol

Pharmacokinetics

Molecular weight (daltons)	811
% Protein binding	99
% Excreted unchanged in urine	35
Volume of distribution (L/kg)	8–27
Half-life – normal/ESRF (hrs)	20/–

Dose in renal impairment GFR (mL/min)

20–50	Dose as in normal renal function
10–20	Dose as in normal renal function
<10	Dose as in normal renal function

Dose in patients undergoing renal replacement therapies

CAPD	Unlikely to be dialysed. Dose as in normal renal function
HD	Unlikely to be dialysed. Dose as in normal renal function. Give post-dialysis on dialysis days
CAV/VVHD	Unlikely to be dialysed. Dose as in normal renal function

Important drug interactions

CYCLOSPORIN

–

POTENTIALLY HAZARDOUS INTERACTIONS WITH OTHER DRUGS

• Phenytoin levels may be reduced

Administration

RECONSTITUTION

• Add 10 mL of diluent to 10-mg vial. May be administered into fast-running drip of sodium chloride 0.9%

ROUTE

• IV

RATE OF ADMINISTRATION

• 1 min

COMMENTS

• Do not dilute with volumes greater than 100 mL or give over long periods (30–60 min) as thrombophlebitis and extravasation may occur

Other information

• Vinblastine is metabolised and excreted principally by the liver. No modification of dosage is recommended in patients with impaired renal function

Vincristine

Clinical use

Antineoplastic agent

Dose in normal renal function

IV:

1.4–1.5 mg/m^2 weekly (maximum 2 mg). Consult relevant local protocol

Pharmacokinetics

Molecular weight (daltons)	825
% Protein binding	75
% Excreted unchanged in urine	12–15
Volume of distribution (L/kg)	8.4
Half-life – normal/ESRF (hrs)	1–2.5/unchanged

Dose in renal impairment GFR (mL/min)

20–50	Dose as in normal renal function
10–20	Dose as in normal renal function
<10	Dose as in normal renal function

Dose in patients undergoing renal replacement therapies

CAPD	Unlikely to be dialysed. Dose as in normal renal function
HD	Unlikely to be dialysed. Dose as in normal renal function
CAV/VVHD	Unlikely to be dialysed. Dose as in normal renal function

Important drug interactions

CYCLOSPORIN

–

POTENTIALLY HAZARDOUS INTERACTIONS WITH OTHER DRUGS

• Phenytoin levels may become raised

Administration

RECONSTITUTION

–

ROUTE

• IV

RATE OF ADMINISTRATION

• Slow bolus

COMMENTS

• May be administered into fast-running drip of sodium chloride 0.9% or glucose 5%

Other information

• Most of an IV dose is excreted into the bile after rapid tissue binding

Vitamin B and C, high dose (Orovite)

Clinical use

Vitamin B and C supplementation

Dose in normal renal function

One daily

Pharmacokinetics

Molecular weight (daltons)	N/A
% Protein binding	N/A
% Excreted unchanged in urine	N/A
Volume of distribution (L/kg)	N/A
Half-life – normal/ESRF (hrs)	N/A

Dose in renal impairment (GFR (mL/min)

20–50	Dose as in normal renal function
10–20	Dose as in normal renal function
<10	Dose as in normal renal function

Dose in patients undergoing renal replacement therapies

CAPD	Dialysed. Dose as in normal renal function
HD	Dialysed. Dose as in normal renal function
CAV/VVHD	Dialysed. Dose as in normal renal function

Important drug interactions

CYCLOSPORIN

–

POTENTIALLY HAZARDOUS INTERACTIONS WITH OTHER DRUGS

–

Administration

RECONSTITUTION

–

ROUTE

• Oral

RATE OF ADMINISTRATION

–

COMMENTS

–

Other information

• Not prescribable on FP10 prescription
• Supplement in HD patients due to loss on dialysis and poor diet
• Each tablet contains:

Vitamin B1 (thiamine)	10 mg
Vitamin B2 (riboflavin)	5 mg
Vitamin B6 (pyridoxine)	5 mg
Nicotinamide	33.3 mg
Vitamin C	100 mg

• Syrup no longer available
• Sachets not equivalent – also contain vitamins A and D

Warfarin

Clinical use

Anticoagulant

Dose in normal renal function

Oral:

daily maintenance: 3–9 mg, dependent on prothrombin time

Pharmacokinetics

Molecular weight (daltons)	330.3
% Protein binding	99.4
% Excreted unchanged in urine	0
Volume of distribution (L/kg)	0.11–0.15
Half-ife – normal/ESRF (hrs)	36–42/unchanged

Dose in renal impairment GFR (mL/min)

20–50	Dose as in normal renal function
10–20	Dose as in normal renal function
<10	Dose as in normal renal function

Dose in patients undergoing renal replacement therapies

CAPD	Not dialysed. Dose as in normal renal function
HD	Not dialysed. Dose as in normal renal function
CAV/VVHD	Not dialysed. Dose as in normal renal function

Important drug interactions

CYCLOSPORIN

• Lowered cyclosporin blood levels, hypercoagulability

POTENTIALLY HAZARDOUS INTERACTIONS WITH OTHER DRUGS

• **There are many significant interactions with warfarin. Prescribe with care with regard to the following:**
• Anticoagulant effect enhanced by alcohol, amiodarone, anabolic steroids, aspirin, azithromycin, aztreonam, cephalosporins, chloramphenicol, cimetidine, ciprofloxacin, clarithromycin, clofibrates, cotrimoxazole, danazol, dextropropoxyphene, dipyridamole, disulfiram, erythromycin, flutamide, fluvoxamine, ifosfamide, imidazoles, metronidazole, NSAIDs, omeprazole, paracetamol, paroxetine, proguanil, propafenone, quinidine, SSRIs, simvastatin, sulphinpyrazone, sulphonamides, tamoxifen, thyroxine, trimethoprim
• Anticoagulant effect decreased by acitretin, aminoglutethimide, barbiturates, carbamazepine, oral contraceptives, phenobarbitone, phenytoin, primidone, rifampicin, sucralfate, vitamin K
• Anticoagulant effects enhanced/reduced by anion-exchange resins, broad-spectrum antibiotics, dietary changes

Administration

RECONSTITUTION

–

ROUTE

• Oral

RATE OF ADMINISTRATION

–

COMMENTS

–

Other information

• Active metabolites are renally excreted and may accumulate in renal impairment
• Reduced protein binding in renal impairment

Zidovudine

Clinical use

Antiretroviral agent

Dose in normal renal function

Oral:

500–600 mg daily in 2–5 divided doses

IV:

1–2 mg/kg every 4 hrs

Pharmacokinetics

Molecular weight (daltons)	267
% Protein binding	10–30
% Excreted unchanged in urine	8–25
Volume of distribution (L/kg)	1.6
Half-life – normal/ESRF (hrs)	1.1–1.4/1.4–3

Dose in renal impairment GFR (mL/min)

20–50	Give 100% of normal dose every 8 hrs
10–20	Give 100% of normal dose every 8 hrs
<10	Give 50% of normal dose every 12 hrs

Dose in patients undergoing renal replacement therapies

CAPD	Not dialysed. Dose as in GFR = <10 mL/min
HD	Not dialysed. Dose as in GFR = <10 mL/min
CAV/VVHD	Not dialysed. Dose as in GFR = 10–20 mL/min

Important drug interactions

CYCLOSPORIN

–

POTENTIALLY HAZARDOUS INTERACTIONS WITH OTHER DRUGS

- Phenytoin levels may be raised or lowered
- Ribavirin antagonises in vitro activity of zidovudine
- Clarithromycin reduces absorption of zidovudine
- Profound myelosuppression with ganciclovir
- Extreme lethargy on administration of IV aciclovir
- Fluconazole increases zidovudine levels

Administration

RECONSTITUTION

- Dilute with glucose 5% infusion to give a final concentration of 2 mg/mL or 4 mg/mL

ROUTE

- IV

RATE OF ADMINISTRATION

- 1 hr

COMMENTS

–

Other information

- Dialysis has little effect on zidovudine, presumably because of rapid metabolism. The glucuronide metabolite (t½ = 1 hr) has no antiviral activity and will be removed by dialysis
- Patients with severe renal failure have 50% higher maximum plasma concentrations
- 90% of a dose is excreted renally, 50–80% as the glucuronide. There is substantial accumulation of this metabolite in renal failure

Zopiclone

Clinical use

Hypnotic

Dose in normal renal function

7.5 mg at night (3.75 mg in elderly patients)

Pharmacokinetics

Molecular weight (daltons)	389
% Protein binding	45–80
% Excreted unchanged in urine	<7
Volume of distribution (L/kg)	100
Half-life – normal/ESRF (hrs)	3.5–6/>7

Dose in renal impairment GFR (mL/min)

20-50	Dose as in normal renal function
10-20	Dose as in normal renal function
<10	3.75–7.5 mg at night

Dose in patients undergoing renal replacement therapies

CAPD	Unknown dialysability. Dose as in GFR = <10 mL/min
HD	Unknown dialysability. Dose as in GFR = <10 mL/min
CAV/VVHD	Unknown dialysability. Dose as in normal renal function

Important drug interactions

CYCLOSPORIN

–

POTENTIALLY HAZARDOUS INTERACTIONS WITH OTHER DRUGS

–

Administration

RECONSTITUTION

–

ROUTE

• Oral

RATE OF ADMINISTRATION

–

COMMENTS

–

Other information

• It is recommended that elderly patients and those with severe renal disease should start treatment with 3.75 mg. However, accumulation has not been observed